ADVANCES IN Ophthalmology and Optometry

Editor-in-Chief
Myron Yanoff, MD

Adjunct Professor, Department of Ophthalmology, University of
Pennsylvania, Chair Emeritus, Drexel University, Former Director
Scheie Eye Institute, Philadelphia, Pennsylvania, USA

ELSEVIER

PHILADELPHIA   LONDON   TORONTO   MONTREAL   SYDNEY   TOKYO

ADVANCES IN
Ophthalmology and Optometry

VOLUMES 1 to 6 (OUT OF PRINT)

Editor: Megan Ashdown
Developmental Editor: Jessica Cañaberal

Reprints: For copies of 100 or more of articles in this publication, please contact the Commercial Reprints Department, Elsevier Inc., 360 Park Avenue South, New York, NY 10010-1710. Tel: 212-633-3874; Fax: 212-633-3820; E-mail: reprints@elsevier.com.

Printed in the United States of America.

Editorial Office:
Elsevier
1600 John F. Kennedy Blvd,
Suite 1800
Philadelphia, PA 19103-2899

International Standard Serial Number: 2452-1760
International Standard Book Number: 13: 978-0-443-12951-3

ADVANCES IN
Ophthalmology and Optometry

Editor-in-Chief

MYRON YANOFF, MD, Adjunct Professor, Department of Ophthalmology, University of Pennsylvania, Chair Emeritus, Drexel University, Former Director Scheie Eye Institute, Philadelphia, Pennsylvania, USA

Section Editors

BHAVNA CHAWLA, MD – Ophthalmic Pathology & Ocular Oncology,
Professor of Ophthalmology, Ocular Oncology Service, RP Center for Ophthalmic Sciences, All India Institute of Medical Sciences, New Delhi, India

GABRIELA MABEL ESPINOZA, MD – Oculoplastics
Clinical Professor, Department of Ophthalmology, Ophthalmic Plastic and Reconstructive Surgery SLUCare Physician Group Saint Louis University School of Medicine, Saint Louis, Missouri, USA

PAUL B. FREEMAN, OD, FAAO, FCOVD – Optometry
Diplomate, Low Vision, Pittsburgh, Pennsylvania, Clinical Professor, Rosenberg School of Optometry, University of the Incarnate Word, San Antonio, Texas, USA

RUSTUM KARANJIA, MD, PhD, FRCSC, DABO – Neuro-ophthalmology
Department of Ophthalmology, David Geffen School of Medicine at UCLA, Los Angeles, California; Doheny Eye Institute, Los Angeles, California, USA; Doheny Eye Institute, Los Angeles, California, Department of Ophthalmology, Ottawa Eye Institute, The Ottawa Hospital, University of Ottawa, Ottawa, Ontario, Canada

RONNI M. LIEBERMAN, MD – Vitreoretinal Disease
Assistant Professor of Ophthalmology, Icahn School of Medicine at Mt. Sinai, Queens Hospital Center, Jamaica, New York, USA

ANN-MARIE LOBO-CHAN, MD, MS – Uveitis
Co-Director, Uveitis Service, Associate Professor, Department of Ophthalmology and Visual Sciences, Illinois Eye and Ear Infirmary, University of Illinois at Chicago, Chicago, Illinois, USA

STEPHEN E. ORLIN, MD – Cornea and External Diseases
Associate Professor, Scheie Eye Institute, University of Pennsylvania, Perelman School of Medicine, Philadelphia, Pennsylvania, USA; Active Medical Staff, Presbyterian Medical Center, Philadelphia, Pennsylvania, USA; Active Medical Staff,

Department of Ophthalmology, Philadelphia VA Medical Center, Director, Cornea Service, Scheie Eye Institute of the University of Pennsylvania Health System, Department of Ophthalmology, University of Pennsylvania Scheie Eye Institute, Philadelphia, Pennsylvania, USA

JOSEPH M. ORTIZ, MD, FRCOphth – Glaucoma
Consultant in Ophthalmology, Abington Memorial Hospital, Abington, Pennsylvania, USA; Formerly Assistant Professor of Ophthalmology, Hahnemann University Hospital, Drexel University School of Medicine, Philadelphia, Pennsylvania, USA

LEONARD J. PRESS, OD, FAAO, FCOVD – Optometry
Press Consulting, P.C, Lakewood, New Jersey; Adjunct Professor, Southern College of Optometry, Memphis, Tennessee, USA

APARNA RAMASUBRAMANIAN, MD – Pediatric Ophthalmology
Director of Retinoblasma and Ocular Oncology, Phoenix Children's Hospital, Phoenix, Arizona, USA

AMY ZHANG, MD – Cataract and Refractive Surgery
Clinical Assistant Professor, University of Michigan, Kellogg Eye Center, Ann Arbor, Michigan, USA

CONTRIBUTORS

DEEPAK AGGARWAL, MCh, Professor, Department of Neurosurgery and Gamma Knife Centre, All India Institute of Medical Sciences, New Delhi, India

ASHRAF AHMAD, MD, Cornea, Cataract and Refractive Surgery, Harvard Eye Associates, Laguna Hills, California, USA

KAMRAN AHMED, MD, University of Arizona College of Medicine, Phoenix Children's Hospital, Creighton University School of Medicine, Mayo Clinic Alix School of Medicine, Phoenix, Arizona, USA

KHOLOUD ALOTAIBI, MD, Department of Ophthalmology, McGill University, Montreal, Canada

TOMAS ANDERSEN, MD, MPH, Scheie Eye Institute, Perelman School of Medicine, University of Pennsylvania, Philadelphia, Pennsylvania, USA

ANVESH ANNADANAM, MD, Department of Ophthalmology, Kellogg Eye Center, University of Michigan, Ann Arbor, Michigan, USA

NOORAN BADEEB, MBBS, Department of Ophthalmology, University of Jeddah, Jeddah, Saudi Arabia

SHERRY J. BASS, OD, FAAO, FCOVD, Dipl. ABO, Associate Clinical Professor, Distinguished Teaching Professor, SUNY College of Optometry, New York, New York, USA

POOJA BHAT, MD, Department of Ophthalmology and Visual Sciences, Illinois Eye and Ear Infirmary, University of Illinois, Chicago, Illinois, USA

WILLY CARPIO-ROSSO, MD, Department of Ophthalmology and Visual Sciences, University of Illinois at Chicago, Chicago, Illinois, USA

LEA CARTER, BS, DO, Candidate, Campbell University School of Osteopathic Medicine, Lillington, North Carolina, USA

BHAVNA CHAWLA, MD, Professor of Ophthalmology, Ocular Oncology Service, RP Centre for Ophthalmic Sciences, All India Institute of Medical Sciences, New Delhi, India

NATALIE CHEUNG, MD, MS, Assistant Professor, Corneal and External Diseases, Ophthalmology, Surgical Services, Louis Stokes Cleveland VA Medical Center, Case Western Reserve University School of Medicine, Cleveland, Ohio, USA

DEVIN COHEN, MD, Scheie Eye Institute, University of Pennsylvania, Philadelphia, Pennsylvania, USA

DAVID A. DAMARI, OD, FCOVD, FAAO, Clinical Professor, The Ohio State University College of Optometry, Columbus, Ohio, USA

DANIEL DAROSZEWSKI, MD, Cornea, Northeast Ohio Eye Surgeons, Stow, Ohio, USA

MAURA DI NICOLA, MD, Department of Ophthalmology and Visual Sciences, University of Illinois at Chicago, Chicago, Illinois, USA

GABRIELA MABEL ESPINOZA, MD, Clinical Professor, Department of Ophthalmology, Ophthalmic Plastic and Reconstructive Surgery SLUCare Physician Group Saint Louis University School of Medicine, Saint Louis, Missouri, USA

ROBERT S. FOX, OD, FCOVD, FCSO, Private Practice, Latham, New York, USA

KUSUMITHA B. GANESH, MD, Senior Resident, Ocular Oncology Service. RP Centre for Ophthalmic Sciences, All India Institute of Medical Sciences, New Delhi, India

ARUJA GANGWANI, MBBS, RP Centre for Ophthalmic Sciences, All India Institute of Medical Sciences, New Delhi, India

SAMUEL GELNICK, MD, Department of Ophthalmology, Northwell Health Eye Institute, Great Neck, New York, USA

ROBIN GINSBURG, MD, Director of Vitreoretinal Surgery, Department of Ophthalmology, Icahn School of Medicine at Mount Sinai, Associate Professor, Department of Ophthalmology, New York Eye and Ear Infirmary at Mount Sinai, New York, New York, USA

SAMANTHA GOLDBURG, MD, Resident Physician, Department of Ophthalmology, Northwell Health Eye Institute, Great Neck, New York, USA

ROSHMI GUPTA, MD, Ophthalmic Plastic Surgery, Orbital Disease and Ocular Oncology, Trustwell Hospital, Bangalore, Karnataka, India

LEON W. HERNDON, MD, Chief of Glaucoma Division, Duke Eye Center, Durham, North Carolina, USA

KYLE HIRABAYASHI, MD, Ophthalmology Resident, Department of Ophthalmology, New York Eye and Ear Infirmary at Mount Sinai, New York, New York, USA

TIFFANY C. HO, MD, Oculoplastic Associates of Texas, Dallas, Texas, USA

JOHN B. HOLDS, MD, Ophthalmic Plastic and Cosmetic Surgery Inc., Des Peres, Missouri, USA; Clinical Professor, Departments of Ophthalmology and

Otolaryngology–Head and Neck Surgery, Saint Louis University, St Louis, Missouri, USA

SHELLEY JELINEO, MD, Ophthalmology Resident, Case Western Reserve University/University Hospitals, Cleveland, Ohio, USA

GEORGE JIAO, MD, Resident Physician, Department of Ophthalmology, Northwell Health Eye Institute, Great Neck, New York, USA

RUSTUM KARANJIA, MD, PhD, FRCSC, DABO, Department of Ophthalmology, David Geffen School of Medicine at UCLA, Los Angeles, California, USA; Doheny Eye Institute, Los Angeles, California, Doheny Eye Institute, Los Angeles, California, Department of Ophthalmology, Ottawa Eye Institute, The Ottawa Hospital, University of Ottawa, Ottawa, Ontario, Canada

RICARDA M. KONDER, BSc, MD, Resident Physician, Department of Neurology, University of Ottawa, Ottawa, Ontario, Canada

SHRUTHI MYSORE KRISHNA, MD, Consultant Ocular Pathologist and In Charge, Center for Ocular Pathology and Education, Narayana Nethralaya, Narayana Health City, Bangalore, Karnataka, India

AJAY KRISHNAMURTHY, MD, Ophthalmic Plastic Surgery, Orbital Disease and Ocular Oncology, Center for Ocular Pathology and Education, Narayana Nethralaya, Narayana Health City, Bangalore, Karnataka, India

ULRICH LACHMUND, MD, Department of Neuroradiology, University of Zürich, Zürich, Switzerland

CHAP-KAY K. LAU, BA, University of Arizona College of Medicine, Phoenix, Arizona, USA

DANIEL LELLI, MD, FRCPC, Assistant Professor of Neurology and Otolaryngology, University of Ottawa, Director, University of Ottawa Neurology Residency Program, Ottawa, Ontario, Canada

ALKIVIADES LIASIS, PhD, Department of Ophthalmology, University of Pittsburgh, UPMC Children's Hospital of Pittsburgh, Pittsburgh, Pennsylvania, USA; Clinical Professor, Department of Basic and Clinical Sciences, University of Nicosia Medical School, Cyprus

RONNI M. LIEBERMAN, MD, Assistant Professor of Ophthalmology, Icahn School of Medicine at Mt. Sinai, Queens Hospital Center, Jamaica, New York, USA

TAYLOR LINABURG, MD, Resident Physician, Scheie Eye Institute, University of Pennsylvania, Philadelphia, Pennsylvania, USA

HENRY LIU, MD, Doheny Eye Center UCLA, Pasadena, California, USA; Department of Ophthalmology, David Geffen School of Medicine at University of California, Los Angeles, California, USA

TIANYU LIU, MD, Scheie Eye Institute, University of Pennsylvania, Philadelphia, Pennsylvania, USA

ANN-MARIE LOBO-CHAN, MD, MS, Co-Director, Uveitis Service, Associate Professor, Department of Ophthalmology and Visual Sciences, Illinois Eye and Ear Infirmary, University of Illinois at Chicago, Chicago, Illinois

HANNA N. LUONG, BS, Mayo Clinic Alix School of Medicine, Scottsdale, Arizona, USA

SAMANTHA MAREK, MD, Resident Physician, Scheie Eye Institute, University of Pennsylvania, Philadelphia, Pennsylvania, USA

EILEEN L. MAYRO, MD, Resident, Flaum Eye Institute, University of Rochester Medical Center, Rochester, New York, USA

MONIQUE MUNRO, MD, FRCSC, Department of Surgery, Section of Ophthalmology, University of Calgary, Calgary, Alberta, Canada

JONATHAN S. MYERS, MD, Glaucoma Service, Wills Eye Hospital, Philadelphia, Pennsylvania, USA

BRIAN J. NGUYEN, MD, Resident Physician, Scheie Eye Institute, University of Pennsylvania, Philadelphia, Pennsylvania, USA

JOSHUA ONG, MD, Michigan Medicine, University of Michigan, Ann Arbor, Michigan, USA

PREETI PATIL-CHHABLANI, MD, Department of Ophthalmology, Associate Professor, University of Pittsburgh, UPMC Children's Hospital of Pittsburgh, Pittsburgh, Pittsburgh, USA

TEJUS PRADEEP, MD, Scheie Eye Institute, Perelman School of Medicine, University of Pennsylvania, Philadelphia, Pennsylvania, USA

VIVIAN QIN, MD, Scheie Eye Institute, Perelman School of Medicine, University of Pennsylvania, Philadelphia, Pennsylvania, USA

RAVNEET S. RAI, MD, Department of Ophthalmology, Northwell Health Eye Institute, Great Neck, New York, USA

APARNA RAMASUBRAMANIAN, MD, Director of Retinoblasma and Ocular Oncology, Phoenix Children's Hospital, Phoenix, Arizona, USA

BETH RAMELLA, PhD, Overbrook School for the Blind, Philadelphia, Pennsylvania, USA

REZA RAZEGHINEJAD, MD, Glaucoma Service, Wills Eye Hospital, Philadelphia, Pennsylvania, USA

DANIELLA RUTNER, OD, MS, MBA, FAAO, FCOVD, Dipl. ABO, Chief, Visual Rehabilitation Service, SUNY College of Optometry, New York, New York, USA

SABHYTA SABHARWAL, MD, Scheie Eye Institute, University of Pennsylvania, Philadelphia, Pennsylvania, USA

ALFREDO A. SADUN, MD, PhD, Doheny Eye Center UCLA, Pasadena, California, USA; Department of Ophthalmology, David Geffen School of Medicine at University of California, Los Angeles, California, USA

ABHISHEK SETHI, BS, Department of Ophthalmology and Visual Sciences, Illinois Eye and Ear Infirmary, University of Illinois, Chicago, Illinois, USA

WESAM SHAMSELDIN SHALABY, MD, Glaucoma Research Center, Wills Eye Hospital, Philadelphia, Pennsylvania, USA; Tanta Medical School, Tanta University Ophthalmology Hospital, Tanta, Gharbia, Egypt

PHILIP SHANDS, MD, Associate Professor, Corneal and External Diseases, Ophthalmology, Surgical Services, Louis Stokes Cleveland VA Medical Center, Case Western Reserve University School of Medicine, Cleveland, Ohio, USA

ALAN SHEYMAN, MD, Department of Ophthalmology, Mount Sinai Health Systems, New York, New York, USA

SAPNA SINHA, MD, Glaucoma Research Center, Wills Eye Hospital, Philadelphia, Pennsylvania, USA

CATHY STERN, OD, FCOVD, FNORA, FCSO, Pappas Rehabilitation Hospital for Children, Canton, Massachusetts, USA

RINA SU, MD, Department of Ophthalmology, Northwell Health Eye Institute, Great Neck, New York, USA

ANGELA J. VERKADE, MD, Department of Ophthalmology, Kellogg Eye Center, University of Michigan, Ann Arbor, Michigan, USA

NANCY WORLEY, MD, Ophthalmology Resident, Department of Ophthalmology, Icahn School of Medicine at Mount Sinai, New York, New York, USA

RACHEL A.F. WOZNIAK, MD, PhD, Associate Professor of Ophthalmology, Flaum Eye Institute, University of Rochester Medical Center, Rochester, New York, USA

DAVID WU, BS, The University of Illinois at Chicago College of Medicine, Chicago, Illinois, USA

MYRON YANOFF, MD, Adjunct Professor, Department of Ophthalmology, University of Pennsylvania, Chair Emeritus, Drexel University, Former Director Scheie Eye Institute, Philadelphia, Pennsylvania, USA

ADVANCES IN
Ophthalmology And Optometry

CONTENTS   VOLUME 8 • 2023

The Americans with Disabilities Act (ADA, 1990) changed
the landscape for individuals with disabilities significantly.
Its ramifications can be seen in the ramps and handicapped
parking spots outside almost every public building in the
United States. This article will give a brief outline of the
components of the ADA Amendments Act (ADAAA,
2008), clarify how disability is defined under that law,
and give the eye-care practitioner guidance on
determining whether a patient qualifies for
accommodations under the ADAAA. We will delineate
the accommodations that would be appropriate for a
patient's impairment, and describe ethical advocacy for a
patient who wants to request accommodations.

The Effects of Modulated Light on the Visual Process   15

Robert S. Fox and Cathy Stern

Photobiomodulation or modulated light therapy is being
used to treat a wide variety of conditions such as wound
healing, brain trauma, Alzheimer's disease, pain
management, and sleep disorders. Today the vision care
community has the opportunity to use devices that
deliver modulated light through the eyes for macular
degeneration, dry eye, myopia control, amblyopia, and
other ocular conditions. In addition, treatment is
available for photosensitivity, migraine headaches and
the sequelae of brain injury. Here, we present an
overview of the latest research and clinical applications
of photobiomodulation both for present use and future applications.

The Differential of Pathological from Functional Vision Loss: The Amblyopia Masqueraders   27

Sherry J. Bass and Daniella Rutner

The failure to differentiate pathological vision loss from
functional vision loss can have significant consequences.
This article will review the diagnostic criteria for
functional vision loss (amblyopia) as well as the standard
examination techniques that should be performed to help
rule out disease. This article also will detail supplemental
testing procedures that may be necessary to help identify

the amblyopia masqueraders. These tests include, but are not limited to, corneal topography, optical coherence tomography, fundus autofluorescence imaging, and electrodiagnostic testing procedures. Specific cases of anterior segment, retinal, optic nerve, and visual pathway diseases that have been "amblyopia masqueraders" are presented.

Pediatric

Correction of Pediatric Aphakia
Kamran Ahmed and Chap-Kay K. Lau

Within the last half century, improvements in the design of spectacles, contact lenses, intraocular lenses, and surgical decision-making and techniques have led to significant advancements in the correction of pediatric aphakia. This article discusses a brief history of pediatric aphakic correction, the present modalities used, and more advanced techniques, such as intraocular lens fixation in the absence of capsular support.

Conjunctival Tumors in Children
Hanna N. Luong and Aparna Ramasubramanian

Conjunctival tumors most commonly are melanocytic or choristomatous in children and the incidence of malignancy is less than 1%. Nevi are the most common conjunctival tumors and typically emerge in the first two decades of life as a darkly pigmented mass in the interpalpebral bulbar conjunctiva. Among the choristomatous conjunctival tumors are dermolipoma and dermoid, and both may be part of Goldenhar syndrome. The literature is deficient on pediatric conjunctival tumors and lot of information must be extrapolated from the adult literature, which is not ideal. Prompt recognition, accurate diagnosis, and appropriate, effective treatment are required.

Update on Cortical Visual Impairment

Joshua Ong, Alkiviades Liasis, Beth Ramella, and Preeti Patil-Chhablani

Cortical visual impairment (CVI), also known as cerebral visual impairment, is one of the leading causes of pediatric blindness. Cause of CVI maybe multifactorial but the commonest causes in developing nations include hypoxic ischemic insults during the perinatal period. The clinical presentation of a child with CVI is highly variable and can range from near total loss of vision to relatively good or preserved central visual acuity with visual field defects and complex higher visual function deficits. Management strategies include prescribing glasses where appropriate, correction of strabismus, and other associated ophthalmic pathology.

Ophthalmic Pathology & Ocular Oncology

Bhavna Chawla, Aruja Gangwani, and Deepak Aggarwal

Gamma Knife Radiosurgery (GKR) is one of the established methods of globe salvage therapies for uveal melanoma. It involves the use of a single large fraction of radiation which is stereotactically directed to the region of interest to obliterate the lesion. The primary advantage is preservation of the globe, with complete or relative sparing of the visual function. GKR also serves as a precious resource where brachytherapy is contraindicated. It has yielded promising results in terms of local tumor control. However, it is not free of complications. Further research is needed to validate its outcomes over other methods of treatment.

Roshmi Gupta, Shruthi Mysore Krishna, and
Ajay Krishnamurthy

Orbital mucormycosis is an opportunistic fungal disease with high morbidity and mortality. Its pathogenesis is a complex interaction between fungal invasive mechanisms and host factors, including cell surface receptors, platelets, phagocytic cells, and serum iron and glucose levels. Angioinvasion and vascular occlusion play key roles in the clinical manifestation of orbital mucormycosis.

Applications of Artificial Intelligence in Ocular Oncology   111
Bhavna Chawla and Kusumitha B. Ganesh

Artificial intelligence (AI) is becoming increasingly relevant in ocular oncology. Recently, several studies have used large clinical databases to develop robust artificial neural network based tumor screening and diagnostic systems. Some clinical applications of AI include the screening and early detection of retinoblastoma, and tumor surveillance after local control to provide recommendations for referral. In uveal melanoma, AI-based tools have been found to be useful in differentiating choroidal melanoma from nevus, assessment of metastatic risks, and predicting the prognosis. Thus, AI has the potential to significantly transform current disease diagnostic patterns and generate a significant clinical impact in the future.

Cataract & Refractive Surgery

Corneal Pathology and Cataract Surgery Considerations   123
Natalie Cheung, Philip Shands, Ashraf Ahmad,
Daniel Daroszewski, and Shelley Jelineo

Various corneal pathology can affect visual outcomes after cataract surgery that need to be taken under careful consideration for each patient undergoing cataract surgery. This review focuses on cataract surgery considerations in patients that have concurrent epithelial basement membrane dystrophy, pterygium, keratoconus, contact lens use, Fuchs' endothelial corneal dystrophy, penetrating keratoplasty or radial keratotomy.

Dropless Cataract Surgery 139

Anvesh Annadanam and Angela J. Verkade

 Video content accompanies this article at http://www.advancesinophthalmology.com.

Cataract extraction is the most common intraocular surgery performed. Routine prophylaxis against postoperative inflammation includes the use of topical steroid and non-steroidal anti-inflammatory drops of varying types, frequencies, and duration. Efforts to decrease the medication burden and improve patient compliance with topical therapy have generated novel approaches utilizing dropless drug delivery methods. Compared with drops, these alternative techniques provide similar efficacy, intraocular pressure elevations, and cystoid macular edema rates. Though few studies compare outcomes between the dropless methods, clinicians can choose their preferred approach based on comfort, availability, and cost.

Three-Dimensional Heads-Up Cataract Surgery 155
Eileen L. Mayro and Rachel A.F. Wozniak

In heads-up cataract surgery, the surgical team views the surgical field on a three-dimensional display screen rather than through a traditional microscope. This allows for better ergonomics and depth perception. Additionally, heads-up cataract surgery has superior educational value than a traditional microscope. In the future, artificial intelligence algorithms could be integrated into heads-up display systems to make cataract surgery even safer and more effective.

Vitreoretinal Disease

Evolution and Advances in Wet Age-Related Macular Degeneration Treatments 165
Samantha Goldburg, George Jiao, and Ronni M. Lieberman

Age-related macular degeneration is a leading cause of vision loss worldwide. Although this is currently an irreversible condition, a growing pool of treatment options exists, particularly when neovascularization occurs. The gold standard of treatment for neovascular macular degeneration is anti-vascular endothelial growth factor therapy, which has drastically improved the prognosis for those affected. However, this treatment comes with several barriers. Many new therapeutic approaches are being investigated, aimed at targeting different pathways involved in the pathogenesis of macular degeneration and improving patient compliance with treatment.

Advances in Pneumatic Retinopexy: Challenges and Innovations

Ravneet S. Rai, Rina Su, Samuel Gelnick, Ronni M. Lieberman, and Alan Sheyman

Pneumatic retinopexy is a method of repairing retinal breaks first described in 1986. It involves the injection of a gas bubble to tamponade the retinal break, use of laser photocoagulation or cryopexy to create permanent adhesions around the break, and postoperative patient positioning to keep the bubble tamponade in place. In the decades since the procedure was first described, it has been utilized for expanded indications, including for inferior retinal breaks. Operative success rates with pneumatic retinopexy compare favorably to other procedures such as pars plana vitrectomy and scleral buckle, and the cost savings are considerable.

Ocular Toxicity of Immunotherapy and Targeted Antineoplastic Agents

Nancy Worley, Kyle Hirabayashi, and Robin Ginsburg

Targeted antineoplastic therapy has improved outcomes in patients with cancer, but it also has been associated with a variety of ocular toxicities, including periorbital edema, dry eye, uveitis, retinopathy, and retinal vein occlusions, to name a few. Knowledge of these associated ocular adverse events and early recognition by oncologists and ophthalmologists as well as close interdisciplinary communication are crucial to provide the best care for these patients.

Glaucoma

Virtual Perimetry   213

Wesam Shamseldin Shalaby, Sapna Sinha, Jonathan S. Myers, and Reza Razeghinejad

Visual field examination is integral to diagnosis and monitoring of glaucoma, optic neuropathies, and some neurologic disorders. Standard automated perimetry is currently the gold standard method for visual field assessment, which has its own limitations. Virtual reality perimetry is a developing technology that has improved affordability and compliance, with wide applications in telemedicine. This review will focus on different types of virtual perimeters, their applications, and limitations.

Minimally Invasive Glaucoma Surgery: Past, Present, and Future

Lea Carter and Leon W. Herndon

 Video content accompanies this article at http://www. advancesinophthalmology.com.

Glaucoma is a chronic disease-causing death to the optic nerve and remains one of the leading causes of blindness today. Many therapies exist for treating glaucoma including medical, laser, and surgical treatments. Traditional glaucoma surgery consists of either trabeculectomy or the insertion of a glaucoma drainage device. The newest group of surgical treatments are procedures termed minimally invasive glaucoma surgery, or MIGS. The rapidly expanding field of MIGS now accounts for the majority of glaucoma procedures being performed and provides a safer surgical option that can be implemented earlier in the course of glaucomatous disease.

Neuro-ophthalmology

Toxic Medications in Mitochondrial Optic Neuropathies   249

Henry Liu and Alfredo A. Sadun

Mitochondrial optic neuropathies are a group of optic nerve disorders caused by mitochondrial dysfunction which may be congenital or acquired. The pathophysiology involves increased accumulation of reactive oxygen species, which can be affected by exposures such as medications. The most common forms of inherited mitochondrial optic neuropathies are Leber's hereditary optic neuropathy and autosomal dominant optic atrophy. While not all patients who carry the mutations for these diseases will be symptomatic, they remain at risk of vision loss. This article reviews the evidence for medications and exposures with potential effects on mitochondrial dysfunction in relation to reactive oxygen species generation.

Ricarda M. Konder and Daniel Lelli

This review provides an in-depth summary of the origins of square wave jerks (SWJs) along with their quantifiable thresholds, neuroanatomic underpinnings, and clinical associations in the context of neuropathology. By reviewing the initial studies that aimed to quantify a "normal" SWJ frequency, we conclude that a cutoff of up to 16 SWJ/min (in light and with fixation) and up to 25 SWJ/min (in darkness) is appropriate. An increase in SWJ frequency does not seem to increase with age in healthy persons. Substantial discordance exists about accepted normal ranges for SWJ amplitude, and further studies are needed for better quantification.

Kholoud Alotaibi, Nooran Badeeb, and Rustum Karanjia

The COVID-19 pandemic has led to the identification of new disease phenotypes associated with infection by the SARS-CoV-2 virus. This includes multiple neuro-ophthalmological sequelae, which have been associated with COVID-19 infection and administration of COVID-19 vaccines. Some of these associations have a plausible pathophysiological link to the infection or vaccination but true causation has yet to be established. We review the literature for associations reported between COVID-19 infection or vaccination and neuro-ophthalmic sequelae and review the potential pathophysiological processes that may underlie these associations.

Cornea and External Diseases

Diagnosis and Management of Ocular Surface Neoplasia   299
Tianyu Liu, Devin Cohen, and Sabhyta Sabharwal

Ocular surface neoplasms include ocular surface squamous neoplasms (OSSNs), melanocytic neoplasms, and lymphoproliferative neoplasms. Diagnosis requires histopathologic examination, although novel imaging modalities including in vivo confocal microscopy, anterior segment optical coherence tomography, and ultrasound biomicroscopy may aid in diagnosis. OSSN and conjunctival melanoma traditionally are treated with surgical excision with wide margins. Low-grade ocular lymphoma typically is treated with radiotherapy and high-grade ocular lymphoma with systemic chemotherapy. Adjuvant therapies including local chemotherapy, immunotherapy, and new radiotherapy regimens may plan an increasing role, whereas new genetic discoveries may yield novel targeted therapies in the future.

Approach to the Diagnosis and Management of the Cloudy Cornea in Neonates and Infants   313
Tomas Andersen, Vivian Qin, and Tejus Pradeep

Corneal opacification in neonates and infants is associated with the risks of amblyopia and vision loss. A wide variety of causes exist for corneal opacification in this age group. Early identification and diagnosis are essential to mitigate the visual morbidity and, in some cases, mortality associated with the implicated diseases. The present review article discusses the approach to the diagnosis and management of corneal opacification in neonates and infants and examines recent and upcoming advances in this exciting field.

Inborn Errors of Metabolism and Their Corneal Manifestations

Samantha Marek, Taylor Linaburg, and Brian J. Nguyen

Inborn errors of metabolism (IEM) disrupt metabolic pathways and lead to accumulation of byproducts that may be pathologic to various systems of the body. This article reviews IEM that have corneal findings with varying degrees of symptoms that may include decreased visual acuity, eye pain, or ocular irritation.

Oculoplastics

Blepharospasm: Review of Current Concepts in Diagnosis and Treatment — 343

Tiffany C. Ho and John B. Holds

Benign essential blepharospasm is a focal dystonia in which patients present with forceful, involuntary closure of muscles surrounding the eyes. Spasms can render these patients functionally blind and can negatively affect patients' quality of life. Although no cure exists for blepharospasm, numerous medical and surgical treatment options have been employed to manage symptoms. This article covers important concepts regarding the clinical diagnosis and manifestations of blepharospasm and discusses important considerations regarding effective management including botulinum toxins, oral medications, and surgical interventions.

Nasolacrimal Duct Obstruction — 357

Gabriela Mabel Espinoza and Ulrich Lachmund

Epiphora is a common problem encountered by eye care providers and is seen in both children and adults. Nasolacrimal duct obstruction (NLDO) is a frequent cause of persistent epiphora and can be due to congenital or acquired changes in the nasolacrimal duct system. Treatment includes conservative methods as well as surgical methods to restore the natural nasolacrimal duct system or to bypass the NLDO and create a new pathway for tears to drain into the nose. We provide a review of the most common etiologies and different medical and surgical treatment modalities used.

Uveitis

Multimodal Imaging in Infectious Uveitis   375
Maura Di Nicola, Pooja Bhat, and Ann-Marie Lobo-Chan

Several infectious processes can involve the eye and cause a variety of clinical manifestations in the context of infectious uveitis. The most common causes of infectious uveitis include herpesvirus infection, syphilis, toxoplasmosis, tuberculosis, bartonellosis, and toxocariasis, among others. The use of multiple imaging modalities including fundus photography, fundus autofluorescence, fluorescein/indocyanine green angiography, optical coherence tomography, optical coherence tomography angiography, and ultrasonography can assist in identifying the correct diagnosis, management, and monitoring the disease.

Inflammatory Choroidal Neovascular Membranes   395

Willy Carpio-Rosso, David Wu, and Pooja Bhat

Inflammatory choroidal neovascularization (CNV) is a rare complication and represents a challenge in diagnosis and management. It frequently presents as a type 2 neovascular membrane, a product of Bruch's membrane alteration secondary to inflammation and inflammatory mediators. Certain uveitic conditions have a higher incidence of CNV; however, it can develop in many other uveitic entities. Alterations in the fundus from the underlying uveitic process may make early detection of inflammatory CNV difficult, and multimodal imaging can facilitate its diagnosis and follow-up. Treatment options include the use of corticosteroids and immunomodulatory therapy to control the underlying inflammation and local antiangiogenic therapy.

Viral Retinitis 411

Abhishek Sethi, Pooja Bhat, Ann-Marie Lobo-Chan, and
Monique Munro

This article discusses the presentation, diagnosis, treatment, and clinical outcomes for two viral retinitis entities that can result in substantial visual morbidity: acute retinal necrosis (ARN) and cytomegalovirus (CMV). ARN is typically caused by the herpes virus family and affects immunocompetent patients whereas CMV is found in immunocompromised individuals. Treatment of viral retinitis includes antiviral therapies, but approaches vary with single or combinations of oral, intravenous, and intravitreal agents. Despite prompt and aggressive treatment, both diseases can cause permanent vision loss given that extensive retinal necrosis may result in retinal breaks and detachments.

ADVANCES IN OPHTHALMOLOGY AND OPTOMETRY

PREFACE

The Experts Speak

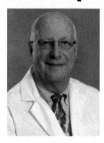

Myron Yanoff, MD
Editor

I n issue 8 of *Advances in Ophthalmology and Optometry*, we again have asked experts in each of the pertinent fields to sift through the current literature to give us insights on the latest developments, such as *The Differential of Pathological from Functional Vision Loss: The Amblyopia Masqueraders; Correction of Pediatric Aphakia; Conjunctival Tumors in Children; Dropless Cataract Surgery; Three-Dimensional Heads-Up Cataract Surgery; Evolution and Advances in Wet AMD Treatments; MIGS: Past, Present, and Future; Neuro-Ophthalmic Complications of COVID-19 Infection and Vaccination; Diagnosis and Management of Ocular Surface Neoplasia; Inborn Errors of Metabolism and their Corneal Manifestations; Blepharospasm: Review of Current Concepts in Diagnosis and Treatment; Nasolacrimal Duct Obstruction; Viral Retinitis*; and much more.

We continue to explore the new ideas, the new treatments, the new ways of doing things to give us a fresh frame of reference to sort through the crush of data and to make sense in a real way of how to proceed.

Myron Yanoff, MD
Department of Ophthalmology
University of Pennsylvania
Drexel University
219 North Broad Street, 3rd Floor
Philadelphia, PA 19107, USA

E-mail address: myanoff4@gmail.com

https://doi.org/10.1016/j.yaoo.2023.04.001
2452-1760/23/© 2023 Published by Elsevier Inc.

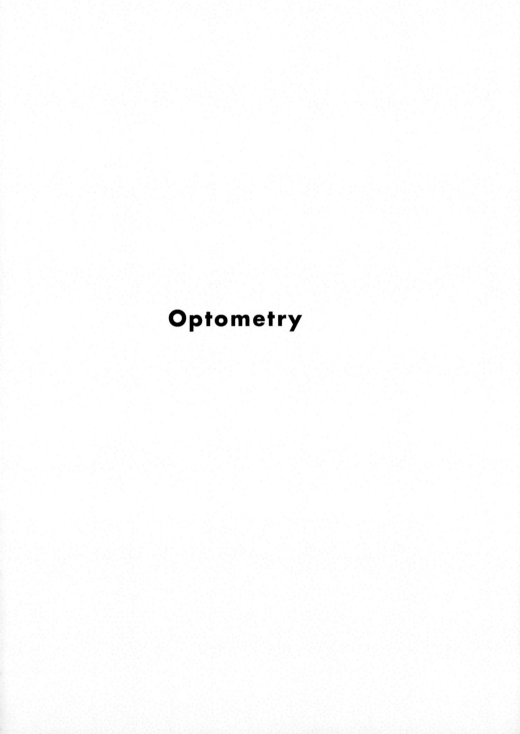

Optometry

Advances in Ophthalmology and Optometry 8 (2023) 1–13

ADVANCES IN OPHTHALMOLOGY AND OPTOMETRY

Visual Disability in the Context of the Americans with Disabilities Act

David A. Damari, O.D, FCOVD

The Ohio State University College of Optometry, 1664 Neil Avenue, Columbus OH 43201, USA

Keywords

• Impairment • Disability • Americans with disabilities amendments act
• Occupational accommodations • Academic accommodations

Key points

- The Americans with Disabilities Act (ADA) (1990), and the subsequent ADA Amendments Act (2008), substantially broadened the definition of what can qualify as a visual disability.
- The ADA definition is based not on acuity, as is the Social Security definition, but on how a visual condition impairs one or more major life activities.
- As binocular, accommodative, and eye movement disorders can impair reading, working on a computer, and other activities, they could be considered disabling in certain circumstances.
- It is important to understand the guidelines provided by your patient's workplace, academic institution, or testing organization to properly advocate for effective accommodations.

INTRODUCTION

The Americans with Disabilities Act (ADA, 1990) significantly changed the landscape for individuals with disabilities. Its ramifications can be seen in the ramps, curb cuts, and handicapped parking spots outside almost every public building in the United States. However, many eye-care practitioners do not realize that the definition of visual disability under the ADA is a significant departure from the old Social Security Act (SSA)/American Medical Association (AMA) definition. In 2008, the ADA was amended by Congress to amplify the definition of disability, further distinguishing its definition of a disability from the SSA

E-mail address: Damari.1@osu.edu

https://doi.org/10.1016/j.yaoo.2023.03.001
2452-1760/23/© 2023 Elsevier Inc. All rights reserved.

definition. This article will give a brief outline of the components of the ADA Amendments Act (ADAAA), clarify how disability is defined under that law, and give eye-care practitioner guidance on determining whether a patient qualifies for accommodations under the ADAAA. The accommodations that would be appropriate for a patient's impairment will be delineated, and ethical advocacy for a patient who wants to request accommodations from an employer, academic institution, or testing organization will be described. However, it should be noted that the author of this article is not an attorney and nothing in this article should be interpreted as or deemed to be legal advice.

After completion of this article, the reader should be able to.

1. Explain the major components of the SSA and the ADAAA;
2. Explain the differences between diagnosis (condition), impairment, and disability.
3. Evaluate components of visual function for impairments as defined by and in the context of the ADAAA;
4. Work with patients to best determine appropriate accommodations; and,
5. Report on patients' visual impairments and disabilities effectively for those who qualify under the ADAAA to obtain accommodations, equal access, and optimal quality of life.

LEGAL CONCEPTS

Laws designed to benefit traditionally or structurally disadvantaged individuals within a population can be roughly divided into two categories: entitlement law and civil rights law. An entitlement law grants some type of compensation to qualified individuals. For the health care professional, the major example of an entitlement law in the United States for almost 90 years has been the Old-Age, Survivors, and Disability Insurance program, otherwise known as the SSA. If a person retires or loses a certain percentage of his physical abilities, as calculated by a formula, then that person is entitled to compensation from the federal government through Social Security payments or income tax credits.

In contrast, a civil rights law does not entitle an individual to direct, government-paid compensation. Civil rights laws are designed to help entire classes or groups of individuals who have been traditionally denied their rights or have been societally disadvantaged by seeking to restore their rights through legal enforcement, accommodation, measures to create more equitable conditions, or some combination of those means. The Civil Rights Act of 1964 is the most well-known example of this type of law [1].

The ADA (now the ADAAA) often is misinterpreted as an entitlement law, but it is a civil rights law. No one is entitled to compensation from the federal government under the ADAAA. However, it is an important law from a public health perspective, because it gives people with disabling health conditions, whether physical, sensory, or mental, equal access to employment opportunities with any employer (Title I), to state and local government services and facilities, and Amtrak (Title II), to the publicly available services and facilities of non-profit organizations and for-profit corporations (Title III), and to broadly available telecommunications (Title IV) within the United States.

CURRENT DISABILITY LAWS IN THE UNITED STATES

The SSA (1935) [2] is an entitlement law that was designed as a "safety net" to financially protect Americans who had retired or who had disabilities that were substantial enough to prevent or limit gainful employment. Therefore, the definition of disability in this law is geared toward the individual's ability, or inability, to remain employed. The disability sections of the law are well-known and quite formulaic. Visual disability was only described as "blindness" in this law, and the law specifically and exclusively named visual acuity loss as the definitive characteristic of blindness. The AMA Guides to the Evaluation of Permanent Impairment now include visual field in the definition of visual impairment. This "blindness provision" of the SSA allows an individual who has been determined to be blind a significant deduction in reportable income for tax purposes. If the individual is not employed or considered only partially employable, the provision allows for financial benefits to be paid monthly.

For many years, the determination of blindness could only be made by "a physician skilled in the diseases of the eye." This provision in the law created a questionable situation in which, by some interpretations, doctors of internal medicine could declare a patient blind, but an optometrist could not. However, in March of 1997, the Social Security Administration determined that optometrists also qualified as an "acceptable medical source" for the assessment of "impairments of visual disorders." [3].

ADAAA: In 1990, the ADA [4], a civil rights law, was enacted. After a series of defining Supreme Court cases in the late 1990s and early 2000s, the law was amplified by the ADAAA [5], which was passed nearly unanimously by the House and Senate and became a law in 2008. Title I of the ADAAA covers employers of every sort, with the notable and specifically cited exceptions of those employers with fewer than 15 employees, the United States government, and "bona fide private membership club[s]." Title II covers access to services of facilities of state and local governments, including public transportation, and Amtrak. It implicitly does not cover Federal government services or facilities, other than Amtrak. Title III covers public access to services and facilities offered by privately held corporations and non-profit organizations. Title IV covers all major telecommunications, such as telephone services, broadcast television or radio, and cable and streaming video services. The ADAAA is first and foremost an employment law, and most of the intent of the 2008 Amendments Act was to close off what some in the disabled community perceived as loopholes being used by the nation's largest employers.

The definition of a disability under the ADAAA has little in common with the SSA. The ADAAA definition has three fundamental aspects.

- "A physical or mental impairment that substantially limits one or more major life activities."

- "a record of such impairment;" or
- "being regarded as having such an impairment."

This is the same language as the original ADA of 1990. Congress largely left it to the courts to decide the meaning of the two major descriptors in the definition: "substantially limits" and "major life activities." The issues raised by these two descriptors became quite contentious and the major cases that came before the Supreme Court on the ADA hinged on the interpretation of both those terms. The Supreme Court's decisions regarding those two descriptors were so offensive to many of the disabled, and to members of Congress, that Congress saw fit to amend the ADA in 2008 to "clarify" the intent of the law. The new law, as amended, attempted to further clarify the two descriptors. In the ADAAA, *major life activities* are defined as including, "but are not limited to, caring for oneself, performing manual tasks, seeing, hearing, eating, sleeping, walking, standing, lifting, bending, speaking, breathing, learning, reading, concentrating, thinking, communicating, and working." It also includes "major bodily functions., including but not limited to functions of the immune system, normal cell growth, digestive, bowel bladder, neurological, brain, respiratory, circulatory, endocrine, and reproductive functions."

The ADAAA also attempts to clarify the definition of the term, *substantially limits*. It specifies that only one major life activity needs to be substantially limited for the individual to be disabled under the ADAAA. Additionally, the effects of mitigating measures, such as medications or "learned behaviors," should not be considered when determining whether an individual is substantially limited, with the specific exception of glasses or contact lenses, but only those glasses or contact lenses that are used "to fully correct visual acuity or eliminate refractive error." Low-vision devices are specifically cited as mitigating measures that should not be considered in determining if an individual is substantially limited by a disabling condition.

The long list of activities that now are considered to be major life activities effectively makes the only issue of contention the definition of what is meant by "substantially limits." The Amendments Act has left this surprisingly vague, especially given Congress's obvious distaste for some of the previous Supreme Court decisions regarding the law.

Title III covers access to almost every eye-care practice today unless that eye-care provider is working directly for an employer and exclusively seeing the employees of that same employer. Therefore, practitioners need to be aware of the provisions of this law. The process for accommodating a disabled individual in one's practice is not straightforward, but it does involve two distinct steps and one caveat.

1. The individual must make the practice aware of the disability and request accommodation. This step is the sine qua non of the entire process. If the practice is not informed beforehand that the patient is disabled, practitioners cannot be held responsible for any diminished access that the patient may later claim.

2. The doctor should review the requested accommodation and determine if it is appropriate and reasonable. The appropriateness of the requested accommodation is key. For example, many hearing-disabled patients request that an American Sign Language (ASL) interpreter accompany them to every doctor's appointment. However, this may not be appropriate for every visual examination in a darkened room with the patient's head in an instrument through most of the examination. Caution should be used in making this determination, however. Almost every time the question has gone to court, the jury has given deference to the patient's viewpoint on the adequacy of an accommodation. When in doubt, one should err on the side of providing the requested accommodation. If it turns out that, by mutual agreement, the provided accommodation was ineffective, the doctor should then work with the patient to come to an understanding of the most appropriate and effective accommodations for future visits.

The caveat is that an eye-care practice must not assume that determining if an accommodation is "reasonable" has anything to do with the cost to the practice of providing that accommodation. Hearing-impaired patients have successfully sued doctors who did not provide what the patients considered a reasonable accommodation of ASL interpreters even though the cost of the interpreter can be up to three times the reimbursement for the examination. The lawsuits often award the plaintiffs hundreds of thousands of dollars, and a practice's tax returns will be part of the discovery documents.

The doctor and office staff should work with the patient during the visit to assure that the quality of care, from the patient's perspective, is at least equivalent to that a non-disabled individual would receive. Doctors should not be afraid to discuss this with their disabled patients, and document everything. This is the key aspect of a practice's compliance with the law. If it can be demonstrated that the patient received care that was of at least the same quality as that offered to non-disabled patients, and that the patient felt at the time of the visit that the standard was met, it will be most likely that the practice will have met the spirit and the letter of the law.

ANALYSIS OF VISUAL IMPAIRMENTS UNDER DISABILITY LAW

For the analysis of visual impairment under the SSA, the practitioner is best served by referring to the AMA Guides to the Evaluation of Permanent Impairment, 6th ed. However, the types of visual conditions most seen in the typical eye-care practice are much more likely to create impairments that will fall under §504 of the Rehabilitation Act or the ADAAA. The new ADAAA has not yet gone through a series of cases that have risen to the level of the Supreme Court, which will help determine what information organizations will look for in evaluations of individuals claiming visual disability. However, the ADAAA encompasses all visual conditions that could substantially limit an individual's ability to read, write, work on a computer or tablet with a display, or perform any of the other activities listed in the Act. This would include visual conditions not traditionally considered disabilities under the typical Social Security analysis. Evaluators, whether those practitioners are optometrists or ophthalmologists, have successfully claimed that visual conditions such as dry-eye disease, vergence disorders, accommodative dysfunctions, and saccadic dysfunction are disabling under the ADA and the ADAAA.

In the ADAAA, the phrase "substantially impaired" has been generally interpreted by the Department of Justice and the Equal Employment Opportunity Commission when compared to the average individual in the general population. Therefore, it is paramount in the evaluation of patients claiming a covered disability, especially those who routinely perform near-point visual activities such as reading or using a computer, that the eye-care practitioner thoroughly evaluate abilities to accommodate, converge, and exhibit controlled reading eye movements through well-standardized methodology. This assessment of near-point visual functioning should include some survey for symptoms of visual disorders, such as the Convergence Insufficiency Symptoms Survey or the College of Optometrists in Vision Development Quality of Life checklist. It also should include well-standardized tests such as Monocular Estimate Method or Nott (dynamic) retinoscopy, near prism vergences, negative and positive relative accommodation, accommodative amplitudes, and, if loss of place or slow reading is a complaint, the Developmental Eye Movement (DEM) test or some type of eye movement recording system, such as the ReadAlyzer, Visagraph, or RightEye. (It should be noted that the norms for reading speed for those tests are not generally recognized, so the evaluator should include the raw clinical data and not simply the z-scores or standard scores.) Tests that are not well-standardized such as the fused cross-cylinder evaluation in a pre-presbyopic patient, Keystone Visual Skills, or the Van Orden Star, often have excellent diagnostic value but should only be used in disability analysis when alternatives with more widely recognized standards are not possible or available.

Deficits in visual information processing (VIP) could also be considered disabling under the ADAAA. Again, the evaluation of VIP disorders should be performed using well-standardized tests that would stand up to rigorous scrutiny. Age norms are notoriously unreliable because they make no account for the standard deviation or standard error of measurement of the test instrument. Therefore, tests that only have age- or grade-normative scores available should be used with the understanding that they may have good clinical value but will be of very little use to disability experts in making a determination of impairment. Instead, test results that include age-adjusted percentile ranks, standard scores, scaled scores, z-scores, or confidence intervals should be used. The author has detailed these considerations elsewhere[6].

Of course, the more traditional impairments of central visual acuity and visual field are still considered disabling under the ADAAA. Once again, the documentation for acuity loss or loss of visual field should be assessed using well-standardized testing. Most testing instruments of visual field released within the last 10 to 15 years have acceptable psychometrics and standards. Visual acuity measured with modern optotypes should be assessed. The Early Treatment of Diabetic Retinopathy Study protocol for visual acuity measurement is currently the gold standard for acuity measurement, but what is more important is that if the patient is claiming a disability of distance vision, a distance visual acuity is acceptable. If, on the other hand, the patient is claiming a disability of activities requiring near vision, a well-standardized measurement of near visual acuity, preferably given in M or logMAR notation, is a necessity.

Standardized methods of testing visual function are critical for determining disability because, by definition, the individual's abilities are being compared to an average individual in the general population for the same age group. Symptom surveys are useful because they help to demonstrate the effect of the impairment on the patient's major life activities, also meeting important elements within the disability definition of the ADAAA.

Finally, the ethical practitioner will consider whether the findings might indicate a less than sincere effort on the part of patients to perform at the highest level of their capability. For one particularly egregious example where this was problematic, the author once received clinical data for a professional healthcare student applying for accommodations on a high stakes licensing examination who performed at the first- or second-grade level on almost all subtests of the Test of Visual Perceptual Skills. There is little likelihood that someone disadvantaged in VIP would be able to pass a course in anatomy or trigonometry, both of which would be required for entry into his professional school.

Once a thorough evaluation of the patient's visual functioning has been performed, how the doctor reports the findings of that evaluation and assessment is critical to allowing a fair analysis by the organization's disability services office. That organization will review the nature of that disability and give recommendations for the most appropriate and reasonable ways to accommodate the disability. They will most often perform that review in consultation with an outside subject-matter expert, typically, but not always, an optometrist or ophthalmologist, or a panel of these experts.

Therefore, the key steps in any examination of a patient who is claiming or desires to claim a visual disability should be:

1. Arrive at a correct, defensible, International Classification of Diseases (ICD)-10 or Diagnostic and Statistical Manual (DSM)-IV diagnosis, preferably giving a salient list of differentials and the means by which the practitioner arrived at the final diagnosis;
2. Establish the functional limitations caused by this diagnosis (the actual impairment); and,
3. Determine what accommodations would most directly and effectively address the specific disability created by the impairment for the tasks required. A thorough discussion with the patient and clear understanding of those tasks are required for completion of this last step.

Keeping in mind the three steps used to determine the appropriate accommodation for a disability is critical to effective report writing. The successful report will contain elements that address at least the first two elements and, in many cases, the third. The inclusion of clinical data and relevant printouts or scans, including a list of the symptoms experienced by the patient, should clearly justify the final diagnosis or diagnoses for the reviewer. In almost every case, those data and symptoms also will establish the extent of the impairment of the patient's visual functioning. Documenting that the condition has significantly reduced some area of the patient's visual functioning to below that of the average American, and that a tangible impact on the patient's daily life exists will show that this impairment meets the definition of disability under the law. Finally, a task analysis should be performed with the patient to describe to the reviewer the specific impact the visual impairment will have on performance in the relevant situation, and what strategies or accommodations would be most effective. This can be based on input from the eye-care practitioner, occupational therapist, speech-language professional, or teachers of the visually impaired.

It is very important for the practitioner to bear in mind that the diagnosis is *not* the disability. This is especially important in those patients who had a condition that responded to some type of rehabilitation or therapy. Under the ADAAA, an organization evaluating a request for accommodation can no longer consider mitigating measures the disabled individual has taken upon herself or with her physician or rehabilitative professional, such as medication for attention deficit/hyperactivity disorder (ADHD) or the use of low-vision devices. However, in many cases, after the patient has undergone a successful regimen of medical management, surgery, or office-based vision therapy, the diagnostic label may still be appropriate, but the nature of the impairment will have changed substantially. The data may indicate that the patient no longer is impaired relative to the average person in the general population, therefore, obviating the need for any accommodation. The determination of an appropriate accommodation must always be decided based on the clinical data and the current impact of the condition on the patient's functioning. In all cases, the practitioner should be aware that a patient may have a condition that causes some impairment, and might be considered disabling under the ADAAA, but does not qualify for requested accommodations either because the patient's level of functioning does not require accommodations, or the requested accommodations are not appropriate to either the impairment or the task.

Times occur in every practice when a patient does have a treatable but disabling condition but chooses not to undergo the recommended treatment or management. In those cases, neither the doctor nor the subject-matter expert can consider the patient's willingness to undergo therapy in analyzing the impact of the disability or the appropriateness of the requested accommodation. Once again, under the laws, the determination of disability must always be decided based on the data and the impact of the condition on the patient's quality of life under the current condition, not under optimal conditions or with mitigating factors or treatment that has not yet occurred.

Disability determination is not difficult, but it does require rigor. The evaluator must perform a dispassionate, logical, data-driven analysis of the patient's visual impairment and document that evaluation and an opinion, based on that evaluation (not on a sense of obligation to the patient), of how the impairment will be disabling during the relevant situation and what could be done to accommodate that visual disability effectively and appropriately.

Finally, it should be noted that, unlike under the SSA, an individual need not be permanently impaired to qualify for accommodations under the ADAAA. Therefore, if a patient is suffering an impairment that is temporary, the doctor should note the expected duration and any variation in the course of the impairment during that period.

DETERMINING APPROPRIATE ACCOMMODATIONS

The determination of appropriate accommodations should have the goal of arriving at an alternate means of accomplishing a task or accessing information that provides an equitable experience or access for an individual who is otherwise qualified for that experience or access. This process can sometimes create conflict because the individual claiming the disability may firmly believe one or more accommodations are appropriate when the actual impairment precludes that accommodation from providing equitable access to an activity. One such example is extended time on a test or other near-point visual activity.

Students and their parents instinctively understand that extra time on standardized tests provides an advantage over those who perform the same test in the standard amount of time, all other things being equal. This was most recently demonstrated in the "Varsity Blues" college admissions scandal of 2019 [7], in which many of the families who were clients of William "Rick" Singer's firms were directed to have their children evaluated by clinical psychologists who provided diagnoses of ADHD or LD to request extended time on the SAT or ACT, and subsequently receive the same accommodation at the college the child attended. This practice of seeking a diagnosis to receive extra time pre-dated Singer's schemes and persists to this day because of the distinct advantage extended time provides on standardized tests [8]. Law firms advertise to parents of means about their ability to obtain extra time for their clients on the SAT, ACT, Law School Admissions Test (LSAT), United States Medical Licensing Examination (USMLE), Comprehensive Osteopathic Medical Licensing Examination (COMLEX), and other standardized and licensing tests [9].

Some small studies demonstrate this instinct is correct. In one study of subjects with either no diagnosis or who had official diagnoses of ADHD or LD, the investigators found that students with no diagnosis or ADHD who had 50% more time on a standardized, timed test performed substantially better than those subjects who had no diagnosis or LD and had to complete the test in the normal time. This indicated that those subjects who had 50% extra time, even those with ADHD, had an unfair advantage over those who did not receive extra time [9]. When the extra time was increased to 100%, even the

LD group showed an advantage over those without a diagnosis who did not receive extended time on the test [9].

However, several other accommodations exist that can be made to give individuals equivalent access to tests and other visual tasks. Among these accommodations are the following:

Extra or extended breaks

Many visual conditions that could be disabling under the ADAAA cause more symptoms the more time the individual spends on a near-point activity, such as reading or working on a computer. For example, convergence insufficiency, dry-eye disease, and accommodative disorders all are exacerbated with extended time on near-point visual tasks. Arguably, extended testing time will only worsen the symptoms, and possibly even the performance, of test-takers with these disorders. A much more effective and equitable option in these cases would be extra breaks during testing.

Enlarged materials and fonts

In some cases, you may determine that enlarging materials may lessen the pressure on the accommodative system and therefore help alleviate symptoms. For example, in the case of a patient with accommodative insufficiency who does not have, nor wishes to obtain, reading eyeglasses, it may be beneficial to enlarge the font to a size that allows the patient to read more comfortably without causing the need for horizontal scrolling. For most testing material, this would be about 16- or 18-point.

Occlusion of one eye

A classic sign of binocular dysfunction in young children is occlusion of one eye when reading. This simple measure also can offer temporary relief during testing and can be an extremely effective accommodation during a test.

Other possible accommodations

If the academic material or test is computer-based, there are often capabilities to reverse the contrast (ie, white type on a black background). Some testing organizations have highly sophisticated computer-driven testing material presentation software so that the test-taker can change the brightness of the screen, alter the contrast ratio between the text and background, or even change the colors of the text and background. Only you, working closely with the patient and after researching to determine what is available, can best determine what accommodation, or combination of accommodations, will be most effective in leveling the playing field for your patient with a visual disability.

Visual conditions occur for which extended time can be an appropriate and justified accommodation. If the patient has 20/80 or worse visual acuities, then the magnification required to comfortably see the examination material will probably require more scrolling and, therefore, 25% to 50% extended time might be appropriate. Also, if the patient has an eye movement disorder that causes a demonstrable problem with tracking (reading eye movements) that can be objectively shown with eye movement recordings or a standardized test such as MNRead (https://mnread.blogspot.com/2019/04/introducing-mnread-blog_36.html) or the DEM, then an accommodation of up to 50% extended time might be deemed appropriate.

CONTENTS OF AN ACCOMMODATIONS REQUEST REPORT

Having performed a thorough evaluation of your patient's visual functioning and worked with the patient to determine the most appropriate accommodation or set of accommodations, it now remains to provide your report and supporting documentation.

THE LETTER

Your report should be in the form of a letter to the testing organization. Before composing the letter, you should review the guidelines for documentation of disability on the organization's website, which they are required to provide under the ADAAA. Assure that your report contains all the elements required under those guidelines. Typically, these include a statement of your diagnosis or diagnoses, the impairment to your patient's visual functioning caused by those conditions, and the recommended accommodations, including a rationale for those accommodations that are specific to the task the patient will be performing or examination she will be taking.

SUPPORTING DOCUMENTATION

The letter itself typically is not sufficient to establish a disability and justify accommodations. The subject-matter expert consulting with the test organization will usually review the documentation for specific clinical findings that both support the diagnoses and demonstrate the severity of impairment. Most often, these findings cannot simply be given in the report, so often, it is best to either provide a copy of the clinical record or include scans, such as eye movement recordings, visual field analysis printouts, and any other supporting materials. All organizations that require this documentation are very cognizant of the patient privacy rights under the Health Insurance Portability and Accountability Act (HIPAA, 1996), so of course you will want to assure that your patient has given permission for the information to be shared.

ADVOCATING FOR A PATIENT WHO CLAIMS A DISABILITY

Most eye-care practitioners today understand the impact that disorders of binocularity, accommodation, and eye movements can have on individuals who spend their day at a computer or doing some other near-point visual activity. They also know that disorders of the vestibular-vision relationship, visual information processing disorders, and other higher order integrative disorders that involve vision, including those that often result from traumatic brain injury, can be extremely disabling. However, not every eye-care practitioner has extensive experience thoroughly evaluating the many elements of visual function above and beyond ocular and neurological integrity or refractive condition.

In an era of increasing economic demand for workers who can gather information from visual displays as an important and extensive portion of their workday, it is important that eye-care practitioners routinely perform more than a structural, ocular health examination of eyes and adnexa. A thorough evaluation of refractive status and visual functioning should be routine for all patients who have academic or occupational visual needs—that is, nearly everyone. These visual function tests should include visual fields, saccadic eye movements (not simply our usual physiological H or rotations, since pursuits are not required for most occupations), and near-point binocular and accommodative testing.

Occasionally, the temptation may occur to shift from advocacy to a desire to actively assist your patient by misrepresenting the extent of the functional limitations she is experiencing. This temptation must be resisted. If you encounter a patient who is insistent that she needs an accommodation for examinations or at work, and that you must write a letter to a school, testing organization, or employer to that effect, two ethical options exist. One, of course, is to plainly refuse. Another option that will do less harm to your relationship of trust with that patient but will not compromise professional ethics is to write the letter stating what the patient is requesting but not stating your support for that request and providing all the clinical findings in a completely transparent manner. Almost all national testing organizations will have subject-matter expert reviewers who will independently evaluate your patient's claim and make an appropriate determination. Unfortunately, many schools and universities do not have as rigorous a review process, and your patient may be accommodated with extra time in many testing situations at that institution. However, when that patient later requests similar accommodations on a national standardized test, the testing organization can and will perform a separate review and may well come to a different conclusion about the propriety of the request. If that happens, please take the opportunity to have a discussion with your patient about the appropriateness of certain accommodations for your patient's actual impairment.

Disabled individuals, with appropriate accommodation under the law, can be fully functional and productive members of the community. Ophthalmologists and optometrists can play an important part in assuring that visually disabled individuals are properly assessed and request effective, appropriate accommodations that will best assure equal access to educational and employment opportunities.

CLINICS CARE POINTS

- The ADAAA has implications for how you accommodate patients seeking services in your practice.
- The ADAAA also has implications for how you must accommodate employees if your practice employs more than 15 people.

- A diagnosis does not typically determine the nature or severity of a patient's visual disability.
- It is important to know the legal distinctions between conditions (diagnoses), impairments, and disabilities under the ADAAA.
- Students and test-takers almost always request extended time as their accommodation of choice for visual problems, but it is very frequently not the most appropriate choice.
- Other possible accommodations that might be more appropriate and effective could include wearing a patch, extra breaks, larger test materials, user-adjustable display characteristics, or the use of eye drops during the exam.
- The eye-care practitioner should be aware that extended time can provide an unfair advantage for a test-taker who is not actually disabled.

DISCLOSURE

The author has nothing to disclose.

References

[1] Available at: https://www.dol.gov/agencies/oasam/civil-rights-center/statutes/civil-rights-act-of-1964. Accessed December 31, 2022.

[2] Available at: ssa.gov. Accessed date 31 December, 2022.

[3] Available at: https://www.ssa.gov/OP_Home/cfr20/404/404-1502.htm. Accessed date 31 December, 2022.

[4] Available at: https://www.congress.gov/101/statute/STATUTE-104/STATUTE-104-Pg327.pdf. Accessed date 31 December, 2022.

[5] Available at: https://www.eeoc.gov/statutes/ada-amendments-act-2008. Accessed date 31 December, 2022.

[6] Damari DA. Visual disability in the vision therapy practice. In: Applied concepts in vision therapy 2.0. Timonium; MD: Press; 2022. p. 491–9.

[7] Available at: https://www.forbes.com/sites/colinseale/2019/08/03/questioning-the-have-money-get-test-taking-accommodations-scandal/?sh=273ccd7b7b77. Accessed date 31 December, 2022.

[8] Lewandowski L, Lambert TL, Lovett BJ, et al. College students' preferences for test accommodations. Can J Sch Psychol 2014;29(2):116–26.

[9] Lewandowski L, Cohen J, Lovett BJ. Effects of extended time allotments on reading comprehension performance of college students with and without learning disabilities. J Psychoeduc Assess 2013;31(3):326–36.

ADVANCES IN OPHTHALMOLOGY AND OPTOMETRY

The Effects of Modulated Light on the Visual Process

Robert S. Fox, OD, FCOVD, FCSO[a],
Cathy Stern, OD, FCOVD, FNORA, FCSO[b],*

[a]Private Practice, Fox Vision Development Center, 1202 Troy Schenectady Road, Latham, NY 12110, USA; [b]Pappas Rehabilitation Hospital for Children, 7 Cedar Drive, Canton, MA 02021, USA

Keywords
- Age-related macular degeneration (AMD) • Amblyopia • Dry eye
- Meibomian gland dysfunction • Migraine • Myopia
- Repeated low-level red-light therapy • Syntonic phototherapy

Key points
- The use of light as medicine is rapidly gaining mainstream acceptance.
- Photobiomodulation promotes healing by way of mitochondrial stimulation.
- The use of light through the eyes effectively treats a wide variety of eye and vision conditions.

INTRODUCTION

Light as medicine may seem like a new concept, but scientists have known since at least the late 1800s that certain wavelengths of light in prescribed doses can be used to heal the tissue [1,2]. For the eye and vision care community, light is being used as Intense Pulsed Light Therapy (IPL) for dry eye, red-light treatment of myopia control, and optometric (Syntonic) phototherapy (OP) for treating visual conditions such as strabismus, amblyopia, and photo-sensitivity following brain trauma.

Photobiomodulation (PBM) is the current term being used to describe light therapy that is non-thermal and utilizes non-ionizing radiation in the visible and near-infrared spectrum. It was formerly called low-level laser (light) therapy or LLLT. Visible light being used and studied is primarily long wavelength red light or short-wavelength blue light (Fig. 1).

Light as medicine is now considered a safe and effective tool and is playing an ever-increasing role in both eye health and general health. The newest

*Corresponding author. E-mail address: doctorstern@gmail.com

https://doi.org/10.1016/j.yaoo.2023.03.009

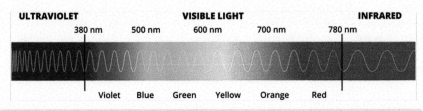

Fig. 1. Color spectrum. (Winwinartlab/123RF.com.)

information, as referenced in each section, is showing light's importance for treatment of dry eye, age-related macular degeneration (AMD), post-cataract surgery, migraine headaches, cognitive enhancement, brain injury, Alzheimer's disease, Parkinson's disease, and other neurodegenerative diseases.

HISTORY OF PHOTOTHERAPY

The modern use of light in medicine generally is credited as beginning with the work of Niels Ryberg Finsen, a Danish physician. He was awarded the Nobel Prize in Medicine in 1903 for his work using ultraviolet light to treat Lupus. This opened the door over the next few decades for others to expand phototherapy. Publications in this era include "Light and Its Rays as Medicine" by Dr Seth Pancoast [3], and "The Principles of Light and Color," by Edwin Babbitt, MD [4]. This book is still referenced today by practitioners of optometric phototherapy.

In the 1920s, optometrist and physician Harry Riley Spitler determined that imbalance in the autonomic nervous (ANS) was responsible for many visual conditions and that specific frequencies of light, delivered,through the eyes, could be used to rebalance the ANS and, thereby, correct many visual dysfunctions at their source. The new science was named "syntonics", meaning to be responsive and in harmony with the environment. In 1933, Spitler founded the College of Syntonic Optometry, and in 1941, he published "The Syntonic Principle." [5] The College of Syntonic Optometry continues to be dedicated to the education, training, and certification of optometrists skilled in the use of modulated light to treat a wide variety of eye and vision conditions.

PHOTOBIOMODULATION

Although it was discovered in the 1960s that treatment with a weak ruby laser could improve wound healing [6], the treatment was maligned for many years until the mechanism was made known through the work of Tiina Karu in Russia [7]. From her work, and with a rapidly growing number of published research studies, the emphasis has now shifted from learning if PBM works to researching how PBM works. Karu identified cytochrome c oxidase in the mitochondrial respiratory chain as a primary chromophore and showed that a brief exposure to light could have an effect on the organism that lasted for hours, days, or weeks. Under stress, such as from disease conditions, the mitochondria produce too much nitric oxide which attaches to cytochrome c oxidase molecules. Cytochrome c oxidase blocks adenosine triphosphate (ATP) synthase from producing ATP. Without ATP, the cell cannot carry out its normal growth and repair. Red and near-infrared light cause the cytochrome c oxidase molecules to release the nitric oxide, allowing the resumption of ATP production. Research has shown measurable improved cellular function within minutes to hours of the application of photobiomodulation (Fig. 2).

For PBM to be successful, a light source is placed in contact with the skin or close to the open eyes allowing the light to penetrate the tissue and interact with chromophores in cells leading to photophysical and photochemical changes that accelerate wound healing, increase circulation, reduce acute inflammation, mitigate acute and chronic pain, and help restore normal cellular function. It may even enhance performance in normal cells and tissue. Although red and near-infrared (650–940 nm) light penetrates most deeply into human tissue, interest is increasing in the use of violet, green, and blue light (430–550 nm) frequencies to also effect positive changes in human physiology [8].

THE VISUAL PATHWAY

Our direct biological response to light is primarily through the visual system. This includes image processing and refractive state along with awareness of day and night. The visual pathway is divided into the ventral and dorsal streams for both detailed perception and direction of action. Our job is to maximize this response through the detection and management of refractive abnormalities and disease processes. Treatment of visual pathway issues may include lenses, prisms, tints, vision therapy or orthoptics, medications, or surgical intervention.

THE NON-VISUAL OCULAR PATHWAY

A third light-sensitive receptor in the retina was identified in 2002. Totally distinct from the rods and cones, they are known as intrinsically photosensitive

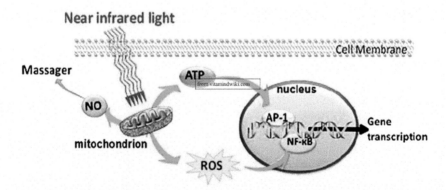

Fig. 2. LLLT. (*From* Chung H, Dai T, Sharma SK, Huang YY, Carroll JD, Hamblin MR. The nuts and bolts of low-level laser (light) therapy. Ann Biomed Eng. 2012;40(2):516-533.)

retinal ganglion cells (ipRGCs). These retinal ganglion cells are associated with the photopigment, melanopsin, and are maximally sensitive to blue light. They number only about 2% of the retinal ganglion cells, and the fibers from these cells bypass the visual cortex and travel to the suprachiasmatic nucleus (SCN) of the hypothalamus to coordinate the body's circadian rhythm [9].

The newfound relationships between blue light, melanopsin, and our sleep–wake system bring new attention to the effects of artificial light sources in our daily lives. Manufacturers of lens coatings, computer hardware, and computer software have quickly jumped on the blue light bandwagon, offering a wide variety of solutions to the blue light "epidemic." [10].

The ipRGCs and their connection to the hypothalamus provide a model for the treatment efficacy of phototherapy. It provides an explanation for some of the effects of low-level light frequencies on human physiology and sets up the introduction of light frequencies through the eyes as a way to institute change in the endocrine system.

CLINICAL PRACTICE AND CURRENT RESEARCH

Photobiomodulation and its action mechanisms have been studied for over 40 years and are finally gaining acceptance for therapeutic applications in optometry and ophthalmology. Optometric (Syntonic) phototherapy may be considered a form of photobiomodulation. As described earlier, the discovery of PBM by cytochrome c oxidase, the role of PBM in activating beneficial antioxidant effects, and the role of selected light frequencies to be therapeutic without adverse effects, have led to scientific discovery and potential treatments for visual and neurological conditions affecting the visual system.

Potential therapeutic applications, current research, and devices now being used in clinical practice are presented by condition to highlight what is available now and what the future holds for us as clinicians.

With few side effects, PBM offers a safer and less invasive alternative to pharmaceuticals and surgical interventions. Indeed, Jacob Liberman, OD, PhD's 1990 book, "Light: Medicine of the Future" has turned out to be extremely accurate in both its title and message [11]. The book discusses the use of light in the treatment of various medical and visual conditions, learning disabilities, and the human immune system.

AGE-RELATED MACULAR DEGENERATION AND NEUROPROTECTION

The retina is vulnerable to mitochondrial dysfunction, especially with increasing age. Retinal photoreceptors and ganglion cells contain a high density of mitochondria and, as such, offer an excellent target for the reduced cell death and mitigation of oxidative stress offered by photobiomodulation (Fig. 3).

Janis Eells, PhD, was an early researcher studying the effect of near-infrared light therapy for retinal healing. Her early studies centered on the loss of vision in laboratory mice following methyl alcohol toxicity. In her experiments, the

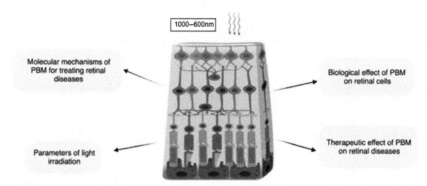

1000–600nm

Molecular mechanisms of
PBM for treating retinal
diseases

Biological effect of PBM
on retinal cells

Parameters of light
irradiation

Therapeutic effect of PBM
on retinal diseases

Fig. 3. Photobiomodulation. (*Adapted from* Zhang C-X, Lou Y, Chi J, Bao X-L, Fan B, Li G-Y. Considerations for the Use of Photobiomodulation in the Treatment of Retinal Diseases. Biomolecules. 2022; 12(12):1811.)

mice were subjected to near-infrared light before being given a toxic dose of methanol. The mice exposed to the light did not demonstrate the loss of vision and retinal damage seen in the untreated mice [12,13].

Photoreceptor neuroprotection was observed by Nora Heinig of the Technische Universität (TU) Dresden, School of Medicine, and colleagues [14]. They were primarily looking at the neuroprotective effects of 670 nm red light and 810 nm near-infrared light on blue light-damaged murine primary photoreceptors. They noted improvement in mitochondrial respiration, reduced retinal inflammation, and reduced mitochondrial-induced apoptosis.

They also referenced earlier work showing that near-infrared light may reduce photoreceptor death by 70%, reduce drusen volume, and can lower intraocular pressure for as long as several months [15]. In 2016, Graham Merry, MBBS, showed that photobiomodulation also reduced drusen volume while improving visual acuity and contrast sensitivity in dry age-related macular degeneration (ARMD) [16].

More recently, Samuel Markowitz, MD, and colleagues led a controlled study on the use of red-light therapy for dry ARMD and found significant acuity improvement in 50% of the patients along with improvement in contrast sensitivity, drusen volume, and central drusen thickness with no adverse effects being reported in the treatment group [17].

LumiThera, which offers AdaptDx Pro for AMD detection (following their recent purchase of Maculogix), is also known for their Valeda Light Delivery System (Fig. 4) which uses photobiomodulation to treat eye disease. Although still considered investigational in the United States, it currently is approved in the European Union for the treatment of ocular damage and disease including inhibition of inflammatory mediators, edema, drusen deposition, improvement of wound healing following ocular trauma or surgery, and increase in visual acuity and contrast sensitivity in patients with degenerative diseases such as dry AMD. In March 2022, LumiThera reported positive findings in its

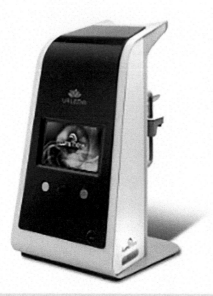

Fig. 4. Valeda Light Delivery System. (*Courtesy of* LumiThera, Inc, Poulsbo, WA.)

LIGHTSITE III clinical trial of the Valeda system for treating dry ARMD [18]. Valeda is designed for ease of use in the clinician's office. Treatments are delivered in a series of nine sessions per eye over a 3 weeks and each treatment session lasts less than 5 minutes per eye.

MEIBOMIAN GLAND DYSFUNCTION AND DRY EYE

Eye doctors have two choices of light therapy for treating inflammatory eye disease. IPL and low-level light therapy or PBM. Although IPL uses light, the light is converted to heat with the chosen wavelengths selectively destroying blood vessels by targeting chromophores within the blood vessels. PBM is nonthermal and involves placing a mask over the face through which the light therapy is released. In the Marco Equinox Low-Level Light Therapy device, the mask covers the patient's forehead, entire eye area, and cheekbones. Although red, yellow, and blue light masks are available, the blue light mask is used to kill bacteria such as in *Staphylococcal blepharitis*. After delivery of the light energy, porphyrin molecules on the cell membrane absorb the blue light generating free radicals that disrupt the cell wall of some gram-positive bacteria leading to cell death. As the cells have a weak defense against the oxygen-induced damage, the treatment is highly effective for dry eye or blepharitis, meibomian gland dysfunction, and chalazion or stye [19–21].

MYOPIA AND RED-LIGHT THERAPY

Slowing myopia progression has become important as we now know that even low levels of myopia increase the risk for glaucoma, macular degeneration, and retinal detachment. Mechanisms for red light suppressing myopia progression suggest that narrow band long wavelength light promotes hyperopia by retarding axial elongation, decreasing elongation of the vitreous chamber, and increasing choroidal thickness [22]. In addition, it has been found that bright light suppresses form-deprivation myopia development by activating dopamine D1 receptor signaling in the retina [23].

Low-level red-light therapy, therefore, is an emerging treatment for slowing myopia progression. In 2022 alone, a number of studies demonstrated positive effects of red-light therapy in reducing myopia, reducing axial length, and being well-tolerated with no adverse effects.

Yu Jiang and colleagues used a home-based desktop light therapy device to administer red light of 650 nm wavelength at an illuminance level of approximately 1600 lux and a power of 0.29 mW for a 4-mm pupil. Treatment was done under parental supervision for 3 minutes per session, twice daily with a minimum interval of 4 hours between sessions. The treatment was administered 5 days per week. Subjects in the experimental group had far less myopic progression and axial length change than the control group that received sham therapy. They reported a mean spherical equivalent refraction change over 6 months of −0.2D, and average axial length change of 0.13 mm in the treatment group versus a refraction change of −0.79D and axial length growth of 0.38 mm in the control group. Results of a 6-month follow-up showed additional positive results; 16% of subjects had reduced myopia and 25% showed reductions in axial length. The therapy was well-tolerated with no adverse effects being reported by test subjects [24].

In another study, Jing Dong and colleagues administered repeated low-level red-light therapy to a group of Chinese children. They also used a desktop red-light device with the experimental group receiving 100% light power and the sham group receiving 10% of the device's power. Treatment was done at home, and they followed a similar schedule of 3-minute sessions twice daily with an interval of at least 4 hours between sessions. Cycloplegic refraction and axial length (AL) were measured at baseline and 6 months. Children in the treatment group had less myopia progression and axial elongation compared to the sham control group. At the final visit, distance visual loss was statistically significantly greater for children with myopia in the sham device group than for those in the red-light therapy group. Visual acuity testing demonstrated a change of 0.076 ± 0.189 logMAR for the treatment group compared to −0.002 ± 0.172 logMAR for the sham treatment group (P =.013). Mean spherical equivalent refraction change over 6 months was 0.06D in the treatment group and −0.11D in the sham device control group. The average AL growth was less 0.02 mm in the treatment group compared with 0.13 mm in the sham control group. The treatment was well-tolerated, and no adverse effects were reported [25].

In a recent literature review [26], it was found that while current recognized treatments for myopia including low-dose atropine, orthokeratology, and defocus-incorporated multiple segment spectacle lenses are 30% to 60% effective in delaying the onset of or progression of myopia, they are not strong enough to restrain AL growth. Lei Zhou and colleagues [27] were able to show that PBM therapy modestly decreases AL for myopia control. In addition, recent studies of red-light irradiation were found to induce hyperopia, therefore, red-light therapy may be a powerful tool in myopia prevention and control. In the literature review, it was noted that red light may be a safe treatment given its protective effect on both the cornea and retina.

In a study of light signaling and myopia, the authors looked at the effects of light wavelength, illuminance, and contrast on the progression of myopia. They note that retinal dopamine secretion is affected by light intensity and different light wavelengths related to the known effect of focus difference between shorter and longer wavelengths called longitudinal chromatic aberration theory [28].

Lei Tian and colleagues investigated the efficacy and safety of 650 nm low-level red light for myopia control in children. The median 6-month change in AL was -0.06 for the treatment group and 0.14 mm for the control group ($P. < 0.001$). The median 6-month spherical equivalent refraction was 0.125D for the treatment group and -0.25 for the control group ($P. < .001$). They concluded that 650 nm low-level red light was an effective and safe treatment. It significantly slowed myopia progression in the children treated, reversed myopia progression in over half the children treated, and no adverse effects were observed [29].

GLAUCOMA AND NEUROPROTECTION

Ongoing glaucoma therapies research includes studies of treatments that are less invasive or with fewer side effects than current surgical and drug treatments. Novel therapeutic targets also are being researched. Photobiomodulation is one therapy being studied as a way to delay glaucoma by slowing down retinal ganglion cell death. PBM's role in targeting mitochondria may offer protection and delay the onset of glaucoma. In addition, PBM may stimulate neural progenitor cells, and therefore, play a role in slowing down retinal ganglion cell death or in part regenerating tissue damaged by glaucoma [30,31].

A current clinical trial, ClinicalTrials.gov Identifier: NCT05309811, is investigating the effect of repeated low-level red-light therapy (RLRL) on existing visual field damage in primary open-angle glaucoma patients. They hope to show that RLRL's ability to improve circulation will have a positive effect on the possible ischemic mechanism of primary open-angle glaucoma and reverse weakened visual function [32].

AMBLYOPIA

BorisIvandic, MD and Tomislav Ivandic, MD researched low-level laser therapy for amblyopia. Adolescent and adult patients with amblyopia ranging from 20/400 to 20/30 were treated for 30 seconds, three to four times per week for 2 weeks with 780 nm light. Although the control patients in the study showed no improvement in visual acuity, the treated patients experienced significant improvement in visual acuity. Of those with ametropia, 90% showed an average acuity increase of three lines while 89% of those with strabismus improved an average of 2.7 lines. The beneficial effect was retained for at least 6 months. Although the exact mechanism of the treatment effect is unknown, the authors speculate that increased cellular metabolism and inter-neuronal communication via promotion of synaptogenesis may be responsible for the improvement in visual acuity [33].

MIGRAINE HEADACHE AND PAIN REDUCTION

Exposing migraine sufferers to a narrow band of green light was found to significantly reduce photophobia and headache severity. This research by Rami Burstein, PhD, of the Harvard Brain Science Initiative was published in 2017 [34]. Before that, he published findings suggesting that patients' experience with color and migraine photophobia may originate in cone-driven retinal pathways, then fine-tuned in relay thalamic neurons outside the main visual pathway, and preserved by the cortex. These findings helped to establish the value of green light for migraine [35,36].

More recently, Dr. Burstein and partners launched a company called Allay Lamp that manufactures and sells a green light lamp that produces the narrow band of green light found to reduce migraine headache sensitivity. They recommend it to be the only light source in the room to be most effective. It is rechargeable, portable, and can be switched between the Allay green mode and regular white light as needed.

In a study presented at the 2022 annual meeting of the American Society of Anesthesiologists, Padma Gulur, MBBS, reported that 34 fibromyalgia patients were assigned to wearing either green, blue, or clear lenses for 4 hours per day for 2 weeks. Those wearing the green lenses reduced their reliance on opioids, were four times more likely to report less pain-related anxiety associated with their fibromyalgia, and they did not want to give up their green lenses at the end of the study [37].

BRAIN INJURY AND PHOTOBIOMODULATION

A recent study of blue light exposure following mild traumatic brain injury (mTBI) provides evidence of the benefits of PBM on functional outcomes following brain injury. Killgore and colleagues provide a well-controlled, double-blind study on the use of blue light treatment. Test subjects received 30-minute pulses of blue light each morning, while control subjects received pulses of amber light. Test subjects showed significant improvements in sleep timing, daytime fatigue, and executive functioning. In addition, MRIs showed increased volume of the posterior thalamus (pulvinar) [38].

A more recent review and meta-analysis of TBI in in vivo mammalian models supports the use of PBM in acute traumatic brain injury. The analysis favored light of 665 nm and 810 nm with no differences found between pulsed or continuous wave light delivery. The review supports antiapoptotic, anti-inflammatory, and pro-proliferative effects, and modulation of cellular metabolism. They concluded that substantial meta-analysis evidence exists for both functional and histological outcomes of traumatic brain injury in in vivo mammalian models [39].

SUMMARY

The use of modulated light to treat visual and systemic conditions now is considered a safe and effective tool. Research has changed its mission from *if* light can heal to *how light* stimulates healing. Initial research concentrated on the effect of modulated light in mitochondria and the cytochrome c oxidase molecule with its ability to allow the release of nitric oxide and assist the cells in increasing ATP production. Now research is expanding to include many other positive effects for light as medicine.

The more recent discovery of intrinsically photosensitive retinal ganglion cells and their connection to hypothalamus support the use of light in the maintenance of health, and the autonomic system balance validates the use of light through the eyes to treat organic and functional vision disorders.

Today, the eye and vision care community has the opportunity to use devices that deliver modulated light through the eyes for macular degeneration, dry eye, myopia control, amblyopia, and other ocular conditions. In addition, we have tools to assist our patients with photosensitivity, migraine headaches, and the sequelae of brain injury.

In the future, there most certainly will be expanded opportunities to use modulated light for Alzheimer's disease, Parkinson's disease, and other neurodegenerative diseases, as well as to prevent or slow ocular conditions resistant to current surgical or drug interventions.

CLINICS CARE POINTS

- Photobiomodulation (PBM) should be considered before pharmaceutical or surgical intervention for Age-related macular degeneration (AMD) as it has been shown to improve visual acuity and contrast sensitivity.
- PBM using blue light can be used to kill bacteria in cases of meibomian gland dysfunction and dry eye.
- PBM should be added to your treatments for myopia control. It is currently the only treatment strong enough to retard and even decrease axial length elongation.

DISCLOSURE

The authors have nothing to disclose.

References

[1] Gottlieb RL, Wallace LB. Syntonic Phototherapy. Photomed Laser Surg 2010;28(4): 449–52.
[2] Pancoast S. Light and its Rays as medicine, kingdom. Philadelphia: Stoddart; 1877.
[3] Babbitt Edwin D. Principles of light and color. Orange, NJ: Babbitt & Co. East; 1878.
[4] Spitler HR. The Syntonic Principle: its relation to health and ocular problems. Eugene, OR: College of Syntonic Optometry; 1941.

[5] Mester E, Szende B, Tota JG. Effect of laser on hair growth of mice. Kiserl Orvostud 1967;19:628–31.

[6] Karu TI, Afanas'eva NI. Cytochrome c oxidase as the primary photoacceptor upon laser exposure of cultured cells to visible and near IR-range light (Russian). Dokl Akad Nauk 1995;342(5):693–5.

[7] Tosini G, Ferguson I, Tsubota K. Effects of blue light on the circadian system and eye physiology. Mol Vis 2016;22:61–72.

[8] Berson DM, Dunn FA, Takao M. Phototransduction by retinal ganglion cells that set the circadian clock. Science 2002;295(5557):1070–3.

[9] Downie LE. Blue-light filtering ophthalmic lenses: to prescribe, or not to prescribe? Ophthalmic Physiol Opt 2017;37(6):640–3.

[10] Liberman J. Light: Medicine of the Future, Bear & Company, Rochester, VT, 1990.

[11] Eells JT, Henry MM, Summerfelt P, et al. Therapeutic photobiomodulation for methanol-induced retinal toxicity. Proc Natl Acad Sci U S A 2003;100:3439–44.

[12] Eells JT, Wong-Riley MTT, VerHoeve J, et al. Mitochondrial signal transduction in accelerated wound and retinal healing by near-infrared light therapy. Mitochondrion 2004;4(5–6): 559–67.

[13] Heinig N, Schumann U, Calzia D, et al. Photobiomodulation Mediates Neuroprotection against Blue Light Induced Retinal Photoreceptor Degeneration. Int J Mol Sci 2020;21(7): 2370.

[14] Albarracin R, Eells J, Valter K. Photobiomodulation protects the retina from light-induced photoreceptor degeneration. Invest Ophthalmol Vis Sci 2011;52:3582–92.

[15] Merry GF, Munk MR, Dotson RS, et al. Photobiomodulation reduces drusen volume and improves visual acuity and contrast sensitivity in dry age-related macular degeneration. Acta Ophthalmol 2016;95(4):e270–7.

[16] Markowitz SN, Devenyi RG, Munk MR, et al. A Double-Masked, Randomized Sahm-Controlled, Single-Center Study with Photobiomodulation for the Treatment of Dry Age-Related Macular Degeneration. Retina 2020;40(8):1471–82.

[17] Kaymak H, Schwahn H. Photobiomodulation as a Treatment in Dry AMD. Retina Today 2020.

[18] Study of photobiomodulation to treat dry age-related macular degeneration (LIGHTSITE III). Case Medical Research 2019; https://doi.org/10.31525/ct1-nct04065490.

[19] Sulek A, Pucelik B, Kobielusz M, et al. Photodynamic Inactivation of Bacteria with Porphyrin Derivatives: Effect of Charge, Lipophilicity, ROS Generation, and Cellular Uptake on Their Biological Activity in Vitro. Int J Mol Sci 2020;21(22):8716.

[20] Park Y, Kim H, Kim S, et al. Effect of low-level light therapy in patients with Dry Eye: A prospective, randomized, observer-masked trial. Sci Rep 2022;12(1); https://doi.org/10.1038/s41598-022-07427-6.

[21] Markoulli M, Chandramohan N, Papas EB. Photobiomodulation (low-level light therapy) and dry eye disease. Clin Exp Optom 2021;104(5):561–6.

[22] Hung LF, Arumugam B, She Z, et al. Narrow-band, long-wavelength lighting promotes hyperopia and retards vision-induced myopia in infant rhesus monkeys. Exp Eye Res 2018;176:147–60.

[23] Chen S, Zhi Z, Ruan Q, et al. Bright Light Suppresses Form-Deprivation Myopia Development With Activation of Dopamine D1 Receptor Signaling in the ON Pathway in Retina. Invest Ophthalmol Vis Sci 2017;58:2306–16.

[24] Jiang Y, Zhu Z, Tan X, et al. Effect of Repeated Low-Level Red-Light Therapy for Myopia Control in Children. Ophthalmology 2022;129(5):509–19.

[25] Dong J, Zhu Z, Xu H, et al. Myopia Control Effect of Repeated Low-Level Red-Light Therapy in Chinese Children: A Randomized, Double-Blind, Controlled Clinical Trial. Ophthalmology 2022.

[26] Huang Z, He T, Zhang J, et al. Red light irradiation as an intervention for myopia. Indian J Ophthalmol 2022;70(9):3198.

[27] Zhou L, Tong L, Li Y, et al. Photobiomodulation therapy retarded axial length growth in children with myopia: evidence from a 12-month randomized controlled trial evidence. Sci Rep 2023;13(1):3321.

[28] Zhang P, Zhu H. Light Signaling and myopia development: A review. Ophthalmol Ther 2022;11:939–57.

[29] Tian L, Cao K, Ma DL, et al. Investigation of the Efficacy and Safety of 650 nm Low-Level Red Light for Myopia Control in Children: A Randomized Controlled Trial. Ophthalmology and Therapy 2022;11(6):2259–70.

[30] Bergandi L, Silvagno F, Grisolia G, et al. The Potential of Visible and Far-Red to Near-Infrared Light in Glaucoma Neuroprotection. Appl Sci 2021;11(13):5872.

[31] Bernstein SL, Guo Y, Kerr C, et al. The optic nerve lamina region is a neural progenitor cell niche. Proc Natl Acad Sci USA 2020;117(32):19287–98.

[32] Zhongshan Ophthalmic Center, Sun Yat-sen University. Effect of Repeated Low-Level Red-Light Therapy on Visual Field Damage in Primary Open-angle Glaucoma: A Randomized Cross-over Clinical Trial. clinicaltrials.gov. 2022. https://clinicaltrials.gov/ct2/show/NCT05309811.

[33] Ivandic BT, Ivandic T. Low-Level Laser Therapy Improves Visual Acuity in Adolescent and Adult Patients with Amblyopia. Photomedicine and Laser Surgery 2012;30(3):167–71.

[34] Burstein R. Reply: Pupil area and photopigment spectral sensitivity are relevant to study of migraine photophobia. Brain 2017;140(1):e3.

[35] Noseda R, Bernstein CA, Nir RR, et al. Migraine photophobia originating in cone-driven retinal pathways. Brain 2016;139(Pt 7):1971–86.

[36] Green Light Exposure May Help Reduce Pain and Headaches. Time. Published October 27, 2022 Available at: https://time.com/6225133/green-light-headaches-pain-relief/. Accessed 3 March, 2023.

[37] Fibromyalgia: How Green Eyeglasses Can Ease Anxiety. Healthline. Published October 23, 2022. Available at: https://www.healthline.com/health-news/fibromyalgia-how-green-eyeglasses-can-help-ease-pain-related-anxiety. Accessed 3 March, 2023.

[38] Killgore WDS, Vanuk JR, Shane BR, et al. A randomized, double-blind, placebo-controlled trial of blue wavelength light exposure on sleep and recovery of brain structure, function, and cognition following mild traumatic brain injury. Neurobiol Dis 2020;134:104679.

[39] Stevens AR, Hadis M, Milward M, et al. Photobiomodulation in Acute Traumatic Brain Injury: A Systematic Review and Meta-Analysis. J Neurotrauma 2023;40(3–4):210–27.

Advances in Ophthalmology and Optometry 8 (2023) 27–44

ADVANCES IN OPHTHALMOLOGY AND OPTOMETRY

The Differential of Pathological from Functional Vision Loss
The Amblyopia Masqueraders

Sherry J. Bass, OD, FAAO, FCOVD, Dipl. ABO[a],*,
Daniella Rutner, OD, MS, MBA, FAAO, FCOVD, Dipl. ABO[a]

[a]SUNY College of Optometry, 33 West 42nd Street, New York, NY 10036, USA

Keywords
- Amblyopia • Keratoconus • Retinal disease • Optic nerve disease
- Visual pathway disease • Ocular imaging technology • Electrodiagnostic testing

Key points

- The misdiagnosis of functional vision loss occurs in the eye care profession, and it is important to establish the criteria for amblyogenic factors before diagnosing functional vision loss (amblyopia).
- Anterior segment disease, retinal disease, and optic nerve and visual pathway disease have been misdiagnosed as functional vision loss sometimes with dire consequences.
- Standard examination techniques are important to support functional vision loss and to rule out the presence of pathological disease and need to be performed.
- Supplemental testing techniques including perimetry, ocular imaging technologies, and electrodiagnostic testing may be crucial to ruling out pathological disease when standard examination techniques are not sufficient.
- The failure to identify amblyopia masqueraders can have significant consequences for both the patient and the eye care practitioner, which can be avoided by adhering to standard examination techniques and ordering supplemental testing procedures when necessary.
- Monitoring the patient for pathological disease should not deter the practitioner from implementing therapeutic procedures to improve functional amblyopia.

*Corresponding author. E-mail address: sbass@sunyopt.edu

https://doi.org/10.1016/j.yaoo.2023.03.002
2452-1760/23/© 2023 Elsevier Inc. All rights reserved.

INTRODUCTION

Amblyopia clinically is defined as a decrease of best-corrected visual acuity of at least one line in one eye or both eyes and is the leading cause of visual impairment in the United States in the absence of obvious organic cause [1]. Whether due to secondary refractive error, strabismus, or visual deprivation, amblyopia results in a failure of cortical visual development with a resultant decrease in vision [2]. Furthermore, amblyopia additionally impacts unsteady or inaccurate monocular fixation, poor tracking ability, reduced contrast sensitivity, and inaccurate accommodative response [2]. Although amblyopia has a reported prevalence of 2% to 4% [3–5], on rare occasions, reduced visual acuity is a result of pathologic condition and can be potentially misdiagnosed as a functional disorder.

Amblyopia is a diagnosis of exclusion. It is important to note that patients with ocular pathologic condition and neurological disease also can have a functional vision disorder. It, therefore, is critical to do a complete assessment of the patients' ocular health to avoid potentially sight-threatening and life-threatening conditions. The malpractice litigation against practitioners for the misdiagnosis of amblyopia, and thereby failure to diagnose disease, have resulted in malpractice jury awards upward of US$9 million [6].

The large settlement and jury awards do not mitigate the potential loss to the patient and loss to the doctor. A potential loss to the doctor's reputation and the impact on the patient can be far costlier [7]. Failure to treat the underlying condition can result in permanent vision loss, with an impact on social and employment opportunities. In addition, the patient diagnosed with amblyopia can experience financial and time loss in search of ineffective treatment. In rare cases, the failure to detect the actual cause of reduced visual acuity can result in paralysis or even death. It, therefore, is the aim of this article to alert the doctor to the potential pitfalls in the misdiagnosis of amblyopia and review ancillary testing that is both necessary and beneficial in ruling out potential sight or life-threatening conditions.

AMBLYOGENIC FACTORS

Refractive amblyopia can be caused by anisometropia or isoametropic high bilateral refractive error. It is important to carefully monitor refractive error over time. Axial lengths seldom shorten. Therefore, if an increase in hyperopia occurs, the potential exists for the presence of a mass pushing behind the eye, resulting in a shortening of axial length. Moreover, changes in astigmatism over time can be the result of lens changes, shifts, or changes in corneal curvature [7,8].

The American Optometric Association published clinical practice guidelines for the detection and treatment of amblyopia [9]. The guidelines listed for amblyogenic factors based on refractive error are listed in Table 1.

The comprehensive eye examination will reveal whether these amblyogenic factors exist. In addition, pupil testing, a thorough slit lamp evaluation, and a dilated fundus examination should help to rule out some disease processes. However, additional testing procedures may be required in some cases, as will be reviewed later in this article.

Table 1		
Amblyogenic refractive errors		
Refractive condition	Anisometropia	Isoametropia
Astigmatism	−1.50D	−2.50D
Hyperopia	+1.00D	+5.00D
Myopia	−3.00D	−8.00D

Significance: exemplary cases

Exemplary cases are presented below in which patients were referred to rule out amblyopia and other causes of functional vision loss. Each case describes the reason for the referral, the clinical findings, and the ancillary testing results, which ultimately enabled the clinician to differentiate a pathological condition from a functional one. A more detailed description of the advanced technologies that were used as an aid in the differential diagnosis is detailed in the section on relevance following the cases.

Case 1: referred for refractive amblyopia

A 13-year-old child presented with a history of eye irritation and rubbing of her eyes. Her first pair of glasses was prescribed at the age of 10 with reports of worsening of visual acuities even with updated glasses prescriptions. She was diagnosed with refractive amblyopia secondary to her high astigmatic spectacle correction, which was OD −0.25 to 4.25 × 45 20/50 OS −0.50 to 3.7 5 × 75 20/70. Given AOA guidelines, one would expect some level of decrease in visual acuity with that magnitude of astigmatism in both eyes. However, the eye with the slightly lower prescription had worse visual acuity, which is not expected. Retinoscopy was performed and scissoring of the retinoscopy reflex was noted in both eyes. The anterior examination of the eyes revealed corneal thinning bilaterally with Fleischer's rings. Corneal topography demonstrated central corneal thinning consistent with keratoconus (Fig. 1). Keratoconus is a noninflammatory, progressive thinning of the cornea resulting in an increased and often irregular astigmatism with vision loss. It starts usually in the second or third decade of life and usually is associated with eye rubbing, atopy, and contact lens use [10–14]. Visual acuity often can be improved with gas permeable contact lenses or scleral lenses that can affect the patient's activities of daily living [15]. Moreover, management of keratoconus with corneal collagen cross-linking can stabilize and prevent the progression of the disease with some reports of improved visual acuity [16].

Case 2: subluxated lens

A 4-year-old boy was referred for refractive amblyopia. The child complained of decreased vision in both eyes, worse in the right eye. Visual acuities were 20/80 in the right eye and 20/30 in the left eye. Manifest refraction was OD +0.50 to 3.25 × 107 VA 20/40 and OS +1.00 to 1.50 × 180 VA 20/ 30. An eye examination through a dilated pupil revealed a subluxated lens

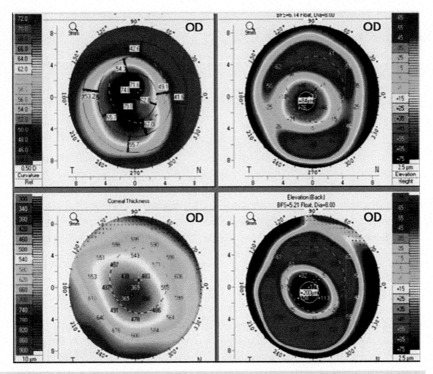

Fig. 1. Corneal topography reveals central thinning consistent with keratoconus.

in the right eye and a tilted lens in the left eye. The child denied any history of trauma. It was recommended that the child be evaluated for collagen vascular disease because of the abnormality in the lenses. A couple of months later, the child's 4-month-old baby brother was referred by his pediatrician for bilateral ectopic lenses. Entering visual acuities were 20/253 OU with Cardiff cards with no resistance to occlusion of either eye. Cycloplegic refraction was OD +1.00 to 7.50 × 60 and OS Plano-6.00 × 80. An examination through a dilated pupil confirmed bilateral ectopic lenses with normal intraocular pressure in each eye. However, since his brother had a similar finding, it leads one to rule out a possible genetic-related disorder that is associated with ectopic lentis. These disorders include Marfan syndrome, homocystinuria, or ADAMTSL4 gene mutation [17,18]. Genetic testing of both parents and 4 children revealed that both parents were carriers of pathogenic variants in the ADAMTSL4 gene. Of the 4 siblings, 3 had 2 copies of the pathogenic variant and had varying levels of ectopic lentis, whereas 1 child was a carrier. This mutation is found in the children of Bukharian Jewish origin and affected individuals present early in life with bilateral isolated ectopic lentis without associated systemic findings such as those found in Marfan syndrome [19]. Often, the lens changes can be subtle, as in one of the children who was brought in, and the best way to perceive a slight shift in the lens is to view it with an ophthalmoscope through a dilated pupil.

Case 3: law student cannot read

A 22-year-old law student presented for evaluation for the inability to read her law school assignments. She was spending hours reading briefs and other related law school documents and found that her eyes were getting fatigued, and she was having trouble seeing some of the letters and words. She was examined by several eye doctors, some of whom told her they could not find anything wrong with her eyes and that she should go for further evaluation to rule out visual skill issues that were causing her to have "eye strain." When she presented for an evaluation to our facility, her best corrected visual acuity, or BCVA was 20/70 in each eye. The anterior examination of the eyes did not reveal any abnormalities. Examination of the fundus revealed mild macular pigment abnormalities in each eye with no foveal reflex (Fig. 2A). Fundus autofluorescence imaging (FAF) revealed symmetric macular hypo-AF (dark areas) surrounded by a brighter ring of hyper-AF (Fig. 2B). Optical coherence tomography (OCT) showed symmetric macular thinning and atrophy (Fig. 2C). Genetic testing revealed a mutation in the ABCA4 gene (G1961 E) associated with a mild form of Stargardt disease. Over the years, the BCVA has decreased to 20/200 in each eye but has not changed since then. Stargardt disease usually causes a gradual loss in central vision in young teenagers and often is associated with flecked lesions filled with lipofuscin (which this patient did not have), which start centrally and expand outwardly. It often is difficult to detect in the early stage when ophthalmoscopic findings are not obvious. This case represents a disease and not a functional problem.

Case 4: rule out "refractive/strabismic amblyopia"

Sometimes, patients present with amblyogenic factors that do not explain the clinical findings. A 16-year-old male patient was referred by an outside provider for reduced BCVA in his right eye due to "refractive and strabismic amblyopia." BCVAs were 20/200 in the OD and 20/40 in the OS. The patient's spectacle Rx was OD: –050 to 3.00 × 30 and OS: +050 to 1.75 × 160. External examination revealed a 10-prism diopter intermittent right hyperesotropia. This case is especially challenging because there are amblyogenic factors but they do not explain all the clinical findings. For example, the OD has 3.00 D of astigmatism on an oblique axis, whereas the OS has –1.75 D of astigmatism, also at an oblique axis. The difference in astigmatism is only –1.25 D between eyes, which does not meet the amblyogenic criteria of –1.50 D between eyes. In addition, the amount of astigmatism does not explain the 20/200 visual acuity in the right eye and the 20/40 visual acuity in the left eye. The patient has an intermittent right hyper esotropia (ET) but an intermittent turn also does not explain the 20/200 visual acuity. Color photos and FAF reveal bone-spicule pigment migration in the periphery and hypo-AF throughout the fundus (Fig. 3A and B). OCT revealed the absence of the photoreceptor integrity

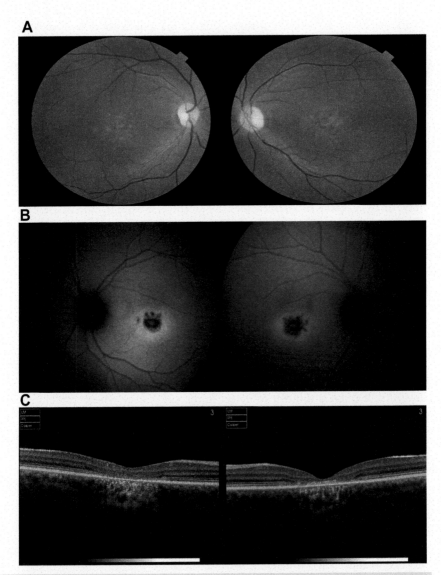

Fig. 2. (**A**) Color photography reveals subtle symmetric macular pigmentary disturbances. (**B**) FAF reveals symmetric macular hypo-AF (dark areas) surrounded by a brighter ring of hyper-AF. (**C**) OCT shows symmetric macular thinning and atrophy consistent with Stargardt disease.

line (PIL) and thinning of the entire outer retina in both eyes, worse in the right eye, which explains the reduced visual acuity in both eyes, worse in the right eye (Fig. 3C). The diagnosis was advanced retinitis pigmentosa, worse in the right eye. This case represents a structural or pathological abnormality with an overlying functional abnormality.

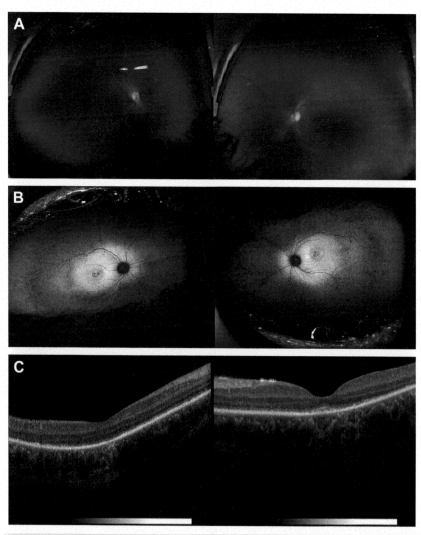

Fig. 3. (**A**) Color photos reveal attenuated arterioles and bone spicule pigmentary changes in the periphery. (**B**) FAF reveals bone-spicule pigment migration in the periphery (hypo-AF) and hypo-AF throughout the peripheral fundus with hyper-AF in the central retina. (**C**) OCT reveals absence of the PIL and thinning of the entire outer retina in both eyes, worse in the right eye.

Case 5: a young teenager with long-standing bilateral reduced visual acuity with no amblyogenic factor

A 13-year-old girl presented for consultation regarding failure to improve visual acuity with vision therapy. BCVAs remained 20/30 in each eye for many years. Refractive errors were OD: −1.50 to 1.25 × 15 and OS: −050 to 1.75 × 180. Even though the astigmatism was less than −2.50, the patient was diagnosed as a refractive amblyope. Ophthalmoscopy revealed the absence of a foveal reflex in each eye (Fig. 4A). All other ocular structures were normal. Visual field testing did not reveal any abnormalities. An OCT was performed, which revealed an absence of the foveal pit in each eye, or foveal plana (Fig. 4B). The diagnosis was isolated foveal hypoplasia or fovea plana, which is a developmental anomaly, unassociated with ocular albinism. Vision therapy would not improve the vision in either eye because this was a structural and not a functional abnormality.

Case 6: vision therapy unsuccessful in an anisometropic myopic amblyope
A 12-year-old boy presented with anisometropic amblyopia and reduced BCVA in the more myopic eye. Refractive error was OD: −6.00 VA 20/40 and OS: Plano. VA 20/20 OS. The patient was diagnosed with refractive anisometropic (myopic) amblyopia OD. The patient underwent several sessions of vision therapy; however, after many months, there was no improvement in the vision of the right eye. Ophthalmoscopy revealed a normal fundus in the left eye; however, examination of the right eye revealed thickened myelinated retinal nerve fibers superiorly and extending less inferiorly (Fig. 5A). In

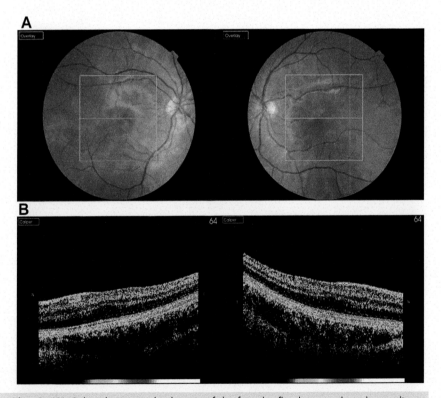

Fig. 4. (A) Color photo reveals absence of the foveal reflex but no other abnormality to explain the reduced visual acuity. (B) OCT through the macula reveals absence of the foveal pit or fovea plana.

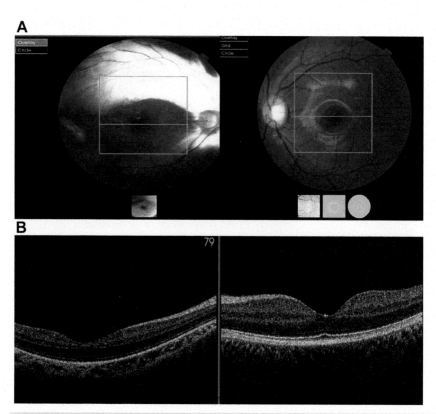

Fig. 5. (A) Fundus photo reveals a normal retina, right eye, and thickened myelinated nerve fibers superiorly and around the disc in the left eye as well as a dysplastic disc. (B) OCT of the macula. The PIL is attenuated in the right eye and is intact in the left eye.

addition, the optic nerve head in the right eye was tilted and hypoplastic. The macula appeared normal in both eyes. However, an OCT revealed attenuation of the PIL–also known as the ellipsoid zone (EZ) in the macula of the right eye, whereas the OCT of the left eye was normal (Fig. 5B). The PIL or EZ represents the interface between the inner and outer segments of the photoreceptors. Attenuation or absence in this layer affects visual function because the integrity of the photoreceptors has been compromised. The diagnosis was a syndrome of disc hypoplasia, myelinated nerve fibers, and myopia. The OCT revealed a structural abnormality in the macula and not a functional abnormality.

Case 7: case of long-standing reduced visual acuity with no amblyogenic factor
This next case reveals the importance in performing visual evoked potential (VEP) testing in questionable cases. A 28-year-old woman presented with a history of poor visual acuity in the left eye for as long as she could remember. Earlier history included examination by a retinal specialist and a neuroophthalmologist, including neuroimaging, but neither of these specialists could explain

why her vision was reduced in the left eye. Refractive errors were OD: −1.00 to 0.50 × 113 VA 20/20 and OS: Plano-1.00 × 90 VA 20/100. Axial lengths were OD: 24.8 mm and OS: 24.5 mm. No measurable strabismus existed. Corneal topography did not reveal any irregular astigmatism. Pupillary responses were normal in each eye, and threshold visual field testing did not reveal any neurological field loss in either eye. Ophthalmoscopic examination of the fundus revealed normal retinas and optic nerves. OCT results revealed normal macular structure and normal retinal nerve fiber layer structure. A Pattern VEP was performed, which revealed normal responses from the right eye and reduced and delayed responses from the left eye (Fig. 6A). A flash (nonpattern) VEP was normal in each eye (Fig. 6B). This case represents a long-term functional abnormality of the left eye, not a disease process.

Relevance: the use of technology in the differential of pathological from functional vision loss

For almost 50 years, practitioners relied solely on keratometry, slit lamp biomicroscopy, ophthalmoscopy, ultrasonography, and fluorescein angiography to detect structural disease conditions of the anterior and posterior segment of the eye. Other testing technologies, such as perimetry and electrodiagnostic testing, were additionally helpful to detect abnormalities in the visual pathways. However, many of the cases presented in this article were misdiagnosed as functional vision disorders because the cause of the reduced vision pathological disease escaped detection by these standard examination techniques.

The development and use of advances in technology have aided the eye care practitioner in ruling out the presence of ocular disease, and the cases presented earlier in this article demonstrate how a combination of standard examination techniques and newer technology have enabled the eye care practitioner to diagnose disease more accurately.

The specific imaging and testing technologies that have aided in the differential of pathological vision loss from functional vision loss, exemplified in the earlier cases are (a) corneal topography, (b) static perimetry, (c) OCT, (d) fundus autofluorescence, and (e) electrodiagnostic testing. These technologies are available to most eye care practitioners and, if not readily available in a private office, the patient can be referred to another eye-care facility. It is important to recognize when these additional technologies are required, and which test is the appropriate test to order.

Corneal topography

Evaluation of corneal curvature has come a long way since the keratometer. The keratometer was able to measure corneal power but only in the central 2 to 3 mm of the cornea. In contrast, today's devices can provide doctors with a vast amount of clinical information in addition to corneal curvature and power, such as typographical maps of the front and back surfaces of the cornea as well as corneal thickness. Case 1 highlights the need for corneal topography in cases of high astigmatism to rule out corneal abnormalities that can be contributory to visual acuity reduction. Furthermore, the

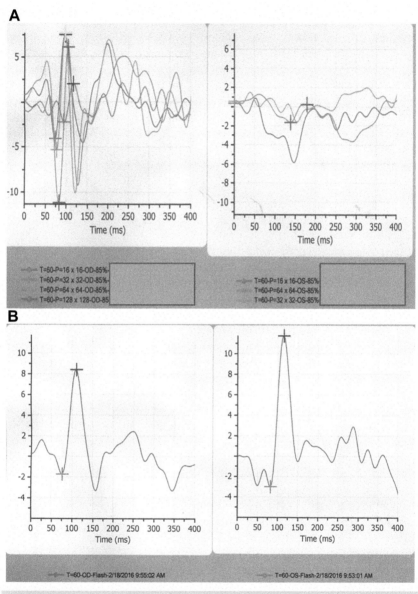

Fig. 6. **(A)** A pattern VEP shows normal responses from the right eye and reduced and delayed responses from the left eye. **(B)** A flash (nonpattern) VEP was normal in each eye.

management with gas permeable contact lenses or scleral lenses will often provide visual acuity improvement, which is critical earlier in life.

Static perimetry
Visual fields test the integrity of the visual pathways from the cornea to the occipital cortex. Amblyopia is a disease of form sense, not light sense. Therefore,

in a visual field test, where the patient responds to various intensities of light, the visual field in amblyopia will not be significantly affected. A generalized depression of the visual field may occur, or a relative central desensitivity or a greater degree of fixation losses in the amblyopic eye but a neurological field loss that respects the vertical meridian will not be evident. Field loss that respects the vertical meridian is suspect for a visual pathway problem and necessitates neuroimaging. Moreover, when testing amblyopic eyes, Goldmann visual fields are preferred to static perimetry in those patients whose visual acuity is less than 20/200 [20,21]. Acuity of worse than 20/400 is very unusual in patients with amblyopia and is often indicative of a disease process.

Optical coherence tomography
One of the most useful technologies in the detection of retinal and optic nerve disease is optical coherence tomography, now well known as OCT. This technology was developed in the early years of the current millennium and has evolved over time to exquisitely image layers of the retina in detail. The history and principles of OCT have been published in detail elsewhere [22]. The basic principle is that OCT uses reflected light to image the retina in depth of about 0.01 mm in living tissue. The resulting cross-sectional views have resolution in current systems that almost equal that achieved by histological slides of the same tissue. The original systems were time domain, or TD-OCTs. Subsequently, systems were designed using spectral domain or SD-OCT technology, which resulted in better resolution. SD-OCTs are universally used today. OCT has many clinical applications and in less than a minute, the mysteries of the various layers in the retina captured within a 6 mm × 6 mm area are revealed. Clinical applications include detection of abnormalities seen in a variety of acquired and hereditary vision disorders affecting the retina as well as disorders affecting the optic nerve, ganglion cell layer, and retinal nerve fiber layer. Several cases presented earlier in this article exemplify how OCT has aided in the differential diagnosis and enabled the detection of a structural abnormality invisible to ophthalmoscopy.

In Case 3, a patient with Stargardt disease was thought to have an accommodative disorder resulting in eye strain. Stargardt disease is a hereditary macular disorder with a prevalence of 1 in 10,000 affecting 30, 000 patients in the United States. [23]. Rando Allekmets demonstrated that Stargardt disease most often is caused by mutations in the ABCA4 gene, which is a retinal transporter gene [24]. Macular degeneration begins early in most forms of Stargardt disease, and patients become symptomatic for vision loss in the first to second decade of life. Often, as in this case, the macular abnormalities are invisible with ophthalmoscopy, and this patient was misdiagnosed for several years. The use of OCT was invaluable in demonstrating the macular atrophy in both eyes of this patient when ophthalmoscopic evidence was lacking.

In Case 4, the OCT revealed absence of the PIL (EZ) throughout the macular scan, worse in the left eye. This finding, combined with the presence of bone-spicule type pigmentation, would make the practitioner suspect retinitis pigmentosa, which can then be confirmed using other testing and imaging techniques.

Case 5 is of a 13-year-old girl had an unexplainable vision loss to the level of 20/30 in each eye. Even though her refractive error was low in sphere and cylinder, she was referred to rule out possible refractive amblyopia because vision therapy had not been helpful. The patient had seen several eye doctors to determine the cause of the reduced vision. Ophthalmoscopy was only noted for an absence of a foveal reflex. However, OCT revealed an absence of the foveal pit. This developmental anomaly also is known as foveal hypoplasia. Foveal hypoplasia is a known feature of ocular and oculocutaneous albinism but no evidence of this disease existed. Negative iris transillumination occurred and no nystagmus was noted. Therefore, the diagnosis in this case was isolated foveal hypoplasia with absence of a foveal pit. Marmor and colleagues [25] published 4 cases where visual acuity ranged from 20/20 to 20/50. They found that central widening of the outer nuclear layer and lengthening of cone outer segments on SD-OCT and adaptive optics imaging (a technology used by few clinical practices) demonstrated normal cone diameters in the central 1° to 2°. Multifocal electroretinogram responses also were normal. The authors, therefore, questioned whether a foveal pit was necessary for normal visual function and suggested that the term be renamed fovea plana because foveal hypoplasia had a negative clinical connotation. However, the absence of the foveal pit could explain the reduced visual acuity. In our patient, vision therapy for "refractive amblyopia" was not helpful because a structural anomaly was not evident on ophthalmoscopy.

In Case 6, the clinical utility of OCT was paramount in helping to explain why a patient with an amblyogenic factor of anisometropic amblyopia failed to improve with vision therapy. She underwent several sessions of vision therapy without any improvement in visual acuity. The refractive error was plano in one eye and −8.00D myopia in the "amblyopic" eye. It is certainly understandable how a clinician would think such a patient could benefit from vision therapy. Fundus examination of the affected eye revealed heavily myelinated nerve fibers along the superior arcade and a tilted disc, but the macula area appeared normal. However, when the visual acuity failed to improve with vision training, an OCT was obtained through the macula, which revealed a significantly attenuated PIL, or EZ.

This case and 2 similar ones were published by one of us (SB) [26] and demonstrate this to be a developmental anomaly in which the patient was born with a syndrome of dysplastic optic nerve head and myelinated nerve fibers, and abnormal photoreceptor integrity. As a result, it is theorized that the development of myopia may have been a sequela of the structural anomaly, in that an eye that does not see well due to a structural anomaly may not have a "stop signal" to prevent additional growth of the affected eye. Animal studies and observational clinical studies have demonstrated that the growth of the eye is influenced by the quality of the retinal image [27]. Failure of vision therapy in this condition has been reported by others [28] in this syndrome but we were the first to demonstrate the macular abnormality in the PIL, which would explain the failure of vision therapy to improve the visual acuity in this condition. The *macular* abnormality was only evident in OCT, not ophthalmoscopy.

Fundus autofluorescence imaging

Fundus autofluorescence imaging, or FAF, is an imaging technology that is currently part of many ophthalmic camera systems. It is a way of imaging a patient's retina in vivo and was developed to topographically map retinal fluorophores that accumulate as lipofuscin, occurring naturally or as part of a pathological process [29]. When disease affecting the outer retina exists, lipofuscin accumulates in the retinal pigment epithelium (RPE) and is visible as hyperautofluorescence (hyper-AF) or bright white areas. Because the outer retina degenerates in progressive outer retinal diseases, the cells degenerate as does the lipofuscin, and this is imaged as hypoautofluorescence (hypo-AF). Clinical applications include the early detection of hereditary retinal disorders and acquired disorders affecting the outer retina such as macular degeneration, central serous choroidopathy, and retinal pigment epitheliopathies.

The 2 cases of hereditary retinal diseases (Stargardt disease and retinitis pigmentosa) that were presented in the earlier section demonstrated abnormalities on the FAF imaging that clearly showed the presence of pathological disease missed in the original examinations of these patients. One was the patient with Stargardt disease, discussed in the section on OCT, but the patient also had abnormalities in FAF, which clearly demonstrated macular hypo-AF indicative of macular atrophy (see Fig. 2B). Another case was the patient with reduced visual acuity in both eyes but worse in the eye with hypotropia and exotropia. Although strabismus can be an amblyogenic cause, no explanation existed for reduced vision in the better eye. FAF clearly demonstrated peripheral hypo-AF and a central hyper-AF ring, findings associated with retinitis pigmentosa. The reduction of visual acuity in the better eye was explained based on not only FAF but also OCT because the PIL (EZ) was almost absent. A young patient like this deserves a diagnosis for career and family planning purposes and to determine future prognosis. Currently, with the development of gene therapies and clinical trials for other medical therapies to treat or slow down progression of these diseases, the accuracy of the diagnosis becomes even more important. For example, an FDA-approved gene therapy exists to replace a defective gene (RPE65) and improve visual function in patients with a night blinding disease, Leber Congenital Amaurosis, who are bi-allelic for RPE65 mutations [30].

Electrodiagnostic testing

Electrodiagnostic testing, namely VEP testing, electroretinography (ERG), and electro-oculography (EOG), are *objective tests* of retinal and visual pathway dysfunction. Apart from static perimetry, the earlier sections reviewed the advanced testing technologies to detect *structural* anomalies of the eye. This section is devoted to objective testing that reveals *functional* anomalies to aid in diagnosis.

The VEP is monitored at the level of the occipital cortex with electrodes and hence tests the patency of the visual pathways. The ERG and EOG are electrical responses that originate from various layers of the retina. Several clinical applications of these testing procedures exist in detecting anomalies in retinal and visual pathway function. These tests are described in detail elsewhere [31,32].

The VEP has many clinical applications and can be used to help to rule out pathological diseases that affect visual acuity in one or both eyes. It also is used to determine the prognosis of acuity improvement with vision therapy in known amblyopia. The test can be performed using both patterned stimulation (usually checkerboard patterns of assorted sizes) and nonpattern (flash) stimulation. Because amblyopia affects form sense, not light sense, an amblyope will have an abnormal response to pattern stimulation but not to the flash stimulation. Therefore, an abnormal response to flash stimulation in a healthy-appearing eye should make the practitioner suspect a pathological problem affecting the visual pathways. The patient in Case 7, with long-standing reduced visual acuity in one eye with no amblyogenic factors, had a reduced VEP to pattern but a normal response to a nonpatterned flash. Because amblyopia is a disease of form sense, not light sense, the presence of an abnormal response to a pattern stimulus with a normal response to a flash stimulus along with the other examination findings and earlier examination history in this case support a diagnosis of amblyopia or functional vision loss in the left eye. Another patient, however, not presented in this article, who was misdiagnosed with refractive amblyopia, had absent VEPs to *both* pattern and flash stimulation. Neuroimaging revealed a large chiasmal glioma (Fig. 7).

The ERG is an electrical response, which comes from the retina (photoreceptors and bipolar cells predominantly). A full-field ERG, which tests the entire retina, is usually ordered to rule out night blinding diseases, such as retinitis pigmentosa, cone and cone-rod dystrophies, and macular dystrophies. Another

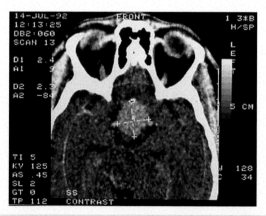

Fig. 7. A large chiasmal lesion was revealed on neuroimaging when no response was present on a pattern or a flash VEP.

type of ERG, the multifocal ERG, is used to determine focal functional loss of outer retinal function, such as is seen in Plaquenil toxicity and sector retinitis pigmentosa. In Case 4, the visual acuities were reduced in both eyes and pigmentary changes occurred in the peripheral retina. The OCT, FAF, and fundus examination were suspicious for retinitis pigmentosa even though the patient had no symptoms of night blindness. The extinguished ERG in this patient, however, confirmed loss of photoreceptor function, which supported the diagnosis of advanced retinitis pigmentosa.

SUMMARY

The misdiagnosis of amblyopia/functional vision loss can have consequences for the patient and for the eye-care practitioner, with the costs to the patient being far greater. Eye-care practitioners need to be aware of the factors that can lead to amblyopia and remember that it is a diagnosis of exclusion once a pathological disease process is ruled out [33]. In the absence of amblyogenic factors, ancillary testing procedures such as corneal topography, static perimetry, OCT, FAF, electrodiagnostic procedures, and neuroimaging must be performed to rule out a disease process. It also is important to recognize that the coexistence of a functional and pathological disorder is possible, and treatment of the functional component is warranted once the disease condition is also addressed. Given that amblyopia results in poorer outcomes on tests of skills required for proficiency in everyday tasks [34], the impact of the functional component should not be overlooked.

CLINICS CARE POINTS

- If a patient has new onset visual loss after the age of 8 years and the stereopsis is normal, perform ancillary vision tests to rule out ophthalmic and/or visual pathway disease.
- If refractive amblyopia is diagnosed, check that the BCVA matches the eye with the worse refractive error in anisometropic cases.
- If the BCVA is worse than 20/20 and the ophthalmoscopic evaluation does not reveal any abnormalities, perform at least a static perimetry test, corneal topography, an OCT of the macula and the optic nerve, and fundus photography with fundus autofluorescent testing.
- If BCVA is reduced and all clinical testing of the eyes does not reveal any abnormality, perform or refer for VEP testing or refer the patient to a neuroophthalmologist for neuroimaging.

DISCLOSURE

The authors have nothing to disclose.

References

[1] Blair K, Cibis G, Gulani AC. Amblyopia. In: StatPearls. Treasure island: StatPearls Publishing; 2022.

[2] Wright KW. Visual development and amblyopia. In: *Handbook of pediatric strabismus and amblyopia*. New York, NY: Springer; 2006. p. 103–37.

[3] Friedman DS, Repka MX, Katz J, et al. Prevalence of amblyopia and strabismus in white and African American children aged 6 through 71 months the Baltimore Pediatric Eye Disease Study. Ophthalmology 2009;116(11):2128–34, e1-2.

[4] DeSantis D. Amblyopia. Pediatr Clin North Am 2014;61(3):505–18.

[5] Pescosolido N, Stefanucci A, Buomprisco G, et al. Amblyopia treatment strategies and new drug therapies. J Pediatr Ophthalmol Strabismus 2014;51(2):78–86.

[6] Jury, decides against optometrist, awards $9.2 million for missed tumor diagnosis, Primary Care Optometry News, 1997.

[7] Espandar L, Meyer J. Keratoconus: overview and update on treatment. Middle East Afr J Ophthalmol 2010;17(1):15–20.

[8] Matsuo T. How far is observation allowed in patients with ectopia lentis? SpringerPlus 2015;4:461.

[9] Optometric Clinical Practice Guidelines. Care of the Patient with Amblyopia. In: American academy of optometry 2004. Available at: https://www.aoa.org/AOA/Documents/Practice%20Management/Clinical%20Guidelines/Consensus-based%20guidelines/Care%20of%20Patient%20with%20Amblyopia.pdf. Accessed 14 December, 2022.

[10] Hashemi H, Heydarian S, Hooshmand E, et al. The Prevalence and Risk Factors for Keratoconus: A Systematic Review and Meta-Analysis. Cornea 2020;39(2):263–70.

[11] Sharma N, Rao K, Maharana PK, et al. Ocular allergy and keratoconus. Indian J Ophthalmol 2013;61:407–9.

[12] Millodot M, Shneor E, Albou S, et al. Prevalence and associated factors of keratoconus in Jerusalem: a cross-sectional study. Ophthalmic Epidemiol 2011;18:91–7.

[13] Georgiou T, Funnell CL, Cassels-Brown A, et al. Influence of ethnic origin on the incidence of keratoconus and associated atopic disease in Asians and white patients. Eye 2004;18:379–83.

[14] McMonnies CW. Abnormal rubbing and keratectasia. Eye Contact Lens 2007;33:265–71.

[15] Kumar M, Shetty R, Lalgudi VG, et al. The effect of scleral lenses on vision, refraction and aberrations in post-LASIK ectasia, keratoconus and pellucid marginal degeneration. Ophthalmic Physiol Opt 2021;41(4):664–72.

[16] Fard AM, Reynolds AL, Lillvis JH, et al. Corneal collagen cross-linking in pediatric keratoconus with three protocols: a systematic review and meta-analysis. J AAPOS 2020;24(6):331–6.

[17] Rødahl E, Mellgren AEC, Boonstra NE, et al. ADAMTSL4-Related Eye Disorders. In: Adam MP, Everman DB, Mirzaa GM, et al, editors. GeneReviews® [internet]. Seattle (WA): University of Washington, Seattle; 2012. p. 1993–2022. Available at: https://www.ncbi.nlm.nih.gov/books/NBK84111/. Accessed 14 December, 2022.

[18] Rahman M, Sharma M, Aggarwal P, et al. Homocystinuria and ocular complications - A review. Indian J Ophthalmol 2022;70(7):2272–8.

[19] Reinstein E, Smirin-Yosef P, Lagovsky I, et al. A founder mutation in ADAMTSL4 causes early-onset bilateral ectopia lentis among Jews of Bukharian origin. Mol Genet Metab 2016;117(1):38–41.

[20] Donahue SP, Wall M, Kutzko KE, et al. Automated perimetry in amblyopia: a generalized depression. Am J Ophthalmol 1999;127(3):312–21.

[21] Kedar S, Ghate D, Corbett JJ. Visual fields in neuro-ophthalmology. Indian J Ophthalmol 2011;59(2):103–9.

[22] Huang D, Tan O, Fujimoto JG, et al. Optical coherence tomography. In: Huang D, Kaiser PK, Lowder CY, et al, editors. Retinal imaging. 1st edition. Philadelphia: Mosby Elsevier; 2006. p. 47–65.

[23] Tanna P, Strauss RW, Fujinami K, et al. Stargardt disease: clinical features, molecular genetics, animal models and therapeutic options. Br J Ophthalmol 2017;101:25–30.

[24] Allekmets R, Singh N, Sun H, et al. A photoreceptor cell-specific ATP-binding transporter gene (ABCR) is mutated in recessive Stargardt macular dystrophy. Nat Genet 1997;15: 236–46.

[25] Marmor MF, Choi SS, Zawadzki RJ, et al. Visual insignificance of the foveal pit: reassessment of foveal hypoplasia as fovea plana. Arch Ophthalmol 2008;126(7):907–13.

[26] Bass SJ, Westcott J, Sherman J. OCT in a Myelinated Retinal Nerve Fiber Syndrome with Reduced Vision. Optom Vis Sci 2016;93(10):1285–91.

[27] Flitcroft DI. The complex interactions of retinal, optical, and environmental factors in myopia aetiology. Prog Retin Eye Res 2012;31:622–60.

[28] Ellis GS Jr, Frey T, Gouterman RZ. Myelinated nerve fibers, axial myopia, and refractory amblyopia: an organic disease. J Pediatr Ophthalmol Strabismus 1987;24:111–9.

[29] Delori FC, Dorey CK, Staurenghi G, et al. In vivo fluorescence of the ocular fundus exhibits retinal pigment epithelium lipofuscin characteristics. Invest Ophthalmol Vis Sci 1995;36: 718–29.

[30] Deng C, Zhao PY, Branham K, et al. Real-world outcomes of voretigene neparvovec treatment in pediatric patients with RPE65-associated Leber congenital amaurosis. Graefes Arch Clin Exp Ophthalmol 2022;260:1543–50.

[31] Sherman J. In: Visual Evoked Potential, In: Terry J.E., *Ocular disease: detection, diagnosis and treatment*. Stoneham, MA: Butterworth Publishers; 1984. p. 495–527.

[32] Sherman J. In: Electroretinography and Electro-Oculography, In: Terry J.E., *Ocular disease: detection, diagnosis and treatment*. Stoneham, MA: Butterworth Publishers; 1984. p. 469–93.

[33] Rutstein RP, Than TP, Hartmann EE, et al. Idiopathic amblyopia: a diagnosis of exclusion. A report of 3 patients. Optometry 2011;82(5):290–7, PMID: 21524600.

[34] Webber AL. The functional impact of amblyopia. Clin Exp Optom 2018;101(4):443–50.

Pediatric

ELSEVIER
MOSBY

Advances in Ophthalmology and Optometry 8 (2023) 45–58

ADVANCES IN OPHTHALMOLOGY AND OPTOMETRY

Correction of Pediatric Aphakia

Kamran Ahmed, MD[a,b,c,d,*], Chap-Kay K. Lau, BA[a]

[a]University of Arizona College of Medicine, Phoenix, AZ, USA; [b]Phoenix Children's Hospital, 1920 East Thomas Road, Phoenix, AZ 85016, USA; [c]Creighton University School of Medicine, Phoenix, AZ, USA; [d]Mayo Clinic Alix School of Medicine, Phoenix, AZ, USA

Keywords

• Pediatric aphakia • Spectacles • Contact lenses • Intraocular lenses • Amblyopia

Key points

• Failure to correct pediatric aphakia in a timely manner can result in permanent visual loss due to amblyopia.

• Correction of pediatric aphakia requires working knowledge of the use of spectacles, contact lenses, and intraocular lenses (IOLs).

• Pediatric aphakia can be associated with other ocular comorbidities, such as glaucoma and structural defects of the eye requiring creative techniques for IOL fixation.

INTRODUCTION

Aphakia, meaning the absence of an intraocular lens (IOL), whether crystalline or artificial, presents a multifaceted problem in the pediatric patient. Without aphakic correction, the resultant defocus of the eye can lead to permanent vision loss due to amblyopia. In addition, pediatric aphakia commonly presents with concurrent ocular morbidities, adding further layers of complexity when formulating a treatment plan. This article discusses the various treatment options available for correcting pediatric aphakia, including the use of spectacles, contact lenses, and IOLs.

HISTORY OF PEDIATRIC APHAKIC CORRECTION

Contact lenses have been the main method of correcting unilateral pediatric aphakia since the 1970s [1]. Advances in contact lens design that allowed for increased oxygen permeability, easy fitting, along with Food and Drug Administration

---

*Corresponding author. E-mail address: kahmed@phoenixchildrens.com

https://doi.org/10.1016/j.yaoo.2023.02.005
2452-1760/23/© 2023 Elsevier Inc. All rights reserved.

(FDA) approval of extended-wear contact lenses made it an ideal choice for the pediatric population [2,3]. Spectacles are used primarily for correcting bilateral aphakia and have limited use for unilateral aphakia due to the significant anisometropia, resulting aniseikonia, and visual distortion [4].

The first IOL placement in an adult patient was done by Sir Harold Ridley in 1949 [5] and soon after, Edward Epstein placed the first IOL in a pediatric patient in 1951 [6]. However, the usage of IOLs in pediatric patients was not widely accepted at the time due to poor postoperative outcomes secondary to limited surgical techniques and lens designs.

IOL use for the pediatric population rose steadily from the 1980s to 1990s due to advances in surgical procedures, safety, lens design, and knowledge of the refractive growth of the eye [7]. IOL implantation in children 2 years of age and older garnered support much sooner than implantation in infants and became a major treatment for aphakia in this age group [8,9].

In 2010, the Infant Aphakia Treatment Study (IATS) compared the visual outcomes and adverse effects between contact lenses and IOLs in the correction of unilateral aphakia in infants' ages 1 to 6 months [10]. The study concluded that no significant difference occurred in the visual acuity between the two groups. However, more adverse effects and additional intraocular operations occurred in the IOL group, so the investigators cautioned against IOL usage in pediatric patients aged 6 months or younger. Extended follow-up of the IATS patients at ages 4.5 years and 10.5 years concluded again that no significant difference in visual acuity occurred between the contact lens and IOL groups [11,12].

CAUSES OF PEDIATRIC APHAKIA

Pediatric aphakia can occur due to congenital causes, ocular trauma, and surgical removal. Congenital primary aphakia is a rare developmental disorder that results in the absence of lens formation during the 4th to 5th week of embryogenesis and can be subdivided histologically into primary and secondary forms depending on the mechanism and severity of ocular defects [13]. In primary aphakia, the failure of induction of the lens placode exists, which is commonly associated with other severe ocular defects such as anterior segment aplasia. In secondary aphakia, normal lens development is disrupted, causing the lens to be resorbed perinatally. Secondary aphakia usually is associated with more moderate ocular defects as compared with primary aphakia. More common causes of pediatric aphakia are cases in which patients are left aphakic during treatment of ocular trauma [14,15], and lens pathology that would necessitate its removal such as cataracts, ectopia lentis, or extremely high refractive errors requiring refractive lens exchange.

MODALITIES OF APHAKIC CORRECTION
Nonsurgical treatment of aphakia
Nonsurgical treatment of aphakia consists of spectacles and contact lenses. The method of choice will depend on whether the aphakia is unilateral or bilateral, infantile onset or later, and even socioeconomic factors.

Aphakic spectacles have several advantages including greater cost-effectiveness and ease of use for infants and their caregivers who are uncomfortable with contact lenses. Their ease of use increases patient compliance, which is important for management of amblyopia in the pediatric population. However, aphakic spectacles have multiple disadvantages. The lenses used are centrally thick and magnify images leading to altered depth perception, ring scotoma, and "pincushion" distortion [7,16]. The lenses also cause the eyes to look highly magnified which can be cosmetically undesirable.

Today's aphakic spectacle lenses are made of CR-39, a plastic material that has several advantages including reduced weight, ultraviolet light absorption, and scratch resistance [16]. As mentioned previously, aphakic spectacles are primarily used for the treatment of bilateral aphakia. However, if the pediatric patient cannot tolerate surgery or contact lenses for aphakic correction, the use of spectacles for unilateral aphakia can still be considered to preserve vision in the aphakic eye. The adult brain can fuse retinal images that differ in size by as much as 8%; the child's brain can handle an even greater disparity [17].

Aphakic contact lenses are used to correct both unilateral and bilateral aphakia and are a suitable choice for all ages, including infants. Similar to aphakic spectacles, aphakic contact lenses have increased central thickness due to the high refractive power, but they do not have the same optical distortions and cosmetic disturbances due to their reduced vertex distance.

Two main types of aphakic contact lenses are used today: silicone elastomer (SE) and rigid gas permeable (RGP) lenses. Currently, the most popular SE lens for the correction of pediatric aphakia in the United States is the SilSoft Super Plus (Bausch & Lomb, Rochester, NY), which is suitable for 30-day extended and overnight wear due to its high oxygen permeability (diffusion coefficient [Dk] = 340). These lenses are advantageous to infants and children who do not tolerate repetitive insertion and removal of lenses. The disadvantages of SilSoft lenses, however, are their limited range of refractive powers (+23, +26, +29, +32 diopters [D]), three base curves (7.5, 7.7, 7.9 mm), and one diameter (11.3 mm). Like other contact lenses, it is associated with adverse events such as microbial keratitis, corneal edema, and corneal scars due to extended wear [18].

In comparison, RGP lenses are highly customizable with more fitting parameters and astigmatic correction. However, the higher customizability of RGP lenses also requires more expertise for the fitting process; other drawbacks include having a lower oxygen permeability compared with SE lenses, risk of breaking in situ, and daily insertion and removal as they cannot be worn overnight [19].

In 2020, the IATS published long-term findings on visual outcomes after the initial IATS study in 2010. Their conclusion, as determined at three different ages (12 months, 4.5 years, and 10.5 years), was that visual acuity was similar in unilateral pseudophakic children and in aphakic children corrected with a contact lens [10,11,20]. In addition, the IATS group found that the subset of children who were left aphakic and continued to wear their contact lenses at age 10.5 years had the best visual outcomes of all the other groups. Though notable, these findings cannot be generalized due to different confounding factors, such as the lenses being provided free of charge until age 5 years, and that continued contact lens use after age 5 years may be associated with families with higher socioeconomic backgrounds who were able to continue purchasing lenses [20,21].

Intracapsular and extracapsular intraocular lens fixation

For pediatric patients undergoing primary or secondary IOL implantation due to aphakia, different methods of IOL fixation can be implemented. The fixation site largely depends on the integrity of the existing lens capsule. Within the posterior chamber, both intracapsular and extracapsular fixation are used. Intracapsular fixation with the IOL haptic and optic in the capsular bag also is known as in-the-bag implantation (Fig. 1A). Extracapsular fixation with the haptic and optic in the iridociliary sulcus (Fig. 1B) is performed as well, especially if there is insufficient support from the posterior capsule. Three-piece IOLs are used for ciliary sulcus implantation and not single-piece acrylic lenses, as these are associated with iris chafing and Uveitis Glaucoma Hyphema syndrome (UGH) syndrome in the ciliary sulcus. Both single-piece and three-piece lenses can be implanted within the capsular bag. Both intracapsular and ciliary sulcus fixation generally are safe when performed with the correct type of IOL [22–25].

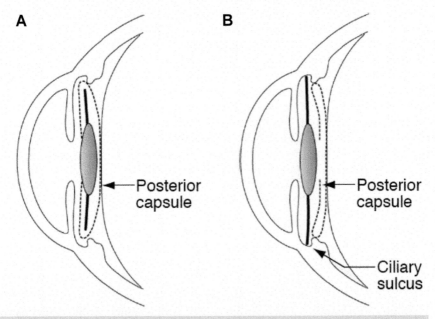

Fig. 1. (A) Intracapsular fixation with haptic and optic in the capsular bag. (B) Extracapsular fixation with haptic and optic in the iridociliary sulcus. (*Reprinted with permission from* Brodie SE, 2022-2023 Basic and Clinical Science Course, Section 3, Clinical Optics and Vision Rehabilitation. American Academy of Ophthalmology, 2022.)

Evidence exists to show that ciliary sulcus implantation without additional fixation such as optic capture may result in long-term IOL decentration and tilt as well as a higher incidence of secondary glaucoma in children [26,27]. Decentration of the three-piece IOL in the ciliary sulcus is thought to be due to the lack of sufficient diameter of the haptics to maintain apposition against the wall of the ciliary sulcus. Therefore, when a three-piece lens is implanted in the ciliary sulcus, central fixation of the lens using optic capture is recommended to prevent long-term decentration of the lens.

Optic capture was originally described by Neuhann and Neuhann in a film, "The Rhexis-Fixated Lens," in 1991. Later in 1994, Gimbel and Debroff published a series of eight pediatric eyes undergoing cataract surgery with posterior optic capture [28,29]. In this series, the haptics of the IOL was in the capsular bag, and the optic was behind the posterior capsule. This resulted in multiple benefits. The IOL was immediately centered and stabilized by the capsular bag, avoiding IOL sundowning, rotation, or changes in effective lens position over time. The anterior and posterior capsular leaflets were in apposition together anterior to the IOL optic, preventing the migration of lens epithelial cells posterior to the optic and significantly reducing posterior opacification. Anterior vitrectomy was not required, because the lens epithelial cells were effectively sealed off from the anterior vitreous face, and a bicameral eye was maintained. Multiple other permutations of optic capture have been developed and all are useful in various situations in the modern correction of pediatric aphakia [30]. The one most commonly used by the author is bicapsular capture in which a three-piece IOL is implanted with haptics in the iridociliary sulcus and optic captured through the anterior and posterior capsulorhexis (Fig. 2).

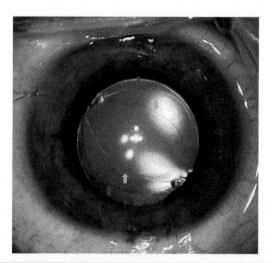

Fig. 2. This intraoperative photo during pediatric cataract surgery by the author shows a three-piece IOL with haptics in the iridociliary sulcus and optic captured through the anterior (*red arrows*) and posterior (*green arrows*) capsulorhexes (bicapsular capture).

Data from the IATS indicate that primary IOL implantation between 1 and 6 months of age has no advantages over aphakia corrected with a contact lens. In fact, primary IOL implantation had a higher rate of adverse events (most commonly, secondary opacities and need for additional surgery) [31]. The risk of developing glaucoma was similar between the primary IOL implantation and contact lens groups. The primary risk factors for developing glaucoma after infantile cataract surgery were younger age at surgery and smaller corneal diameter [32]. Beyond 6 months of age, primary IOL implantation has favorable visual outcomes and a low rate of adverse events, such as glaucoma, lens reproliferation, and IOL dislocation [33]. In the IATS, 53 eyes had primary IOL implantation, whereas 23 eyes had secondary IOL implantation. An analysis of the visual outcomes after secondary IOL implantation performed at a median age of 5.4 years compared with primary IOL implantation found a significant difference in mean refraction at age 10.5 years: -3.2 ± 2.7 D in the secondary IOL group compared with -5.5 ± 6.6 D in the primary IOL group ($P = 0.03$). The investigators concluded that postponing IOL implantation until after age 5 years resulted in the reduced risk of high myopia due to greater predictability of axial elongation [31].

Anterior chamber intraocular lenses

Anterior chamber IOLs (ACIOLs) are typically angle-supported, meaning that the S-shaped haptics rests in the iridocorneal angle (Fig. 3). In a retrospective study in 2005 of eight eyes of pediatric patients with Marfan syndrome who had undergone pars plana lensectomy, vitrectomy, and primary ACIOL placement, follow-up was a mean of 12.7 months. None of the patients experienced corneal decompensation, increased intraocular pressure, persistent inflammation, IOL displacement, or explantation during the follow-up period [34]. In a more recent study in 2021 of ACIOL implantation in 35 eyes of 22 children with a median age of 10.6 years, 12 eyes required additional surgery for ACIOL repositioning or IOL exchange with an Artisan iris-enclavated lens (Ophtec BV, Groningen, the Netherlands). Therefore, the investigators recommended avoiding the use of angle-supported ACIOLs in children [35]. The current, general consensus is that other forms of IOL fixation are preferred over ACIOLs for children.

Iris-fixated intraocular lenses

The iris-enclavated Artisan lens has commonly been used for the correction of pediatric aphakia in Asia and Europe and more recently in the United States. The Artisan lens clips onto the anterior surface of the iris using two claws that pinch the iris stroma for fixation, also known as enclavation (Fig. 4). Although the lens shown in Fig. 4A is a biconcave lens for the correction of myopia, this diagram illustrates the positioning of all types of Artisan lenses within the anterior chamber. The Artisan aphakia lens (see Fig. 4B) is biconvex for the correction of aphakic hyperopia [36]. The lens is made of polymethyl methacrylate, and its vaulted design allows for aqueous flow through the pupil, though a peripheral iridectomy is still performed at the time of implantation. The feasibility

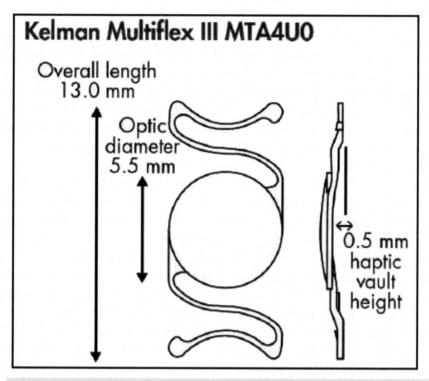

Fig. 3. Dimensions of the anterior chamber intraocular lens (ACIOL) with S-shaped haptics, which press against the iridocorneal angle. (*Reprinted with permission from* Chang DF. Advanced IOL Fixation Techniques: Strategies for Compromised or Missing Capsular Support. Thorofare, NJ: SLACK Incorporated; 2019.)

of such a lens is limited by the need for sufficient aqueous depth (AQD), the distance from the central corneal endothelium to the central anterior lens capsule or iris plane. The Artisan lens requires an AQD of 3.2 mm. In children who tend to have smaller eyes than adults, the AQD plays an important role in choosing the method of aphakic correction. Implantation of an Artisan lens in the setting of insufficient AQD can result in angle-closure glaucoma, accelerated corneal endothelial cell loss, subclinical inflammation, and pigmentary dispersion [37]. Therefore, it is critical for the pediatric ophthalmologist to check the patient's AQD, white-to-white distance, and corneal endothelial health before implantation to ensure that the appropriately sized lens is used.

Currently, in the United States, implantation of the Artisan aphakia lens is undergoing a multicenter clinical trial for patients' ages 2 to 21 years old. Its power ranges from +10.0 to +30.0 D [38]. Implantation of the Artisan aphakia lens in aphakic children lacking capsular support has been shown to improve best corrected visual acuity about 0.45 Log of Minimum Angle of Resolution (logMAR) with minimal postoperative complications [39]. The Artisan lens

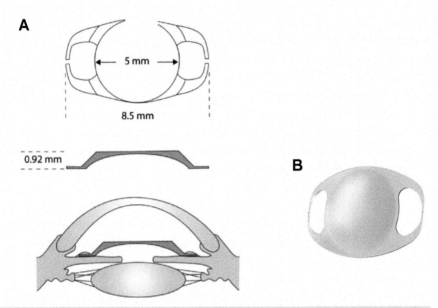

Fig. 4. (A) Dimensions and anatomic position of the Ophtec-Artisan myopia lens, which has a biconcave optic, in the anterior segment. (B) The Ophtec-Artisan aphakia lens has a biconvex optic. ([A] This article was published in Journal of American Association for Pediatric Ophthalmology and Strabismus, 25, Nicholas Faron DO, James Hoekel OD, Lawrence Tychsen MD(s), Visual acuity, refractive error, and regression outcomes in 169 children with high myopia who were implanted with Ophtec-Artisan or Vision phakic IOLs, 27.e1-27.e8, Copyright Elsevier 2021; [B] *Courtesy of* Ophtec BV, Sunrise, FL.)

comes in optic sizes of 5.0 and 6.0 mm diameter. Typically, the 5.0 mm diameter optic is used in children, which requires a corneal incision of 5.2 mm for insertion. The overall length of the lens including the haptics is 8.5 mm [40,41]. De-enclavation of the Artisan lens from the iris can occur, usually in the setting of trauma. In a study of the Artisan aphakia lens with 25 aphakic eyes followed for 1 year, the average age of the patients was 7 years. Eight percent of patients developed traumatic dislocation of the lens [39]. In a study of retropupillary iris enclavation in pediatric eyes, three out of eight eyes experienced haptic de-enclavation [42]. Therefore, in the author's opinion, retropupillary fixation of the Artisan lens as sometimes performed in adults is not recommended in children, because traumatic de-enclavation of the lens will cause the lens to fall posteriorly into the vitreous chamber.

Suturing of a three-piece IOL to the posterior surface of the iris is usually performed with 10-0 polypropylene suture in the setting of insufficient capsular support. In a study of 12 pediatric eyes, dislocation of the iris-sutured IOL occurred in four eyes, and no suture breakage was detected [43]. In another retrospective study of 17 pediatric eyes, seven iris-sutured IOLs became dislocated at a mean of 12 months after surgery [44]. In both studies, the investigators indicated that sutures were intact at the time of dislocation, and it was likely rotational instability of the lens that led to the haptics slipping out of the suture tunnels. Owing to the high rate of IOL dislocation in some studies, iris-sutured IOLs in children should be reserved for situations where other fixation methods are not possible.

Scleral-fixated intraocular lenses

In recent years, a variety of methods have been developed for fixation of IOLs to the sclera. They fall into two broad categories: suture fixation and haptic fixation. In suture-fixation, the entire IOL is within the eye, and suture is used to fixate the IOL to the scleral wall. Typically, polypropylene (Prolene-Ethicon Inc, Raritan, NJ) or polytetrafluoroethylene (GORE-TEX–Gore Medical, Newark, DE) sutures are used. In haptic fixation, the haptics of the IOL passes through the scleral wall and maintain centration of the optic. Three-piece IOLs are used that have haptics made of polymethylmethacrylate (PMMA) or polyvinylidene fluoride (PVDF) (Fig. 5).

The risks of scleral fixation of an IOL include suture or haptic erosion [45], suture breakage or slippage, IOL decentration or tilting, iris capture of the IOL optic [46], reverse pupillary block ocular hypertension [47], intraocular hemorrhage due to passage of suture through uveal tissue [48], and other complications associated with intraocular surgery. Suture or haptic erosion can occur through the conjunctiva, which increases the risk of "suture wick" endophthalmitis, because the suture provides a tract through the scleral wall for pathogens to migrate. The exposed haptic or suture can be treated with repair of the conjunctiva, and placement of a patch graft over the protruding haptic or suture. A novel technique of the use of an autologous scleral flap adjacent to the exposed haptic or suture has been described [49]. IOL decentration can be prevented by

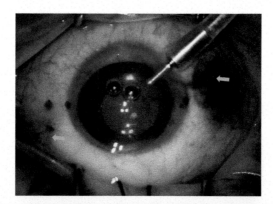

Fig. 5. In this figure, the author demonstrates intrascleral haptic fixation of a three-piece IOL with PVDF haptics in a pediatric patient. The haptic bulbs (*green arrows*) have been created by using low-temperature cautery to melt the tips of the haptics. This prevents the bulbs from sliding through the scleral tunnels. The bulbs can then be pushed into the sclera and buried to prevent overlying conjunctival erosion.

ensuring that the points of scleral fixation are symmetrically placed along a central meridian through the visual axis. IOL tilt in the intrascleral haptic fixation technique can be prevented by ensuring that needle tracts through the sclera are of sufficient length to prevent the haptics from angulating due to their inherent elasticity (Fig. 6). An alternative method is to use a 4-point scleral fixation method that significantly reduces the risk of IOL tilt (Fig. 7). The risk of iris capture and reverse pupillary block can be reduced by creating a peripheral iridectomy at the time of surgery. Last, the risk of intraocular hemorrhage due to needle passes through the iris root or pars plicata of the ciliary body can be reduced by placing the point of scleral fixation 1.0 to 1.5 mm posterior to the surgical limbus, also known as the end of the blue zone. Also, the needle should be oriented perpendicular to the sclera until entering the eye to prevent laceration of the iris root.

Scleral fixation is useful in the absence of capsular support for an IOL and becomes the only method of IOL-fixation when concomitant lack of iris tissue for an iris-fixated IOL exists. The position of scleral-fixated lenses behind the iris reduces the risk for corneal endothelial damage and has the optical benefit of proximity to the nodal point of the eye [50].

The various types of IOLs have been used for suture fixation including single-piece PMMA, single-piece acrylic, and three-piece. In a retrospective case series of 33 eyes of 26 children undergoing scleral fixation of an IOL, the use of 10-0 polypropylene resulted in suture breakage occurring at a mean of 5.11 years after surgery (3.5–9 years) in children [51]. The investigator of the study, therefore, recommended alternative suture material or size for

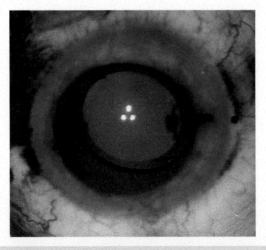

Fig. 6. This pediatric patient had significant tilting of the three-piece IOL due to scleral tunnels which were too short. This patient also had Marfan syndrome, which is associated with atypical scleral rigidity. The haptics became angulated due to their inherent elasticity, resulting in high levels of lenticular astigmatism due to the tilted IOL.

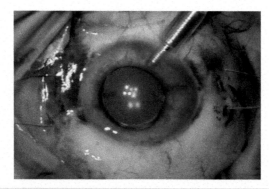

Fig. 7. The patient in Fig. 6 had the tilted intrascleral haptic-fixated IOL removed. Then, four-point fixation of an AO60 lens was performed using 6-0 prolene suture. Once the lens was centered, the prolene sutures were cut, and bulbs were created at the tips using low-temperature cautery. The bulbs were then buried into the sclera to prevent overlying conjunctival erosion. The end result was a stable and well-centered IOL without tilt.

suture fixation. The preferred lens of the investigator for suture fixation is the Akreos AO60 (Bausch & Lomb, Rochester, NY), which can be fixated with 6-0 polypropylene or 7-0 polytetrafluoroethylene suture through the haptic eyelets. The use of polypropylene allows for fixation through the conjunctiva without performing a conjunctival peritomy. Once the suture is passed through the conjunctiva and sclera, the IOL can be fixated with the ends of the suture fashioned into bulbs using low-temperature cautery and buried into the sclera to prevent overlying conjunctival erosion. The thicker size of the suture should provide longer durability; however, long-term studies have not been completed at this point.

Intrascleral haptic fixation is advantageous in that it avoids the concerns of suture material for IOL fixation and generally is a quicker surgery. The haptics of the IOL can be affixed to the sclera using glue or by melting the tips of the haptics to make bulbs which can be buried into the sclera. In a retrospective study of intrascleral haptic fixation in 40 eyes of 25 children with ectopia lentis, patients were followed for a median of 12 months (12–62 months). There was one case of IOL subluxation, which required refixation (2.5%), and five eyes developed intraocular hemorrhage (12.5%) without any long-term sequelae [52]. The long-term studies of intrascleral haptic fixation in children are needed, as this is a relatively new technique.

SUMMARY

In summary, pediatric aphakia can present difficulties in management, as it is frequently associated with other ocular comorbidities, such as glaucoma, amblyopia, and structural defects of the eye requiring creative techniques for IOL fixation. Each patient presents unique challenges, and an understanding of the treatment modalities outlined in this article allows for customized care of pediatric aphakia.

CLINICS CARE POINTS

- Nonsurgical treatment of unilateral, pediatric aphakia is usually best performed with contact lenses. Bilateral aphakia is usually treated with spectacles, though contact lenses are also an option.
- Use bicapsular optic capture to fixate a three-piece intraocular lens placed in the iridociliary sulcus to prevent long-term decentration, reduce the risk of posterior capsular opacification, and avoid the need for anterior vitrectomy.
- If capsular support is not available, fixate the intraocular lens using iris enclavation or scleral fixation. Avoid angle-supported anterior chamber intraocular lenses in children.

DISCLOSURE

The authors have nothing to disclose.

References

[1] Gurland JE. Use of silicone lenses in infants and children. Ophthalmology 1979;86(9): 1599–604.
[2] McMahon TT, Zadnik K. Twenty-five years of contact lenses. Cornea 2000;19(5):730–40.
[3] Baker JD. Visual rehabilitation of aphakic children II. Contact lenses. Surv Ophthalmol 1990;34(5):366–71.
[4] Levin AV, Edmonds SA, Nelson LB, et al. Extended-wear contact lenses for the treatment of pediatric aphakia. Ophthalmology 1988;95(8):1107–13.
[5] Ridley H. Intra-ocular acrylic lenses. Br J Ophthalmol 1952;36(3):113.
[6] Letocha CE, Pavlin CJ. Follow-up of 3 patients with ridley intraocular lens implantation. J Cataract Refract Surg 1999;25(4):587–91.
[7] Zhang X, Zeng J, Cui D, et al. Rigid gas permeable contact lenses for visual rehabilitation of unilateral aphakic children in China. Contact Lens Anterior Eye 2019;42(5):502–5.
[8] Zwaan J, Mullaney PB, Awad A, et al. Pediatric intraocular lens implantation surgical results and complications in more than 300 patients. Ophthalmology 1998;105(1):112–9.
[9] BENEZRA D, COHEN E, ROSE L. Traumatic cataract in children: correction of aphakia by contact lens or intraocular lens. Am J Ophthalmol 1997;123(6):773–82.
[10] Group IATS, Lambert SR, Buckley EG, et al. A Randomized clinical trial comparing contact lens with intraocular lens correction of monocular aphakia during infancy: grating acuity and adverse events at age 1 year. Arch Ophthalmol 2010;128(7):810–8.
[11] Lambert SR, Lynn MJ, Hartmann EE, et al. Comparison of contact lens and intraocular lens correction of monocular aphakia during infancy: a randomized clinical trial of HOTV optotype acuity at age 4.5 years and clinical findings at age 5 years. Jama Ophthalmol 2014;132(6):676–82.
[12] Lambert SR, Plager DA, Buckley EG, et al. The infant aphakia treatment study: further on intra- and postoperative complications in the intraocular lens group. J Am Assoc Pediatric Ophthalmol Strabismus 2015;19(2):101–3.
[13] Manschot WA. Primary Congenital Aphakia. Arch Ophthalmol 1963;69(5):571–7.
[14] Brophy M, Sinclair SA, Hostetler SG, et al. Pediatric eye injury–related hospitalizations in the United States. Pediatrics 2006;117(6):e1263–71.
[15] Parikakis E, Batsos G, Kontomichos L, et al. Traumatic aniridia and aphakia management with iris reconstruction lens using gore-tex sutures, an Ab-Externo approach. Am J Case Reports 2020;21:9247066-1-e924706-5.

[16] Repka MX. Visual rehabilitation in pediatric aphakia. Dev Ophthalmol 2016;57:49–68.
[17] American Academy of. Ophthalmology. 2017-2018 Basic and Clinical Science Course (BCSC), Section 03: Clinical Optics. American Academy of Ophthalmology; 2017.
[18] Lambert SR, Kraker RT, Pineles SL, et al. Contact lens correction of aphakia in children a report by the american academy of ophthalmology. Ophthalmology 2018;125(9): 1452–8.
[19] Russell B, DuBois L, Lynn M, et al. The infant aphakia treatment study contact lens experience to age 5 years. Eye Contact Lens Sci Clin Pract 2017;43(6):352–7.
[20] Lambert SR, Cotsonis G, DuBois L, et al. Long-term effect of intraocular lens vs contact lens correction on visual acuity after cataract surgery during infancy. Jama Ophthalmol 2020;138(4):365–72.
[21] Repka MX. Visual acuity outcome at age 10.5 years for treatment of monocular infantile cataract—it is worth the effort. Jama Ophthalmol 2020;138(4):372–3.
[22] Awad AH, Mullaney PB, Al-Hamad A, et al. Secondary posterior chamber intraocular lens implantation in children. J Am Assoc Pediatric Ophthalmol Strabismus 1998;2(5):269–74.
[23] Biglan AW, CHENG KP, DAVIS JS, et al. Secondary intraocular lens implantation after cataract surgery in children. Am J Ophthalmol 1997;123(2):224–34.
[24] Biglan A, Cheng K, Davis J, et al. Results following secondary intraocular lens implantation in children. Am J Ophthalmol 1997;123(3):437.
[25] DeVaro JM, Buckley EG, Awner S, et al. Secondary posterior chamber intraocular lens implantation in pediatric patients. Am J Ophthalmol 1997;123(1):24–30.
[26] Zhao Ye, Gong XH, Zhu XN, et al. Long-term outcomes of ciliary sulcus versus capsular bag fixation of intraocular lenses in children: An ultrasound biomicroscopy study. PLoS One 2017;12(3):e0172979.
[27] Shenoy BH, Mittal V, Gupta A, et al. Complications and visual outcomes after secondary intraocular lens implantation in children. Am J Ophthalmol 2015;159(4):720–6.e2.
[28] Gimbel HV, DeBroff BM. Posterior capsulorhexis with optic capture: Maintaining a clear visual axis after pediatric cataract surgery. J Cataract Refract Surg 1994;20(6):658–64.
[29] Gimbel HV. History of posterior continuous curvilinear capsulorhexis and optic capture. Cataract Refractive Surgery Today Europe 2019;40–2.
[30] Gimbel HV, DeBroff BM. Intraocular lens optic capture. J Cataract Refract Surg 2004;30(1): 200–6.
[31] VanderVeen DK, Drews-Botsch CD, Nizam A, et al. Outcomes of secondary intraocular lens implantation in the Infant Aphakia Treatment Study. J Cataract Refract Surg 2021;47(2): 172–7.
[32] Freedman SF, Lynn MJ, Beck AD, et al. Glaucoma-Related adverse events in the first 5 years after unilateral cataract removal in the infant aphakia treatment study. Jama Ophthalmol 2015;133(8):907–14.
[33] Struck MC. Long-term results of pediatric cataract surgery and primary intraocular lens implantation from 7 to 22 months of life. Jama Ophthalmol 2015;133(10):1180–3.
[34] Morrison D, Sternberg P, Donahue S. Anterior chamber intraocular lens (ACIOL) placement after pars plana lensectomy in pediatric marfan syndrome. J Am Assoc Pediatric Ophthalmol Strabismus 2005;9(3):240–2.
[35] Wilson ME, Adams C, Alex A, et al. Long-term outcome of angle-supported anterior chamber intraocular lens implantation for pediatric aphakia. J Am Assoc Pediatric Ophthalmol Strabismus 2021;25(4):e11.
[36] Faron N, Hoekel J, Tychsen L. Visual acuity, refractive error, and regression outcomes in 169 children with high myopia who were implanted with Ophtec-Artisan or Visian phakic IOLs. J Am Assoc Pediatric Ophthalmol Strabismus 2021;25(1):27.e1–8.
[37] Arne JL. Posterior chamber phakic intraocular lens. In: Azar D, editor. *Refractive surgery.* 3rd edition. Amsterdam, Netherlands: Elsevier; 2019. p. 412–20.
[38] Artisan Aphakia Lens for the Correction of Aphakia in Children. Available at: https://clinicaltrials.gov/ct2/show/NCT01547442. Accessed June 26, 2021.

[39] Gawdat GI, Taher SG, Salama MM, et al. Evaluation of Artisan aphakic intraocular lens in cases of pediatric aphakia with insufficient capsular support. J Am Assoc Pediatric Ophthalmol Strabismus 2015;19(3):242–6.

[40] Ophtec. Artisan myopia model 206. Available at: https://www.ophtec.com/products/refractive-surgery/p-iols/artisan-myopia-model-206. Accessed June 20, 2021.

[41] Ophtec. The ARTISAN® Phakic IOL Clinical Study and Post-Approval Study (PAS) I & II Results. 2019. Available at: https://www.ophtec.com/product-overview/refractive/artisan-myopia-206.

[42] Shuaib AM, Sayed YE, Kamal A, et al. Transscleral sutureless intraocular lens versus retropupillary iris-claw lens fixation for paediatric aphakia without capsular support: a randomized study. Acta Ophthalmol 2019;97(6):e850–9.

[43] Kopel AC, Carvounis PE, Hamill MB, et al. Iris-sutured intraocular lenses for ectopia lentis in children. J Cataract Refract Surg 2008;34(4):596–600.

[44] Yen KG, Reddy AK, Weikert MP, et al. Iris-fixated posterior chamber intraocular lenses in children. Am J Ophthalmol 2009;147(1):121–6.

[45] Cheung CS, VanderVeen DK. Intraocular lens techniques in pediatric eyes with insufficient capsular support: complications and outcomes. Semin Ophthalmol 2019;34(4):293–302.

[46] Bardorf CM, Epley KD, Lueder GT, et al. Pediatric transscleral sutured intraocular lenses: efficacy and safety in 43 eyes followed an average of 3 years. J Am Assoc Pediatric Ophthalmol Strabismus 2004;8(4):318–24.

[47] Bharathi M, Balakrishnan D, Senthil S. "Pseudophakic reverse pupillary block" following yamane technique scleral-fixated intraocular lens. J Glaucoma 2020;29(7):e68–70.

[48] Epley KD, Shainberg MJ, Lueder GT, et al. Pediatric secondary lens implantation in the absence of capsular support. J Am Assoc Pediatric Ophthalmol Strabismus 2001;5(5):301–6.

[49] Alameri AH, Stone DU. Autologous scleral flap technique to repair exposed sutures after transscleral suture fixation of an intraocular lens. Middle East Afr J Ophthalmol 2018;25(1):47–8.

[50] Jürgens I, Rey A. Simple technique to treat pupillary capture after transscleral fixation of intraocular lens. J Cataract Refract Surg 2015;41(1):14–7.

[51] Buckley EG. Hanging by a thread: the long-term efficacy and safety of transscleral sutured intraocular lenses in children (an American Ophthalmological Society thesis). Trans Am Ophthalmol Soc 2007;105:294–311.

[52] Kannan N, Kohli P, Pangtey BPS, et al. Evaluation of sutureless, glueless, flapless, intrascleral fixated posterior chamber intraocular lens in children with ectopia lentis. J Ophthalmol 2018;2018:3212740.

Advances in Ophthalmology and Optometry 8 (2023) 59–73

ADVANCES IN OPHTHALMOLOGY AND OPTOMETRY

Conjunctival Tumors in Children

Hanna N. Luong, BS[a],
Aparna Ramasubramanian, MD[b],*

[a]Mayo Clinic Alix School of Medicine, 13400 East Shea Boulevard, Scottsdale, Az 85259, USA;
[b]Phoenix Children's Hospital, 1920 East Cambridge Avenue, Phoenix, AZ 85016, USA

Keywords
- Pediatric • Conjunctiva • Nevus • Melanoma • Primary acquired melanosis
- Dermoid • Dermolipoma • Lymphoma

Key points
- Nevi are the most common conjunctival tumors and typically emerge in the first two decades of life.
- Primary acquired melanosis is a brown to light brown patchy lesion that has a risk of transformation to melanoma dependent on the degree of atypia.
- Dermolipoma and dermoids are choristomatous lesions that can be associated with Goldenhar syndrome.
- Among lymphoid conjunctival tumors, it is critical to distinguish between benign reactive lymphoid hyperplasia and lymphoma.
- Newer diagnostic tools such as optical coherence tomography, ultrasound biomicroscopy, and in vivo confocal microscopy can be utilized for diagnosis and management.

INTRODUCTION

Conjunctival tumors in the pediatric population have varied presentations with limited coverage in the literature. They originate from melanocytic, choristomatous, vascular, epithelioid, and lymphoid tissue, each possessing distinct clinical features and management strategies. Most are of melanocytic or choristomatous origin, and the most common conjunctival tumor is nevi [1].

No financial interest associated with article.
No funding support.
This article, or parts of it, have not been presented at any meetings.

*Corresponding author. E-mail address: aramasubramanian@phoenixchildrens.com

https://doi.org/10.1016/j.yaoo.2023.02.006
2452-1760/23/© 2023 Elsevier Inc. All rights reserved.

Overall, the incidence and progression of malignant lesions in pediatric populations is less than 1% [1,2]. Several benign tumors can transform into their malignant phenotypes, including primary acquired melanosis (PAM) to melanoma and benign reactive lymphoid hyperplasia (BRLH) to lymphoma. Specific patient risk factors and clinical features increase the suspicion of malignancy. Melanoma typically occurs in those of greater age. It is more likely to be located in the fornix and tarsus [3] and has a larger basal diameter and thickness [4], lacks intralesional cysts [4], features prominent feeder and intrinsic vessels [5], and hemorrhage [4]. Lymphoma tends to have a larger basal dimension with diffuse, inferior, or superior locations (vs nasal) compared with BRLH [5]. Malignancy rates are higher in those with immunodeficiency or xeroderma pigmentosum [1,2,5].

Ophthalmologists monitor benign conjunctival lesions annually [6]. New noninvasive imaging techniques, such as optical coherence tomography (OCT), ultrasound biomicroscopy (UBM), and in vivo confocal microscopy (IVCM), are promising new avenues to investigate the conjunctiva and enhance diagnostic accuracy. Indications for removal are varied, including suspicion of malignancy [7], functional disturbance [6], and cosmesis [8]. Surgical excision is highly recommended for lesions in the setting of immunodeficiency or xeroderma pigmentosum [2]. Biologic therapies are emerging to combat malignancies based on genetic analyses.

This article describes the characteristics of the most common pediatric conjunctival tumors and malignancies as well as their current and upcoming diagnostic and management strategies. Enhanced awareness and anticipation of conjunctival tumor presentations can prevent life-altering or vision-altering outcomes.

SIGNIFICANCE
Melanocytic conjunctival tumors
Melanocytic proliferations account for the highest proportion of conjunctival tumors with reports ranging from 23% to 83% [1,6,9,10]. They can be benign, premalignant, and malignant. Several subtypes have been identified: nevus, melanosis, and melanoma.

Nevus
Conjunctival nevi are the most common melanocytic tumor [1]. They most commonly emerge within the first two decades of life and present in the interpalpebral bulbar conjunctiva as a darkly pigmented (65%), lightly pigmented (19%), or completely nonpigmented (16%) mass [1]. They can be classified similarly to cutaneous nevi into compound, junctional, or deep, of which compound is the most prevalent [8,11]. Both the level of pigmentation and size can change in 5% and up to 8% of cases, respectively [3]. Fifty percent of cases show globules with dots and structureless pigmentation [11], and 40% to 82% can demonstrate fine clear cysts [1,8,11] (Fig. 1); 75% can have some degree of inflammation, called inflammatory conjunctival nevi, which is associated with allergic or vernal conjunctivitis [12]. Despite rapid growth, they have benign histology [8].

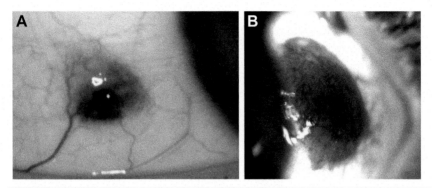

Fig. 1. (A) Conjunctival nevus with feeder vessel and multiple cysts. (B) Large conjunctival nevus with no clinical cysts.

Management is with serial ophthalmologic examination typically with lesion measurements and photographic comparisons annually [6]. Surgical excision is recommended if growth or functional impairment occurs [6]. During surgery, the entire mass is removed and, if adherent to the globe, it is followed by removal of the thin lamella of underlying sclera [1]. The conjunctival margins of the lesion are treated with standard double freeze–thaw cryotherapy [1,6]. The aim is to prevent recurrence of either the nevus or potential melanoma, depending on post-histopathologic analysis [1]. Once excised, the diagnosis of nevus is made if nests of well-defined, round melanocytes are visualized within the stroma near basal epithelial layers [1]. Immunohistochemical (IHC) staining for specific cellular antigens also is recommended, which can differentiate between benign conjunctival nevus and malignant melanoma; specifically, human melanoma black-45 (HMB-45) monoclonal antibody is characteristic of the latter [6].

Several additional features can aid in the determination of benign nevus versus malignant melanoma: age, location, and appearance. First, nevi is usually present during puberty or early adult life whereas melanoma spawns in the early fifties and rarely develops in the first two decades [4,6]. Among the few documented incidences when this has occurred, it has been in older children 10 to 15 years old [4]. Second, whereas nevi are located in the interpalpebral bulbar conjunctiva, melanoma often resides and invades the cornea, palpebral conjunctiva, plica, or caruncle [1]. Third, nevi tend to be solitary, well-demarcated, smaller in size and in base/elevation, less intensely and evenly pigmented, cystic, and are freely movable over the episclera relative to melanoma [1,6]. Less than 1% of conjunctival nevi transform into malignant melanoma [3,13].

Melanosis

Conjunctival melanosis can be racial or acquired. Racial melanosis more commonly occurs in darker-pigmented individuals and presents bilaterally and/or symmetrically [14]. This lesion is located on the limbus and, rarely, on the bulbar conjunctiva and limbal cornea [7]. It is usually of a dark brown pigment [7]. It rarely transforms into melanoma; the recommended management is observation [1].

PAM also is a benign conjunctival pigmented condition. It is the second largest group of melanocytic conjunctival tumors behind nevi [14]. On slit lamp examination, PAM is flat and contains dots that could be confluent in a structureless pattern [11]. Histopathologically, PAM is characterized by the proliferation of abnormal melanocytes in the basal layers of the epithelium [1]. As opposed to racial melanosis, PAM almost always is unilateral [1], exhibits a patchy and brown to light brown pigmentation [11], more often occurs in fair-skinned individuals [1], and has a much higher risk of converting to malignant melanoma [1].

Therefore, management depends on the extent of involvement as that helps govern the risk of melanoma. If PAM occupies a small area–which has been defined as less than three clock hours of the conjunctiva [7,14]–, either serial observation or excisional biopsy and cryotherapy are reasonable options [7]. If PAM occupies a larger area of more than three clock hours of the conjunctiva, incisional map biopsy of all four quadrants of the lesion plus double freeze–thaw cryotherapy afterward is necessary [7]. Complete excision is warranted if the patient has a history of melanoma or there are features (eg, nodularity or vascularity) present [7] suspicious of melanoma. Excision beyond clinically observed margins is emphasized to prevent recurrence [15]. Management also should be informed by histopathological risk assessment.

Every effort should be made to ascertain if melanocytes are typical or atypical based on nuclear features and growth patterns. The Armed Forces Institute of Pathology (AFIP) has established criteria to grade atypia from mild to severe based on histologic characteristics (eg, basilar hyperplasia, basilar nests, pagetoid involvement) and cell types (eg, small epithelioid cells, epithelioid cells, spindle cells) [15]. In addition to grade, several parameters, in particular, appear to be predictive of progression to melanoma: one, the presence of epithelioid cells [15]; two, growth in a predominant pattern other than basilar hyperplasia [15]; and three, extent of involvement in clock hours of the conjunctiva [14]. To date, zero cases of PAM with no and mild cytologic atypia have progressed to melanoma [14]. However, PAM recurrence in non-atypical and mildly atypical lesions is 11% and 26%, respectively [14]. In contrast, PAM with severe atypia has a recurrence rate of 50% [14]. It has been reported to carry a 13% to 46% risk of malignant melanoma [14,15] and is the predisposing lesion in up to 75% of melanoma cases [16]. The risk is compounded with larger lesion size [14]. The average interval between PAM and the development of malignant melanoma is 2.5 to 3.3 years [14,15]. It is unclear if PAM without atypia is a precursor lesion to PAM with atypia, and no consistent clinical characteristics have emerged to differentiate the two [15]. There appears to be a low risk of developing malignant melanoma from PAM with atypia after 10 years of follow-up [15].

Between PAM and malignant melanoma, several differences have been identified. PAM is more likely to occur in younger age groups and individuals of female sex [5]. PAM presents with smaller basal diameter and thickness and does not have feeder or intrinsic vessels and hemorrhage [5]. On slit lamp examination, PAM are mainly light brown in color and display the "flag sign," [11] in which stretching the conjunctiva nearest to the PAM causes the epithelium to form multiple pigmented folds, leaving a nonpigmented area behind; this suggests that PAM involves only the conjunctiva and not the episclera and sclera, such as can occur in malignant melanoma.

Melanoma
Conjunctival melanoma can arise from PAM (which occurs approximately 50% to 76% of the time) [6,17], de novo (approximately 12% to 26%) [6], or a preexisting nevus (1% to 20%) [5,6,17] with increased risk in individuals with chronic solar radiation exposure [5]. It accounts for 5% of ocular melanoma and 1% to 2% of all eye malignancies [6]. It peaks in incidence in the fifth decade of life [6], and only an estimated 1% occurs in children [1].

Their presentation is highly variable. Though the most common sites are the limbic area and bulbar conjunctiva [16], they also have been found in the forniceal and palpebral conjunctiva [5]. Most typically, they are characterized as dark-brown pigmented lesions organized in irregular dots, but all growths have been found to have more than one color [11], including pink [1], yellow [1], and gray [11]. Higher prevalence of gray color is a particular distinguishing feature from conjunctival nevi; presence of gray color was observed in 63% of melanoma cases and has been surmised to represent melanocytic invasion of the underlying stroma [11]. Neo-angiogenesis is an additional element key to melanoma growth. In a series of 147 conjunctival lesions evaluated by three dermatologists and three ophthalmologists, all 8 melanomas diagnosed featured linear vessels directly feeding the lesions [11]. The vessels feeding malignant lesions were thicker in diameter and tortuous compared with those feeding benign lesions [11] and increased in prominence with raised tumors [6]. In a large study of 601 malignant melanomas, 48% possessed feeder vessels and 33% had intrinsic vessels [18].

The behavior of conjunctival melanoma is similarly variable. Some can demonstrate nodular growth whereas others display aggressive invasion into the globe and even posterior to the orbit leading to proptosis and metastatic disease [6]; 40% have shown local tumor recurrence over a mean of 2.4 years [17]. Systemic metastasis occurs in 19% of melanomas on average over 3.4 years [17]. Common sites are regional lymph nodes (eg, preauricular or submandibular nodes), the brain, lungs, and liver [17].

The American Joint Committee on Cancer (AJCC) has both clinical and pathology classification criteria for conjunctival melanomas based on size, location, extent of invasion, and extent of metastasis. In a large retrospective chart review performed by Shields and colleagues, [19] AJCC staging was predictive of prognosis. Compared with melanomas staged as T1, those staged as

T2 and T3 had higher rates of local recurrence, regional lymph node and distant metastasis, and mortality [19].

The current standard of care dictates wide local excision of the corneal and conjunctival components using the "no-touch" technique [5], which is a philosophy that involves zero direct manipulation of the lesion to avoid tumor seeding. Alcohol corneal epitheliectomy is used to remove the corneal component of the tumor [5], taking care not to disrupt the Bowman membrane. The conjunctival part is excised with 2 to 3 mm margins [5]. Partial lamellar scleroconjunctivectomy releases the tightly adherent limbal region, then double freeze–thaw cryotherapy is directed at the lesion's margins and the bare sclera afterward [5]. Closure [5], rotational flap [5], conjunctivoplasty [6], or placement of an amniotic membrane transplant [5] with or without insertion of a symblepharon ring [5,17] can reconstruct lost tissue following. Sentinel lymph node biopsy can be considered if the tumor thickness exceeds 2 mm or if there is a concern for local recurrence [17].

Additional management options exist in cases of non-excizable lesions, local recurrence, or metastatic disease. Local recurrence and metastatic disease typically are associated with tumors in the conjunctival caruncle, fornix, or tarsal regions [6]; those that demonstrate corneal involvement or have been incompletely excised [6]; and lesions with positive margins on histopathology [5]. Local recurrence and lymph node involvement can be treated with local excision and radiotherapy with cobalt or radium [6]. Diffuse melanoma has been treated with a combination of local excision, cryotherapy, and mitomycin C [17]. Reported adjuvant therapies range from topical chemotherapy (eg, mitomycin C, interferon alpha-2b), focal cryotherapy, external or proton beam radiotherapy, and brachytherapy [17]. Exenteration may be required if melanoma has invaded the orbit, but it has not demonstrated improved survival rates [20,21]. In any case of conjunctival melanoma, an ocular and/or systemic oncologist should be consulted due to the high risk of metastasis [17].

Choristomatous conjunctival tumors

A choristoma (Fig. 4A) is a mass of histologically normal tissue located in an abnormal anatomic location.

Dermolipoma

The second most common conjunctival tumor in children is dermolipoma, which comprises approximately 5% [1]. It is hypothesized to be congenital and may be apparent in the setting of Goldenhar syndrome, which is a rare disorder characterized by hemifacial microsomia and defects in the ears, eyes, and spine; the incidence of dermolipomas in patients with Goldenhar syndrome ranges from 47% to 75% [22,23].

In dermolipoma, adipose tissue with dermis-like, collagenous connective tissue is situated in the superotemporal conjunctival fornix [24]. Clinically, it can present as a soft yellow sessile mass with fine hairs superficially [1,25] (Fig. 2A). Most lesions do not require surgical treatment; excision is reserved for larger, symptomatic dermolipomas or cosmetic reasons [1,25].

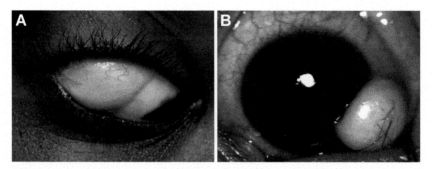

Fig. 2. (A) Temporal conjunctival lipodermoid. (B) Limbal dermoid.

The preferred surgical approach varies. Both complete and subtotal excisions have been undertaken. The entire orbito-conjunctival lesion can be removed through a conjunctival forniceal approach [1], which more completely can relieve irritation or cosmetic concerns [26]. Or, just anterior (to the lateral orbital rim) debulking of the dermolipoma can be performed, as posterior extension is rare [1]. Care must be taken as complications of blepharoptosis, keratoconjunctivitis sicca, and diplopia have been reported secondary to damage to adjacent ocular adnexal structures during removal [27].

Dermoid
Dermoids are congenital small to large growths comprised of ectodermal and mesodermal tissue that typically reside in the inferotemporal quadrant [1,28] (Fig. 2B). They can occur in isolation, but more commonly occur with other manifestations such as upper eyelid coloboma, dermolipoma, auricular skin appendages, and vertebral anomalies as part of Goldenhar syndrome [29]. Limbal dermoids are categorized into three grades [30]: Grade I entails a superficial lesion, confined to the limbus, that is less than 5 mm in diameter, Grade II includes larger lesions deep to the corneal stroma up to Descemet's membrane, and Grade III are lesions that involve the entire cornea and/or extend to the anterior segment structures.

No overarching consensus exists on the optimal timing of surgery or surgical technique(s). For smaller, visually asymptomatic lesions, management is with observation [31]. Generally, surgical intervention is indicated in cases with increased growth with encroachment on the visual axis, amblyopia, high astigmatism, dellen, and poor cosmesis [31]. The standard surgical options of simple excision and lamellar keratoplasty are recommended for Grades II and III lesions [32]. Concerns or complications have arisen in the literature for each method in isolation. These include the possibility of residual epithelial defect, scar development, incomplete excision, corneal vascularization, pseudopterygium, and accidental corneal perforation for simple excision and microperforation, delayed re-epithelialization, graft rejection, staphyloma, high cost, and requirement of a corneal donor for lamellar keratoplasty [32].

Therefore, some have suggested that these techniques be performed in combination or have proposed novel approaches [31]. Regardless, long-term followup and treatment of amblyopia should be anticipated [1].

Lymphoma. The second most common conjunctival malignancy behind melanoma is lymphoma [1]. An estimated 2% of extranodal lymphomas are ocular lymphomas, and 49% are conjunctival in children [33]. Risk factors include BRLH and immune deficiency or dysfunction [5]. Its four main subtypes are extranodal marginal zone lymphoma (EMZL), follicular lymphoma, mantle cell lymphoma, and diffuse large B-cell lymphoma [5]. It most often presents as a raised salmon pink mass sometimes with feeder vessels within the substantia propria of the conjunctival fornix [5].

As BRLH is far more common than lymphoma in children [1], care must be taken to distinguish the two conditions. Clinically, BRLH is typically smaller in size, more discrete, and more likely to be found in the nasal conjunctival fornix; in contrast, lymphoma has a predilection for inferior and superior locations [5]. Differences in biopsy with histopathology–reactive hyperplasia appear as large interfollicular zones of variable shapes and sizes–and genetic markers, such as bcl-2 specific to follicular lymphoma, also are valuable [34].

Treatment spans surgery, cryotherapy, radiotherapy, systemic chemotherapy, or selective anti-B-cell therapy (rituximab) [5,34]. For local disease, complete resection is ideal with or without external beam radiotherapy [5]. Rituximab can be used for more extensive lesions [5]. If invasion past the orbit or systemic lymphoma occurs, treatment with R-CHOP or similar chemotherapy regimens (eg, R-CVP) is advised [33]. Although most prognostic information available pertains to adult conjunctival lymphoma [34], recent data within the pediatric population have shown that histologic subtype is the main outcome predictor, and that EMZL is the most common conjunctival lymphoma with a very favorable prognosis [5]. Follow-up after 35 years yielded no second primary malignancies in any children [35].

SIGNIFICANCE AND FUTURE DIRECTIONS

Only a handful of large series exists that describe conjunctival tumors in children. Other studies have been single case reports or descriptive in nature only. Most of the remaining literature pertains to adults, such as pathology series from AFIP, Wilmer Eye Institute, Wills Eye Hospital, and the Singapore Cancer Registry [5]. It is difficult to extrapolate from adult conjunctival tumors to children, especially in which substantial differences in tumor incidence (eg, conjunctival melanoma) are present. But many epidemiological considerations, tumor features, and malignancy risk differ between these age groups and are important to keep in mind.

For one, tumor types differ. Though melanocytic lesions composed by far the largest proportion of conjunctival tumors diagnosed in both children and adults (67% [1] and 52% [36], respectively), children had greater numbers of choristomatous and vascular growths whereas adults had more squamous

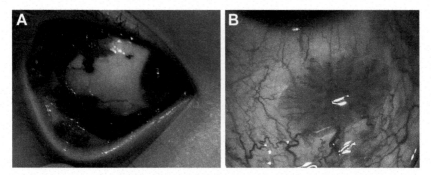

Fig. 3. (A) Extensive congenital conjunctival hemangioma. (B) Conjunctival papilloma.

epithelial lesions [4]. Indeed, the most common malignancy in adults was ocular surface squamous neoplasia (OSSN) [5] compared with melanoma and lymphoma in children [1]. Malignancy rates themselves are extremely low in children relative to adults. In a comprehensive series of 5002 conjunctival tumors, 30% of tumors were found to be malignant in adults compared with 3% in children [18]. In subgroup analyses, malignancies in children occurred at mean age 14 years with relative frequency of 1% to 3% between 0 and 15 years and 7% between 15 and 21 years [4], suggesting even more granular risk stratification.

Whether benign or malignant, tumors may be vision-threatening. For example, delayed or absent ophthalmic examination for melanocytic lesions has been associated with refractive amblyopia [6]. Therefore, recognition of the broad range of conjunctival tumors is important. Beyond the most common conjunctival tumors and malignancies described in this article, there are a variety of vascular (Fig. 3A), epithelial (Fig. 3B), and even nonneoplastic lesions simulating a tumor. The last category has been demonstrated to make up a striking 9.5% to 30% of conjunctival tumors identified [1,4]. These include epithelial inclusion cyst, pingueculum, pterygium, foreign body, keloid, vernal conjunctivitis, pyogenic granuloma (Fig. 4B), nonspecific granuloma, and others [1]. Awareness of tumor types and salient features of malignancy combined with history, examination, and histopathology can allow for prompt and accurate diagnosis and prevention of long-term vision impairment.

Recently, several new tools and techniques have been developed, which can aid in the recognition of these rare tumors. OCT, ultrasound biomicroscopy (UBM), and in vivo confocal microscopy (IVCM) are noninvasive imaging techniques that have shown exceptional promise in investigating the conjunctiva. OCT was first used to image the anterior segment in 1994 [37]. Ultra-high-resolution OCT devices have resolutions of less than 5 microns and can scan to depths of 2 to 7 mm [38]. OCT has added significant value to the management of nevi (Fig. 5), melanoma, lymphoma, and OSSN. For instance, Tran and colleagues [39] discovered that 17% of patients with apparent clinical

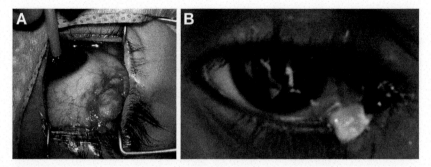

Fig. 4. (A) Osseous choriostoma presenting as an inflamed subconjunctival mass. (B) Postoperative pyogenic granuloma following strabismus surgery.

resolution of OSSN still had the residual disease as detected by high-resolution OCT; this prompted additional cycles of treatment with no recurrences in an average of 2-year follow-up. For melanoma and lymphoma, OCT allows for detailed assessment of the epithelium and subepithelium, including the characterization of tissue infiltrates, reflectivity, and thickness, which distinguish melanomas from PAM and lymphomas from BRLH [38,40]. In addition, OCT angiography can map vessel structure and density to discriminate between the more tortuous, interlesional pattern present in melanomas from the fine vessels present in PAM, nevi, and normal conjunctiva [40]. From a surgical standpoint, OCT has been deployed preoperatively to accurately outline the margins of OSSN lesions and intraoperatively to help position grafts in endothelial procedures and inform depth in lamellar keratoplasty [38], a standard treatment in dermoid removal [28]. Emerging polarization-sensitive "micro" OCT possesses the highest resolution known to date–1.5 × 1.5 × 1 μm–[38]which will presumably yield even further progress.

UBM is another technique that does not possess as high resolution as OCT, but can scan greater depths (approximately 4–6 mm [38]) without deterrence from shadowing. Its technology involves the use of high-frequency ultrasound transducers of 35 to 50 MHz to obtain cross-sections of the anterior segment, anterior chamber, ciliary body, iris, angle, and other structures [38,40]. This has made it especially useful for detecting intraocular involvement of ocular surface tumors. For example, both melanomas and lymphomas are present as large, thick lesions. When imaging with OCT, shadowing and obscuration have prevented proper assessment of deeper subepithelial tissues [40]. The addition of UBM has been helpful to assess the full extent of these lesions, including posterior margins and intraocular invasion [38,40]. In a case series of seven patients with OSSN, intraocular involvement was detected in four only through the use of UBM (vs clinically in the remaining three) [41]. The strengths and limitations of these two techniques have been corroborated elsewhere in the literature. In a comparison of OCT and UBM for conjunctival nevi in 21 patients, cysts were detected in 8 through slit lamp examination,

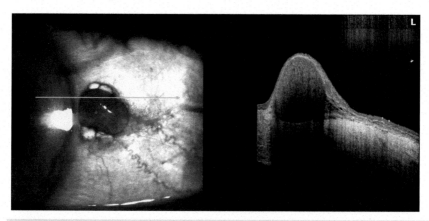

Fig. 5. Anterior segment OCT showing the elevation of a nevus with imaging of the contents of the lesion and the depth of involvement.

12 through OCT (4 had subclinical cysts), and 6 through UBM [42]. However, all posterior margins were visible via UBM but occluded due to shadowing via OCT. Thus, OCT appears to be superior in visualizing finer details, but UBM can serve as a valuable complement through its penetrative power that is relatively unimpaired by shadowing.

Finally, IVCM can help diagnose and differentiate conjunctival tumors from their benign counterparts on a cellular level [40]. IVCM uses pinhole apertures, point-by-point illumination, and blockage of stray light for up to 800x magnification of ocular surface microstructure [38]. These high-resolution, high-contrast images have revealed the unique morphologies of melanocytic conjunctival tumors especially well [40]. Images of melanoma show hyperreflective cells with abnormally large nuclei, nucleoli, and tumor vessels in a background of inflammation [40]. In comparison, PAM with atypia typically has networks of large (>20 microns) pagetoid dendritic cells and hyperreflective epithelial granules [40]. IVCM has demonstrated 89% sensitivity and 100% specificity for diagnosing conjunctival melanomas as well as 100% sensitivity and 96% specificity for diagnosing PAM with atypia, though these results have only been drawn from small cohorts thus far [40]. Less available data exist on the use of IVCM in lymphoma, but results appear to closely correspond to histopathology findings: small, round, tightly packed cells in cystic spaces or nests representing stromal lymphocytes [40]. IVCM would likely be maximally beneficial in conjunction with OCT imaging to narrow the differential diagnoses for possible tumors. The findings of these imaging modalities could augment the prognostic value of established grading systems, such as those of the AJCC, or newer proposed schemes, such as the visual scoring system for limbal dermoid [43].

In addition to new imaging tools, novel medical therapies exist. Growing associations of conjunctival lymphoma with chronic inflammation (eg, *Helicobacter pylori, Chlamydia psittaci* infection) [5] pave the way for potential antibiotic treatment approaches. Evidence is mounting that conjunctival melanomas share genetic markers with cutaneous melanoma [17]. BRAF mutations, in particular, have a high level of concordance between cutaneous and conjunctival melanoma [17], and they have been found in approximately 22% to 50% of conjunctival melanomas. Concomitantly, the efficacy of vemurafenib and dabrafenib, highly selective BRAF-kinase inhibitors FDA-approved for the treatment of metastatic and unresectable melanoma, are currently being studied. A single case report of conjunctival melanoma from 2020 demonstrated complete response to combination dabrafenib and trametinib, though other reports have had varying results [44]. Other potential genetic targets to which new biological therapies may emerge include mitogen-activated protein kinase (a pathway that relays extracellular signals to cell nuclei), KIT (a gene that encodes the receptor tyrosine kinase CD117, which is involved in growth and survival and has been mutated in acral and mucosal melanomas), and NRAS (a gene within the Ras superfamily that encodes a GTPase that regulates cell division) [17].

Throughout any management plan, interdisciplinary care is crucial. Histopathology remains the gold standard in diagnosis despite the advent of advanced imaging techniques [38], which are currently costly and limited to specialized centers [11]. Timely involvement of oncology, genetics, and possibly immunology is critical to identify comorbid disorders (such as systemic lymphoma, Goldenhar syndrome, or xeroderma pigmentosum) and tailor therapies, especially biologic therapies on the horizon. More clinical trials, especially specific to pediatric populations, are needed on the efficacies of these treatment options.

SUMMARY

Conjunctival tumors in children are highly variable and rarely malignant. The most common tumors are melanocytic and choristomatous in tissue origin, and the most common malignancies are melanoma and lymphoma [1]. The incidence of malignant lesions is less than 1% [1], though both benign and malignant tumors can cause long-lasting vision impairment. Therefore, prompt recognition, accurate diagnosis, and appropriate, effective treatment are required.

Overall, the literature remains limited on conjunctival tumors, especially in children. What is known about adult tumors can be difficult to extrapolate to pediatric populations, but key differences, namely in tumor types and incidence of malignancy, are well-established. The conjunctival tumors discussed in this article scratch the surface of the variety that have been discovered to date, including epithelial and vascular lesions. New noninvasive imaging techniques of OCT, UBM, and IVCM offer striking resolution, penetration, and cellular morphologic characterization that have already shown value in the recognition, accurate diagnosis, and management of conjunctival tumors. Coupled with genetic tumor analyses and biologic therapies, further advancement can only be anticipated, pending the increased availability of these imaging modalities and additional clinical trials.

CLINICS CARE POINTS

- Nevi are the most common conjunctival lesions in children and are differentiated from other lesions by slit lamp examination and other ancillary tests like OCT and UBM.
- Prompt recognition, diagnosis, and treatment are important in the management of pediatric conjunctival lesions.

References

[1] Shields CL, Shields JA. Conjunctival tumors in children. Curr Opin Ophthalmol 2007;18(5): 351–60.

[2] Zimmermann-Paiz MA, García de la Riva JC. Conjunctival tumors in children: histopathologic diagnosis in 165 cases. Arq Bras Oftalmol 2015;78(6):337–9.

[3] Shields CL, Fasiuddin AF, Mashayekhi A, et al. Conjunctival nevi: clinical features and natural course in 410 consecutive patients. Arch Ophthalmol 2004;122(2):167–75.

[4] Shields CL, Sioufi K, Alset AE, et al. Clinical features differentiating benign from malignant conjunctival tumors in children. JAMA Ophthalmol 2017;135(3):215–24.

[5] Shields CL, Chien JL, Surakiatchanukul T, et al. Conjunctival tumors: review of clinical features, risks, biomarkers, and outcomes–the 2017 J. Donald M. Gass Lecture. Asia Pac J Ophthalmol (Phila) 2017;6(2):109–20.

[6] Ciuntu RE, Martinescu G, Anton N, et al. Conjunctival melanocytic tumors in children - a challenge in diagnosis and treatment. Rom J Morphol Embryol 2018;59(1):317–22.

[7] Shields CL, Shields JA. Tumors of the conjunctiva and cornea. Indian J Ophthalmol 2019;67(12):1930–48.

[8] Negretti GS, Roelofs KA, Damato B, et al. The natural history of conjunctival naevi in children and adolescents. Eye 2021;35(9):2579–84.

[9] Beby F, Kodjikian L, Roche O, et al. [Conjunctival tumors in children. A histopathologic study of 42 cases]. J Fr Ophtalmol 2005;28(8):817–23; https://doi.org/10.1016/s0181-5512(05)80999-4, Tumeurs de la conjonctive bulbaire de l'enfant. Résultats de l'examen histologique de 42 lésions opérées.

[10] Cunha RP, Cunha MC, Shields JA. Epibulbar tumors in children: a survey of 282 biopsies. J Pediatr Ophthalmol Strabismus 1987;24(5):249–54.

[11] Cinotti E, La Rocca A, Labeille B, et al. Dermoscopy for the diagnosis of conjunctival lesions. Dermatol Clin 2018;36(4):439–49.

[12] Zamir E, Mechoulam H, Micera A, et al. Inflamed juvenile conjunctival naevus: clinicopathological characterisation. Br J Ophthalmol 2002;86(1):28–30.

[13] Gerner N, Nørregaard JC, Jensen OA, et al. Conjunctival naevi in Denmark 1960-1980. A 21-year follow-up study. Acta Ophthalmol Scand 1996;74(4):334–7.

[14] Shields JA, Shields CL, Mashayekhi A, et al. Primary acquired melanosis of the conjunctiva: experience with 311 eyes. Trans Am Ophthalmol Soc 2007;105:61–71 [discussion: 71-2].

[15] Folberg R, McLean IW, Zimmerman LE. Primary acquired melanosis of the conjunctiva. Hum Pathol 1985;16(2):129–35.

[16] Novais GA, Fernandes BF, Belfort RN, et al. Incidence of melanocytic lesions of the conjunctiva in a review of 10 675 ophthalmic specimens. Int J Surg Pathol 2010;18(1):60–3.

[17] Wong JR, Nanji AA, Galor A, et al. Management of conjunctival malignant melanoma: a review and update. Expert Rev Ophthalmol 2014;9(3):185–204.

[18] Shields CL, Alset AE, Boal NS, et al. Conjunctival tumors in 5002 cases. Comparative analysis of benign versus malignant counterparts. The 2016 James D. Allen Lecture. Am J Ophthalmol 2017;173:106–33.

[19] Shields CL, Kaliki S, Al-Dahmash SA, et al. American Joint Committee on Cancer (AJCC) clinical classification predicts conjunctival melanoma outcomes. Ophthal Plast Reconstr Surg 2012;28(5):313–23.

[20] Papandroudis AA, Dimitrakos SA, Stangos NT. Mitomycin C therapy for conjunctival-corneal intraepithelial neoplasia. Cornea 2002;21(7):715–7.

[21] Missotten GS, Keijser S, De Keizer RJ, et al. Conjunctival melanoma in the Netherlands: a nationwide study. Invest Ophthalmol Vis Sci 2005;46(1):75–82.

[22] Baum JL, Feingold M. Ocular aspects of Goldenhar's syndrome. Am J Ophthalmol 1973;75(2):250–7.

[23] Feingold M, Baum J. Goldenhar's syndrome. Am J Dis Child 1978;132(2):136–8.

[24] Fry CL, Leone CR Jr. Safe management of dermolipomas. Arch Ophthalmol 1994;112(8):1114–6.

[25] Ferri S, Shinder R. Inferomedial dermolipoma with ectopic lacrimal gland. Ophthal Plast Reconstr Surg 2013;29(2):e43–4.

[26] Maeng H-S, Lee LK-M, Woo K-I, et al. A Unique case of dermolipoma located in the lower eyelid. Ophthal Plast Reconstr Surg 2010;26(4):288–9.

[27] McNab AA, Wright JE, Caswell AG. Clinical features and surgical management of dermolipomas. Aust N Z J Ophthalmol 1990;18(2):159–62.

[28] Pant OP, Hao JL, Zhou DD, et al. Lamellar keratoplasty using femtosecond laser intrastromal lenticule for limbal dermoid: case report and literature review. J Int Med Res 2018;46(11):4753–9.

[29] Singh M, Kaur M, Grewal AM, et al. Ophthalmic features and management outcomes of 30 children having Goldenhar syndrome. Int Ophthalmol 2020;40(3):667–75.

[30] Pirouzian A. Management of pediatric corneal limbal dermoids. Clin Ophthalmol 2013;7:607–14.

[31] Abdulmannan DM. Successful management of limbal dermoid in infancy and childhood: a case series. Cureus 2022;14(3):e22835.

[32] Promelle V, Lyons CJ. Management of limbal dermoids by simple excision in young children. J Pediatr Ophthalmol Strabismus 2021;58(3):196–201.

[33] Kirkegaard MM, Rasmussen PK, Coupland SE, et al. Conjunctival lymphoma—an international multicenter retrospective study. JAMA Ophthalmology 2016;134(4):406–14.

[34] AlSemari MA, Maktabi A, AlSamnan MS, et al. Conjunctival pediatric follicular lymphoma: case report and literature review. Ophthal Plast Reconstr Surg 2020;36(1):e14–5.

[35] Moustafa GA, Topham AK, Aronow ME, et al. Paediatric ocular adnexal lymphoma: a population-based analysis. BMJ Open Ophthalmol 2020;5(1):e000483.

[36] Shields CL, Demirci H, Karatza E, et al. Clinical survey of 1643 melanocytic and nonmelanocytic conjunctival tumors. Ophthalmology 2004;111(9):1747–54.

[37] Izatt JA, Hee MR, Swanson EA, et al. Micrometer-scale resolution imaging of the anterior eye in vivo with optical coherence tomography. Arch Ophthalmol 1994;112(12):1584–9.

[38] Alvarez OP, Galor A, AlBayyat G, et al. Update on imaging modalities for ocular surface pathologies. Curr Ophthalmol Rep 2021;9(2):39–47.

[39] Tran AQ, Venkateswaran N, Galor A, et al. Utility of high-resolution anterior segment optical coherence tomography in the diagnosis and management of sub-clinical ocular surface squamous neoplasia. Eye Vis (Lond) 2019;6:27.

[40] Venkateswaran N, Sripawadkul W, Karp CL. The role of imaging technologies for ocular surface tumors. Curr Opin Ophthalmol 2021;32(4):369–78.

[41] Meel R, Dhiman R, Sen S, et al. Ocular surface squamous neoplasia with intraocular extension: clinical and ultrasound biomicroscopic findings. Ocul Oncol Pathol 2019;5(2):122–7.

[42] Vizvári E, Skribek Á, Polgár N, et al. Conjunctival melanocytic naevus: diagnostic value of anterior segment optical coherence tomography and ultrasound biomicroscopy. PLoS One 2018;13(2):e0192908.

[43] Zhong J, Deng Y, Zhang P, et al. New grading system for limbal dermoid: a retrospective analysis of 261 cases over a 10-year period. Cornea 2018;37(1):66–71.

[44] Kim JM, Weiss S, Sinard JH, et al. Dabrafenib and trametinib for BRAF-mutated conjunctival melanoma. Ocul Oncol Pathol 2020;6(1):35–8.

Advances in Ophthalmology and Optometry 8 (2023) 75–89

ADVANCES IN OPHTHALMOLOGY AND OPTOMETRY

Update on Cortical Visual Impairment

Joshua Ong, MD[a], Alkiviades Liasis, PhD[b,c],
Beth Ramella, PhD[d], Preeti Patil-Chhablani, MD[b,*]

[a]Michigan Medicine, University of Michigan, Ann Arbor, MI, USA; [b]Department of Ophthalmology, University of Pittsburgh, UPMC Children's Hospital of Pittsburgh, 4401 Penn Avenue, Pittsburgh, PA 15224, USA; [c]Department of Basic and Clinical Sciences, University of Nicosia Medical School, Cyprus; [d]Overbrook School for the Blind, Philadelphia, PA, USA

Keywords
- Cortical visual impairment • Neuroimaging • Electrophysiology • Low vision

Key points
- Cortical visual impairment is a diverse clinical entity, children may present with a vast variety of visual symptoms and the clinician must be aware of the potential causes to make a diagnosis
- While CVI remains a clinical diagnosis, investigations such as visual field testing, electrodiagnostics and OCT aid in reaching clinical decisions
- Management of CVI must involve a team approach, with the clinicians and teachers for the visually impaired playing important roles

UPDATE ON CORTICAL VISUAL IMPAIRMENT

CVI, also known as cerebral visual impairment, is one of the leading causes of pediatric blindness [1,2]. It is estimated that CVI accounts for around 27% of blindness in the pediatric population [3] and in the United States. CVI is the most common diagnosis in individuals that attend schools for the blind [4]. The term CVI refers to a vast and heterogeneric group of causes that lead to blindness in the pediatric population where vision loss is not primarily caused by an ocular etiology but rather stems from cortical-related abnormalities or injuries.

Causes

As an overarching umbrella term, CVI encompasses various broad subgroups of pathology including infectious etiologies (eg, bacterial meningitis [5]),

*Corresponding author. E-mail address: drpreetipatil@gmail.com

https://doi.org/10.1016/j.yaoo.2023.02.018
2452-1760/23/© 2023 Elsevier Inc. All rights reserved.

metabolic/genetic disorders (eg, Rett syndrome [6], copper storage disorder [7], and maple syrup urine disease [8]), structural cerebral abnormalities/malformations (eg, schizencephaly [9], porencephaly [10], polymicrogyria [11], and cortical dysplasia [12]), hypoxic-ischemic encephalopathic sequelae (eg, periventricular leukomalacia [PVL] [13]), environmental and natural toxins (eg, mercury [14] and snake bite [15]), drug toxicity (eg, metronidazole [16]), and perinatal/postnatal complications (eg, twin-twin transfusion syndrome [17] and pediatric cardiac arrest [18]). The inciting etiology of CVI also may be multifactorial. The commonest causes, however, are hypoxic ischemic insults and a stormy perinatal course, which results in a hypoxia, hypoglycemia, or both [19]. Depending on the time of insult, these influences can result in different patterns of injury [20]. In babies born full term, hypoxic insults tend to damage the striate and peristriate cortex, whereas in preterm babies, injury involves the subcortical white matter, including the optic radiations. At term, the cerebral blood supply has watershed zones at the interfaces between the major cerebral arteries, and hypoxic injury in this period can result in watershed infarctions in the parieto-occipital and parasagittal cortex, resulting in cortical visual loss.

Nomenclature and terminology
Given the broad spectrum of etiologies that can cause CVI, discussion exists around the nomenclature of using "cortical" versus "cerebral" in the "C" of CVI. The historical clinical definition of CVI has been described as visual impairment from insult to cerebral structures and retrochiasmatic visual pathway without ocular or anterior visual pathway injury [21].

Although the terminology is often viewed as interchangeable even in the medical setting, the distinction between "cortical" and "cerebral" in CVI carries multiple implications. "Cortical" is the most commonly used in the United States [22,23]. However, "cerebral" encompasses a larger range of causes compared with "cortical." "Cerebral" in CVI also has its limitations, including exclusion of the cerebellum [21,22]. Literature exists to support the reassessment of the definition of blindness from brain structure insult [23]. The term "brain-based vision impairment" has been used, and it encompasses a broader etiology [23].

Although common clinical presentations occur for CVI, no standard consensus criteria currently exist for diagnosis [3,24]. Because CVI continues to increase in prevalence, inclusion of patients with suspected CVI is critical. It is well described that CVI often is underdiagnosed [25]. This underdiagnosis leads to difficulty for children to adapt and/or receive specialized vision services to develop and receive necessary support during critical, formative years.

CLINICAL FEATURES OF CORTICAL VISUAL IMPAIRMENT
Ophthalmic findings and clinical examination
Visual symptoms in children with CVI vary tremendously and can range from total/near total visual impairment to relatively preserved visual acuity with

complex visual processing deficits. Children with CVI can have reduced visual acuity, defects in visual fields, and other visual functional deficits. These may vary with time of day and presence of other systemic issues such as concurrent illnesses. Children with CVI can have difficulty with contrast recognition, "visual crowding," which refers to difficulty in viewing multiple objects at once, especially against a patterned background, difficulty with facial recognition, spatial orientation and depth assessment, and detection of motion [26].

Visual field defects are one of the primary clinical features in CVI. Hemianopias maybe present, especially with neonatal strokes, preferential involvement of the inferior visual fields also is seen in children with PVL.

Although the clinical features of CVI revolve around a child's vision, it is important to note that CVI is associated with various comorbidities, including learning disabilities, thus achieving a diagnosis often can be challenging and may require a range of tests [27]. Typical ophthalmic examination findings in CVI include decreased visual acuity, fixation defects, visual field defects, strabismus, and nystagmus [3].

Visual acuity assessment often is difficult in children with CVI. Depending on the age of the child, various tests may be used. In very young children, one may only be able to test the ability to fix and follow light/bright objects and toys. These children often find the human face very interesting and just following the examiner as he/she moves into different visual fields may be a method to judge visual response. In children aged older than 6 months, preferential looking tests such as Teller Acuity Charts maybe used to estimate vision. Other tests such as Cardiff optotypes, Lea symbols, and Allen pictures can be used in older children. Sometimes moving objects are better appreciated by children with CVI than stationary targets. Using objects such as lighted spin toys is helpful.

Various studies have shown that strabismus is quite commonly present in children with CVI (ranging from 30% to 90%) [28]. Esodeviation and exodeviation have been reported in children with developmental delay and CVI [29]. Congenital exotropia often is associated other neurologic deficits, and in a child presenting with congenital exotropia, a detailed history and review of developmental milestones would be prudent. Other forms of strabismus, such as dissociated vertical deviation (DVD) and pattern strabismus, have been described.

Nystagmus is a common association. Studies report a prevalence ranging from 11% to 92% [28]. In children with severe PVL and cerebral palsy, nystagmus may be absent [30], which may be attributed to extensive disruption of oculomotor organization and loss of fixation. Oculomotor apraxia and saccadic and pursuit abnormalities also have been described in children with severe PVL.

Refractive errors often are present. Myopia, hyperopia, and astigmatism have been reported. Myopia frequently is present in premature children, especially those with history retinopathy of prematurity. Deficiency of accommodation has been noted in children with cerebral palsy and possible CVI [31]. A dynamic retinoscopy before dilation is recommended, and a good cycloplegic refraction is a must in these children in order to adequately manage the refractive errors associated.

Fundus examination maybe completely normal, even in children with severe visual impairment, with normal optic nerves and macula. Children with CVI may have varying degrees of optic nerve pallor, optic nerve hypoplasia, and optic nerve cupping (Figs. 1 and 2) [32]. Optic atrophy reflects damage to the anterior visual pathways, which may coexist with posterior pathway insult. In scenarios where the insult occurs in the early prenatal period, optic nerve hypoplasia may be present. Pseudoglaucomatous cupping is thought to reflect transsynaptic degeneration, resulting in a reduced number of axons in an optic disc, which is "normal" in size.

Investigations

CVI remains a clinical diagnosis; however, tests may aid the clinician in determining the severity and extent of the deficits. Visual field testing, fundus photography, and optical coherence tomography (OCT) are some of the routinely used testing modalities for obtaining additional information, which may aid management. Visual field testing often may need to be done clinically versus using a formal perimetry machine because most children with CVI are unable to reliably complete testing. Where possible, a Goldmann kinetic perimeter may be more accurate than automated perimetry. The severity of visual field defects varies, ranging from partial field defects to severe visual field constriction [3]. OCT has become a more recent ophthalmic imaging modality for aiding the diagnosis and helping the prognosis in children with CVI. OCT can demonstrate retinal nerve fiber layer (RNFL) thinning and ganglion cell (GCL) thinning in children with optic atrophy. Focal GCL thinning has been found to predict visual field function, as well as serves a potential way to detect CVI [33]. In PVL, a cause of CVI, disc cupping is a common imaging finding [34], and OCT can help monitor the cup disc ratio and RNFL and GCL thinning in these cases.

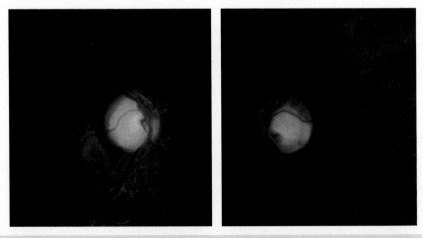

Fig. 1. Bilateral optic atrophy and segmental optic nerve hypoplasia in a 10-year-old boy with CVI.

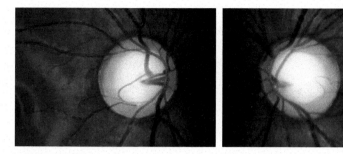

Fig. 2. Bilateral optic disc cupping, with normal intraocular pressure, in an 8-year-old boy, born prematurely, with developmental delay, CVI, and epilepsy.

Electrophysiology

Visual electrodiagnostic tests (EDTs) are useful in young infants or those who are not able to comply with normal testing of visual function and are particularly useful in determining the cause of decreased visual function because of retinal and or optic nerve dysfunction [35–38]. The common clinical EDTs carried out include the full field electroretinogram (ERG) and pattern electroretinogram (PERG); sweep visual evoked potentials (sVEPs) using checkerboard or gratings (sVEP); and transient visual evoked potentials (tVEPs), using pattern reversal, pattern appearance, and flash stimulation.

The ERG is a mass response from the retina in response to typically a short luminance stimulus (Fig. 3A). In the dark-adapted eye, the ERG to a bright

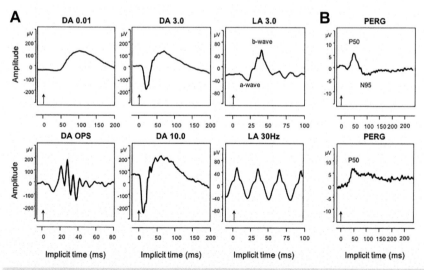

Fig. 3. (A) Representative 6 ISCEV standard ERGs recorded from a corneal electrode. The stimuli are defined by their state of adaption (DA = Dark adapted and LA = Light adapted), and flash strength in cd/s/m² [2]. **(B)** Pattern ERG to 50' test check, top = normal, bottom trace revealing degraded N95 component.

flash consists of 2 components: the a-wave, a negative component reflecting photoreceptor hyperpolarization, followed by a positive b-wave originating predominantly from ON-bipolar cells.

The pattern ERG is typically evoked using a high-contrast checkerboard and reflects the central retina [39] (Fig. 3B). The N95 of the PERG is generated in the retinal ganglion cells, while, although the origins of the P50 have not been confirmed, three-quarters of the amplitude is associated with ganglion cell activity. The PERG is therefore valuable for identifying either macula, ganglion cell/optic nerve dysfunction [29,40].

VEPs are recorded from the scalp positioned over the occipital region [41] and can be used to investigate the integrity of the chiasm, optic tracts, and radiations. The combination of the VEP and PERG helps determine if visual dysfunction is located before or after chiasm.

sVEP can be used to obtain an electrophysiological measure of visual acuity and have been found to provide better estimates of visual function compared with behavioral measures in those aged younger than 12 months.

tVEPs employ stimuli at a slower rate, resulting in waveform components, which can be measured and compared with normative data [42]. Stimuli typically consist of flash and reversing black and white checkerboard (Fig. 4) with pattern reversal responses typically having a well-defined maturation time course with the majority of the P100 changes occurring during the first 7 months of life [43]. Multichannel recordings of tVEPs help identify and differentiate general cerebral dysfunction, chiasmal, and unilateral hemisphere dysfunction.

Electrophysiology in cortical visual impairment

The most common findings in patients with CVI on clinical assessment is a reduction in visual acuity, and as a result, the sVEP is particularly useful in

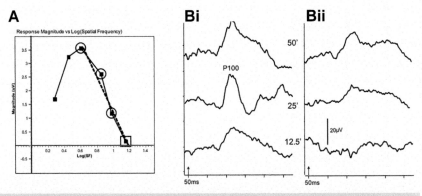

Fig. 4. (A) Normal Sweep VEP of a normal subject amplitude in μV against Log (SF). Analysis calculates a visual acuity of 20/23 (15.47 CPD, Log(SF) 1.19). Values within circles are significant and those in a box are not. **(B)** Pattern reversal VEPs in a normal 4-month-old (Bi) and a 4-month-old with CVI (Bii) to differing test check sizes. Note the degraded VEPs to the smaller checks in the case of CVI.

determining visual acuity in nonverbal children or those unable to generate an oculomotor response [44–47].

As mentioned, tVEPs are evoked by stimuli at a much slower rate that sVEP, and, as a result, individual components can be analyzed for amplitude and latency [48,49]. Flash tVEPs can be used in children with CVI who are not able to take up fixation to pattern stimuli and, despite not providing any information regarding macula function, have been shown to prognosticate visual acuity in children with CVI [50,51].

Pattern reversal tVEPs also are reported to be predictive of future visual acuity in children with CVI [52,53] but have also been reported as normal to absent [54,55], most probably reflecting the diverse range of children that are labeled as having CVI. The advantage of pattern stimulation over flash is that it reflects macula pathway function and in subjects who can maintain fixation, the crossing and noncrossing pathways can be stimulated individually enabling the identification of unilateral hemisphere dysfunction [56–59]. The presence of a normal clinical sVEP or tVEP, however, does not exclude CVI as in many cases of CVI, the site of dysfunction is after primary visual cortex [60,61]. In these cases, complex stimuli can be used to evoke electrophysiological responses reflecting higher cognitive visual function [62–64].

Neuroimaging

MRI allows for clinicians to further understand the cause of CVI (Fig. 5). In retrospective studies, MRI of patients with CVI were rarely read as normal, with one study reporting only 14% of CVI patients with MRI scans were reported as normal [3]. Given the broad range of causes of CVI, there are various MRI features including white matter abnormalities (eg, PVL) and anatomic abnormalities (dysplasia of the corpus callosum, lissencephaly) [3], and infarction. Studies have looked at correlating neuroimaging findings with severity of CVI

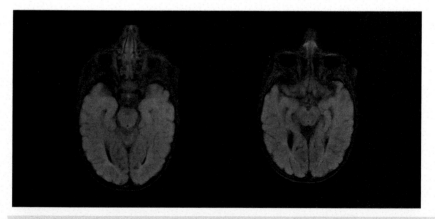

Fig. 5. Axial T2—FLAIR MR images, of a 2-year-old girl, with perinatal hypoxic-ischemic injury, with developmental delay and CVI, showing volume loss involving the bilateral parietal and occipital convexities with periventricular gliosis.

and the results have not been conclusive [48], generally, the presence of severe cystic encephalomalacia is thought to be associated with a poorer prognosis.

It is important for clinicians to note that structural neuroimaging that is read as normal does not exclude CVI. Causes of CVI also may develop from genetic abnormalities or seizures, which may not necessarily show up on neuroimaging [28]. Advances in functional neuroimaging allow for further insights in CVI, particularly in the setting of normal structural neuroimaging. These imaging modalities include single-photon emission computerized tomography, functional MRI (fMRI), and positron emission tomography (PET) [28,65]. In an fMRI study with infants with PVL, CVI was found in 75% of study patients [65].

Imaging of white matter tracts has been attempted using diffusion MR imaging techniques [48]. Additional advances in neuroimaging techniques include fractional anisotropy and high-angular-resolution diffusion imaging (HARDI), which allow for imaging of white matter tracts [28,66]. Bauer and colleagues reported 2 cases of CVI evaluation with the HARDI technique to assess the organization of white matter in the extrageniculo-striate visual pathway [67]. Although these advances in neuroimaging modalities and techniques are not currently a routine part of the standard workup of a child with CVI, these techniques may help to provide further insights in cases where structural neuroimaging is nonrevealing of the diagnosis.

Functional assessment in children

A functional vision evaluation examines how a student who is visually impaired uses vision in day-to-day activities at home, in school, and in the community [68]. Functional vision assessment is a process of gathering information through observation, interviews, and formal testing. Ideally, a teacher of the visually impaired (TVI) spends time reviewing ophthalmologic examinations, neuroimaging, and medical records as part of the comprehensive assessment. Following the records review, the TVI interviews with the parent and/or student with CVI to gather perceptions on the student's use of vision. Although the TVI often is the educational assessment coordinator for a child with CVI, the child's parents are the best reporters on their child's use of vision [69].

The functional vision evaluation determines what and where the student sees best, as well as identifies what helps or hinders the student's visual performance [68]. Throughout the assessment process, careful considerations should be paid to observing the lighting in the room, noise levels, environments free from visual clutter, positioning of the student, fatigue, and the use materials such as real objects versus pictures or line drawings [69].

Few evaluations or checklists for measuring the functional vision of a student with CVI exist. Two of the vision assessments created specifically for students with CVI and most familiar to TVIs are the Insight Inventory and the CVI range assessment. Developed by Dr. Gordon Dutton, the Insight Inventory consists of 52 questions that refer to visual–perceptual and visuo–motor difficulties that children with CVI may experience [70]. These questions are grouped into 6 domains: (1) visual search, (2) visual fields, (3) visual attention, (4) perception of movement,

(5) visual guidance of movement, and (6) recognition/navigation. For each item, caregivers rate how often the problem develops for their child on a 5-point scale (0, never; 1, rarely; 2, sometimes; 3, often; 4, always). Mean scores can be calculated for each of the 6 domains and the total. Christine Roman-Lantzy, PhD, created the CVI range assessment, an assessment used to determine the degree of effect of CVI on a 0 to 10 scale. The CVI range assessment is an evaluative instrument used to determine the degree of impact of CVI [69]. Following a continuum of visual functioning, the child is assessed using a 0 (no detectable vision) to a 10 (vision comparable to a typically developing, sighted peer) scale. In addition to parent interviews and the assessor's observation of the child, 2 ratings are used to get a score. Rating I is used to determine the extent to which CVI interferes with the child's functional vision. Rating II is used to examine each characteristic and the effect on functional vision. On completion of ratings, I and II, the evaluator can produce a score and create a guideline for interventions. The CVI range is structured to measure the behavioral characteristics displayed most often by children with CVI. These characteristics are color, movement, visual field preferences, latency, difficulties with visual complexity, light (need for), difficulty with distance viewing, atypical visual reflexes, difficulty with the novelty of new objects, and lack of visual-motor match [69].

Additional testing
Outside of ophthalmic testing and neuroimaging, additional testing and workup may be indicated in CVI. These include genetic testing, evaluation of systemic and metabolic disorders, and utilization of multidisciplinary teams for evaluation can provide further understanding of the etiology of CVI for individual patients. Referral grading criteria also have been developed to assess for CVI [71]. As many patients with CVI will have intellectual disability and other comorbidities, systemic evaluation, and the use of multidisciplinary teams for evaluation will be beneficial. These multidisciplinary teams may include clinical geneticists, ophthalmologists, neurologists, pediatricians, neuroradiologists, obstetricians, and other health-care professionals.

MANAGEMENT
Although the specific management of CVI varies based on cause, early detection is universally understood as a critical aspect of CVI management. Various screening programs and referral guidelines have been made for CVI [71,72]. These include questionnaires, specialist-based assessments, neuro-radiologic findings, neurologic signs, and functional assessment of visual orienting functions [72–74]. Because screening the entire pediatric population in geographic areas is likely still an ongoing area of development, screening targeted at populations most at risk (eg, children born preterm) may be most effective. Because CVI is a leading cause of pediatric blindness, population-based screening for CVI is being developed and assessed [74].

Once detected, various strategies exist to manage CVI. Given that CVI may present with a myriad of visual dysfunctions, including strabismus and nystagmus, ophthalmic management may be useful for many patients with CVI. High refractive errors have been reported in patients with CVI, thus corrective lenses may be worn to help with ocular comorbidity. Use of bifocals in children with hypoaccomodation is of significant benefit.

Strabismus has been found to spontaneously resolve in CVI [75]; however, persistent strabismus needs to be treated. Surgical management in these cases is reported to have a variable success rate, and under and over corrections are reported frequently. Dose adjustments may be needed to avoid over corrections [76,77]. Botulinum toxin injection is another option to treat strabismus in these patients. This often is helpful because it is a quick, less permanent treatment option and can be repeated if required [78].

Comorbidities also may affect the effectiveness of certain management strategies. West and colleagues reported that patients with CVI with cerebral palsy had worse outcomes compared with patients with CVI without cerebral palsy. Thus, it is critical to consider all comorbidities in CVI when managing visual dysfunction in CVI.

Educational support and stimulation

Following the functional assessment, individualized interventions must be created based on the student's use of vision, strengths, needs, interests, and routines at home/school. Recommendations for a child who has very emerging vision may include the use of black backgrounds to eliminate visually complex environments; materials chosen based on the child's preferred color and presented in his/her best visual field; and use shiny or moving light to direct vision. As the child demonstrates greater use of functional vision, materials and targets can be presented on a light box or backlit device (Fig. 6), may produce sound, may be more than one color, use backlighting to access a communication device, and may continue to use color to draw their visual attention. For children who have more developed vision, print work (such as worksheets) can be adapted to include less on a page or by covering some of the visual information

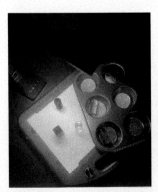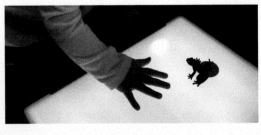

Fig. 6. A light box being used to help teach visual skills. The light box can be used to create a high-contrast background and to create an awareness of light, color, contrast, and objects.

by using a typoscope or line marker, with visually clean fonts, well-spaced between words and lines of print; learning materials presented on a backlit device such as a tablet or computer screen; presented upright on a reading stand; long passages made accessible through the use of screen readers or braille; and using color to draw attention to permanent landmarks for mobility purposes. For all students with CVI, attention must be given to visual fatigue and frequent visual breaks may be required [79].

Optimization and accommodation of the surrounding environment for patients with CVI also has been found to be helpful. Tailoring management strategies and making teachers and families aware of how a patient with CVI can be accommodated is crucial. Various strategies have been identified, including having family and instructors wear the nonsimilar bright clothing, so that the child can identify daily individuals based on colors [28]. Special schools are available that can further accommodate a child's needs to low vision.

SUMMARY

CVI is a dynamic brain-based visual disorder with a myriad of etiologies. It is one of the most common causes of vision loss in the pediatric population and early detection and management are critical. An ongoing discussion on CVI is the terminology and nomenclature to ensure optimized inclusion and treatment of patients affected by CVI. Current research is focused on optimizing imaging, screening, and management for CVI patients. These interventions may help to detect and treat patients with CVI to rehabilitate vision and allow for optimized vision during years of development.

CLINICS CARE POINTS

- A high suspicion for CVI must be maintained while examining children with history of prematurity, prolonged neonatal intensive care unit (NICU) stays, perinatal hypoxia, seizure disorders, and so forth.

- Asking parents/caregivers specific questions about visual behavior, such as preference for light, issues with color/contrast recognition, facial recognition, difficulty with mobility, and so forth, will help determine functional deficits.

- A complete ophthalmic examination is the key to determine the presence of any other conditions that can be treated.

- A team approach, with the involvement of pediatricians, ophthalmologists, teachers for visually impaired, occupational and physiotherapists, and rehabilitation specialists, is needed to optimize the visual function and improve quality of life for these children.

FUNDING

Acknowledgement of Funding - Buncher Foundation, Pittsburgh, PA.

References

[1] Pehere N, Chougule P, Dutton GN. Cerebral visual impairment in children: Causes and associated ophthalmological problems. Indian J Ophthalmol 2018;66:812–5.

[2] Ozturk T, Er D, Yaman A, et al. Changing trends over the last decade in the aetiology of childhood blindness: a study from a tertiary referral centre. Br J Ophthalmol 2016;100: 166–71.

[3] Bosch DG, Boonstra FN, Willemsen MA, et al. Low vision due to cerebral visual impairment: differentiating between acquired and genetic causes. BMC Ophthalmol 2014;14:59.

[4] Kong L, Fry M, Al-Samarraie M, et al. An update on progress and the changing epidemiology of causes of childhood blindness worldwide. J AAPOS 2012;16:501–7.

[5] Thun-Hohenstein L, Schmitt B, Steinlin H, et al. Cortical visual impairment following bacterial meningitis: magnetic resonance imaging and visual evoked potentials findings in two cases. Eur J Pediatr 1992;151:779–82.

[6] von Tetzchner S, Jacobsen KH, Smith L, et al. Vision, cognition and developmental characteristics of girls and women with Rett syndrome. Dev Med Child Neurol 1996;38:212–25.

[7] Gasch AT, Caruso RC, Kaler SG, et al. Menkes' syndrome: ophthalmic findings. Ophthalmology 2002;109:1477–83.

[8] Burke JP, O'Keefe M, Bowell R, et al. Ophthalmic findings in maple syrup urine disease. Metab Pediatr Syst Ophthalmol (1985) 1991;14:12–5.

[9] Good WV, Jan JE, Burden SK, et al. Recent advances in cortical visual impairment. Dev Med Child Neurol 2001;43:56–60.

[10] Khetpal V, Donahue SP. Cortical visual impairment: etiology, associated findings, and prognosis in a tertiary care setting. J AAPOS 2007;11:235–9.

[11] Good WV. The spectrum of vision impairment caused by pediatric neurological injury. J AAPOS 2007;11:424–5.

[12] Good WV, Jan JE, DeSa L, et al, Cortical visual impairment in children, Surv Ophthalmol 1994;38:351–64.

[13] Jacobson LK, Dutton GN. Periventricular leukomalacia: an important cause of visual and ocular motility dysfunction in children. Surv Ophthalmol 2000;45:1–13.

[14] Bose-O'Reilly S, McCarty KM, Steckling N, et al. Mercury exposure and children's health. Curr Probl Pediatr Adolesc Health Care 2010;40:186–215.

[15] Dhaliwal U. Cortical blindness: an unusual sequela of snake bite. Indian J Ophthalmol 1999;47:191–2.

[16] Chang MY, Borchert MS. Cortical Visual Impairment Treated by Plasmapheresis in a Child With Metronidazole-Induced Encephalopathy. J Neuro Ophthalmol 2021;41:e66–8.

[17] Good WV, Brodsky MC, Angtuaco TL, et al. Cortical visual impairment caused by twin pregnancy. Am J Ophthalmol 1996;122:709–16.

[18] Weinberger HA, Van Der Woude R, Maier HC. Prognosis of cortical blindness following cardiac arrest in children. JAMA 1962;179:126–9.

[19] Chhablani PP, Kekunnaya R. Neuro-ophthalmic manifestations of prematurity. Indian J Ophthalmol 2014;62:992–5.

[20] Brodsky MC, Fray KJ, Glasier CM. Perinatal cortical and subcortical visual loss: mechanisms of injury and associated ophthalmologic signs. Ophthalmology 2002;109:85–94.

[21] Bennett CR, Bauer CM, Bailin ES, et al. Neuroplasticity in cerebral visual impairment (CVI): Assessing functional vision and the neurophysiological correlates of dorsal stream dysfunction. Neurosci Biobehav Rev 2020;108:171–81.

[22] Cortical Visual Impairment vs. Cerebral Visual Impairment. CVI Now. 2019. Available at: https://www.perkins.org/cortical-visual-impairment-vs-cerebral-visual-impairment/. Accessed January 18 2023.

[23] Kran BS, Lawrence L, Mayer DL, et al. Cerebral/Cortical Visual Impairment: A Need to Reassess Current Definitions of Visual Impairment and Blindness. Semin Pediatr Neurol 2019;31:25–9.

[24] Sakki H, Bowman R, Sargent J, et al. Visual function subtyping in children with early-onset cerebral visual impairment. Dev Med Child Neurol 2021;63:303–12.
[25] Moon JH, Kim GH, Kim SK, et al. Development of the Parental Questionnaire for Cerebral Visual Impairment in Children Younger than 72 Months. J Clin Neurol 2021;17:354–62.
[26] Jan JE, Groenveld M, Sykanda AM, et al. Behavioural characteristics of children with permanent cortical visual impairment. Dev Med Child Neurol 1987;29:571–6.
[27] McConnell EL, Saunders KJ, Little JA. What assessments are currently used to investigate and diagnose cerebral visual impairment (CVI) in children? A systematic review. Ophthalmic Physiol Opt 2021;41:224–44.
[28] Chang MY, Borchert MS. Advances in the evaluation and management of cortical/cerebral visual impairment in children. Surv Ophthalmol 2020;65:708–24.
[29] Holder GE. Electrophysiological assessment of optic nerve disease. Eye 2004;18:1133–43.
[30] Lanzi G, Fazzi E, Uggetti C, et al. Cerebral visual impairment in periventricular leukomalacia. Neuropediatrics 1998;29:145–50.
[31] Leat SJ. Reduced accommodation in children with cerebral palsy. Ophthalmic Physiol Opt 1996;16:385–90.
[32] Holder GE. Electrophysiological assessment of optic nerve disease. Eye 2004;18:1133–43.
[33] Jacobson L, Lennartsson F, Nilsson M. Ganglion Cell Topography Indicates Pre- or Postnatal Damage to the Retro-Geniculate Visual System, Predicts Visual Field Function and May Identify Cerebral Visual Impairment in Children - A Multiple Case Study. Neuro Ophthalmol 2019;43:363–70.
[34] Pilling RF, Allen L, Bowman R, et al. Clinical assessment, investigation, diagnosis and initial management of cerebral visual impairment: a consensus practice guide. Eye 2022; https://doi.org/10.1038/s41433-022-02261-6.
[35] Mohapatra M, Rath S, Agarwal P, et al. Cerebral visual impairment in children: Multicentric study determining the causes, associated neurological and ocular findings, and risk factors for severe vision impairment. Indian J Ophthalmol 2022;70:4410–5.
[36] Robson AG, Nilsson J, Li S, et al. ISCEV guide to visual electrodiagnostic procedures, Doc Ophthalmol, 136, 2018, 1–26.
[37] Pompe M, Liasis A, Hertle R. Visual electrodiagnostics and eye movement recording - World Society of Pediatric Ophthalmology and Strabismus (WSPOS) consensus statement. Indian J Ophthalmol 2019;67; https://doi.org/10.4103/ijo.IJO_1103_18.
[38] Yap GH, Chen LY, Png R, et al. Clinical value of electrophysiology in determining the diagnosis of visual dysfunction in neuro-ophthalmology patients. Doc Ophthalmol 2015;131:189–96.
[39] Bach M, Brigell MG, Hawlina M. ISCEV standard for clinical pattern electroretinography (PERG): 2012 update. Doc Ophthalmol 2012;126:1–7.
[40] Lois N. Phenotypic Subtypes of Stargardt Macular Dystrophy–Fundus Flavimaculatus. Arch Ophthalmol 2001;119; https://doi.org/10.1001/archopht.119.3.359.
[41] Odom JV, Bach M, Brigell M, et al. ISCEV standard for clinical visual evoked potentials: (2016 update), Doc Ophthalmol, 133, 2016, 1–9.
[42] Sokol S. Measurement of infant visual acuity from pattern reversal evoked potentials. Vis Res 1978;18:33–9.
[43] Lenassi E, Likar K, Stirn-Kranjc B, et al. VEP maturation and visual acuity in infants and preschool children. Doc Ophthalmol 2008;117:111–20.
[44] Good WV. Development of a quantitative method to measure vision in children with chronic cortical visual impairment. Trans Am Ophthalmol Soc 2001;99:253–69.
[45] Lim M, Soul JS, Hansen R, et al. Development of visual acuity in children with cerebral visual impairment. Arch Ophthalmol 2005;123:1215–20.
[46] Bane MC, Birch EE. VEP acuity, FPL acuity, and visual behavior of visually impaired children. J Pediatr Ophthalmol Strabismus 1992;29:202–9.

[47] Sokol S, Moskowitz A. Comparison of pattern VEPs and preferential-looking behavior in 3-month-old infants. Invest Ophthalmol Vis Sci 1985;26:359–65.

[48] Sokol S. Visually evoked potentials: Theory, techniques and clinical applications. Surv Ophthalmol 1976;21:18–44.

[49] Walsh P. The clinical role of evoked potentials. J Neurol Neurosurg Psychiatr 2005;76: ii16–22.

[50] Clarke MP, Mitchell KW, Gibson M. The prognostic value of flash visual evoked potentials in the assessment of non-ocular visual impairment in infancy. Eye 1997;11(Pt 3):398–402.

[51] Iinuma K, Lombroso CT, Matsumiya Y. Prognostic value of visual evoked potentials (VEP) in infants with visual inattentiveness. Electroencephalogr Clin Neurophysiology Evoked Potentials Sect 1997;104:165–70.

[52] Howes J, Thompson D, Liasis A. Prognostic value of transient pattern visual evoked potentials in children with cerebral visual impairment. Dev Med Child Neurol 2021;64:618–24.

[53] Taylor MJ, McCulloch DL. Visual Evoked Potentials in Infants and Children. J Clin Neurophysiol 1992;9:357–72.

[54] Quintiliani M, Ricci D, Petrianni M, et al. Cortical Visual Impairment in CDKL5 Deficiency Disorder. Front Neurol 2022;12; https://doi.org/10.3389/fneur.2021.805745.

[55] Kamino D, Almazrooei A, Pang EW. Abnormalities in evoked potentials associated with abnormal glycemia and brain injury in neonatal hypoxic-ischemic encephalopathy. Clin Neurophysiol 2021;132:307–13.

[56] Maccolini E, Andreoli A, Valdé G, et al. Hemifield pattern-reversal visual evoked potentials (VEPs) in retrochiasmal lesions with homonymous visual field defect. Ital J Neurol Sci 1986;7:437–42.

[57] Kuroiwa Y. Visual Evoked Potentials With Hemifield Pattern Stimulation. Arch Neurol 1981;38; https://doi.org/10.1001/archneur.1981.00510020044005.

[58] Arruga J, Feldon SE, Hoyt WF, et al. Monocularly and binocularly evoked visual responses to patterned half-field stimulation. J Neurol Sci 1980;46:281–90.

[59] Handley SE, Šuštar M, Tekavčič Pompe M. What can visual electrophysiology tell about possible visual-field defects in paediatric patients. Eye 2021;35:2354–73.

[60] Kelly JP, Phillips JO, Saneto RP, et al. Cerebral Visual Impairment Characterized by Abnormal Visual Orienting Behavior With Preserved Visual Cortical Activation. Investigative Opthalmology & Visual Science 2021;62; https://doi.org/10.1167/iovs.62.6.15.

[61] Weiss A. The infant who is visually unresponsive on a cortical basis. Ophthalmology 2001;108:2076–87.

[62] Czigler I. Visual Mismatch Negativity. J Psychophysiol 2007;21:224–30.

[63] Tales A, Newton P, Troscianko T, et al. Mismatch negativity in the visual modality. Neuroreport 1999;10:3363–7.

[64] Flynn M, Liasis A, Gardner M, et al. Can illusory deviant stimuli be used as attentional distractors to record vMMN in a passive three stimulus oddball paradigm? Exp Brain Res 2009;197:153–61.

[65] Yu B, Guo Q, Fan G, et al. Assessment of cortical visual impairment in infants with periventricular leukomalacia: a pilot event-related FMRI study. Korean J Radiol 2011;12:463–72.

[66] Hagmann P, Jonasson L, Maeder P. Understanding diffusion MR imaging techniques: from scalar diffusion-weighted imaging to diffusion tensor imaging and beyond. Radiographics 2006;26(Suppl 1):S205–23.

[67] Bauer CM, Heidary G, Koo BB. Abnormal white matter tractography of visual pathways detected by high-angular-resolution diffusion imaging (HARDI) corresponds to visual dysfunction in cortical/cerebral visual impairment. J AAPOS 2014;18:398–401.

[68] Kaiser JT, Herzberg TS. Procedures and Tools Used by Teachers When Completing Functional Vision Assessments with Children with Visual Impairments. J Vis Impair Blind (JVIB) 2017;111:441–52.

[69] Roman-Lantzy C. Cortical visual impairment: an approach to assessment and intervention. Second Edition. New York, NY: AFB Press; 2018.

[70] Macintyre-Beon C, Young D, Calvert J. Reliability of a question inventory for structured history taking in children with cerebral visual impairment. Eye 2012;26:1393.

[71] Boonstra FN, Bosch DGM, Geldof CJA, et al. The Multidisciplinary Guidelines for Diagnosis and Referral in Cerebral Visual Impairment. Front Hum Neurosci 2022;16:727565.

[72] Ortibus E, Laenen A, Verhoeven J. Screening for cerebral visual impairment: value of a CVI questionnaire. Neuropediatrics 2011;42:138–47.

[73] Kooiker MJG, van Gils MM, van der Zee YJ. Early Screening of Visual Processing Dysfunctions in Children Born Very or Extremely Preterm. Front Hum Neurosci 2021;15:729080.

[74] Gorrie F, Goodall K, Rush R, et al. Towards population screening for Cerebral Visual Impairment: Validity of the Five Questions and the CVI Questionnaire. PLoS One 2019;14: e0214290.

[75] Binder NR, Kruglyakova J, Borchert MS. Strabismus in patients with cortical visual impairment: outcomes of surgery and observations of spontaneous resolution. J AAPOS 2016;20:121–5.

[76] Pickering JD, Simon JW, Lininger LL, et al. Exaggerated effect of bilateral medial rectus recession in developmentally delayed children. J Pediatr Ophthalmol Strabismus 1994;31: 374–7.

[77] Bang GM, Brodsky MC. Neurological exotropia: do we need to decrease surgical dosing? Br J Ophthalmol 2013;97:241–3.

[78] Salvin, J. H. & Hendricks, D. in Cerebral Palsy Ch. Chapter 77-1, 1-7 (2018).

[79] McDowell N. A review of the literature to inform the development of a practice framework for supporting children with cerebral visual impairment (CVI). Int J Incl Educ 2021;1–21.

Ophthalmic Pathology & Ocular Oncology

ADVANCES IN OPHTHALMOLOGY AND OPTOMETRY

Gamma Knife Radiosurgery for Uveal Melanoma

Bhavna Chawla, MD[a,*], Aruja Gangwani, MBBS[a],
Deepak Aggarwal, MCh[b]

[a]Ocular Oncology Service, RP Centre for Ophthalmic Sciences, All India Institute of Medical Sciences, New Delhi 110029, India; [b]Department of Neurosurgery & Gamma Knife Centre, All India Institute of Medical Sciences, New Delhi 110029, India

Keywords
• Uveal melanoma • Stereotactic radiosurgery • Gamma Knife
• Globe salvage therapy

Key points

• Uveal melanoma is the most common primary intraocular malignancy in adults.

• The management of uveal melanoma has developed a trend toward globe salvage therapies; Stereotactic Radiosurgery using Gamma Knife is one of the established methods.

• Gamma Knife has yielded promising results in terms of local tumor control; however, it is not free of complications.

INTRODUCTION

Uveal melanoma is the most common primary intraocular malignancy in adults [1]. Among these tumors, more than 90% arise from the choroid (Fig. 1), 5% to 8% arise from the ciliary body, and 3% to 5% arise from the iris [2].

The annual incidence of uveal melanoma is 0.2 to 6.3 cases per million population and shows significant racial differences [1,2]. Several predisposing factors have been reported, ranging from patient factors, including light skin color, light eye color, oculodermal melanocytosis, dysplastic nevus syndrome, iris nevus, and choroidal nevus, to environmental factors, such as UV light exposure [2].

Uveal melanomas are broadly grouped into small, medium, and large (Table 1), depending on the tumor dimensions [3]. The management of uveal

---

*Corresponding author. E-mail address: bhavna2424@hotmail.com

https://doi.org/10.1016/j.yaoo.2023.02.001
2452-1760/23/© 2023 Elsevier Inc. All rights reserved.

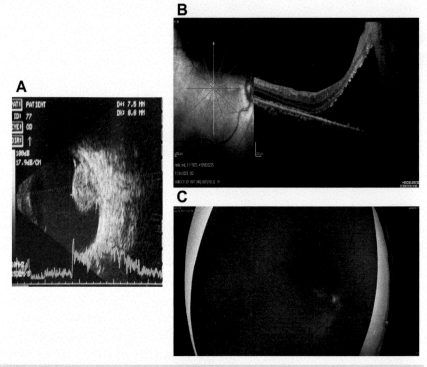

Fig. 1. (A) B scan ultrasonography of a patient with RE choroidal melanoma showing a dome-shaped choroidal mass. (B) SS-OCT image and (C) fundus photograph of the mass. RE, right eye; SS-OCT, swept source optical coherence tomography.

melanoma has improved significantly, with a trend toward globe salvage and preservation of vision, whenever possible. Enucleation, which was historically the preferred treatment, is now reserved for tumors too large to treat with conservative radiation or for painful, blind eyes [2]. At present, several globe salvage therapies are available, which include transpupillary thermotherapy, plaque

Table 1
COMS classification for uveal melanoma

Collaborative ocular melanoma study (COMS) classification	Tumor size
Small	1.5-mm to 2.4-mm apical height 5- to 16-mm basal diameter
Medium	2.5-mm to 10-mm apical height <16-mm basal diameter
Large	>10-mm apical height >16-mm basal diameter

Data from Refs. [5–7].

brachytherapy, proton beam radiotherapy, and stereotactic radiosurgery (SRS). The selected approach depends on several clinical factors, such as the tumor size, its location (choroid, ciliary body, or iris), and extent, as well as on the status of the fellow eye, the patient's age, general health, and psychological status [4].

SRS refers to the use of a single large fraction of radiation for treatment. The radiation is stereotactically directed to the region of interest in order to obliterate the lesion. Gamma Knife is one of the established forms of SRS.

PRINCIPLE OF STEREOTACTIC RADIOSURGERY

SRS uses the principle of directing a single large fraction of radiation to the region of interest to obliterate the lesion. This technology has evolved over the years into the use of multiple radiation sources oriented at a variety of angles, thus permitting the creation of various treatment target shapes. This allows for nonopen surgical treatment of pathologic conditions, which significantly decreases the risk of morbidity. The destruction of pathologic tissue following radiosurgery is a stepwise process that involves a number of different stages, beginning with the necrotic stage, followed by the resorption stage, and concluding with the scar formation stage. Currently, a number of different delivery methods of SRS exist, including linear accelerators, Gamma Knife units, and charged particle methods (Bragg-peak and plateau-beam) [8].

Gamma Knife radiosurgery is the most established form of SRS. With this approach, no incision is needed; instead, it uses MRI or other high-resolution imaging to make a 3-dimensional (3D) picture of the targeted part. The area is treated with many small beams of radiation delivered with robotic precision, instead of a scalpel.

The 201 gamma beams from the cobalt 60 sources of the Gamma Knife intersect within 0.3 mm, and it is possible to align the selected target point with the focal point within a mechanical accuracy of 0.5 mm. The technical specifications of the Gamma Knife make it possible to safely produce sharply circumscribed lesions in a single session with superior accuracy and precision. Gamma Knife surgery is a 4-step neurosurgical procedure, including the application of a stereotactic frame to the patient's head, stereotactic image acquisition, treatment planning, and the delivery of radiation. The system allows stereotactic acquisition of images from computed tomography (CT), magnetic resonance tomography, cerebral angiography, and PET scans.

TECHNICAL SPECIFICATIONS

Six current versions of the Leksell Gamma Knife (Elekta Instrument, AB, Stockholm, Sweden) (Models U, B, C, 4C, Perfexion, and ICON) (Fig. 2) exist. Although the physical appearances of the models differ, the internal design leads to dose profiles that differ only slightly. Each system consists of 6 components: the radiation unit; the beam-focusing technology; the patient couch; an electric bed system; the control console; and the planning computer system. The newer Perfexion and ICON units use an internal collimation system with 4-, 8-, or 16-mm isocenters and 192 Cobalt 60 sources [9].

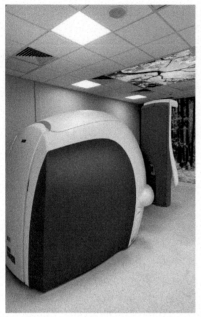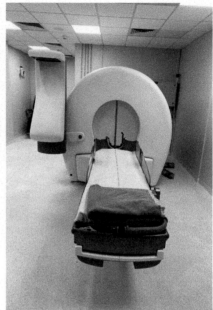

Fig. 2. Gamma Knife unit.

Movement of the patient couch in and out of the radiation unit, and opening of the shielding door are performed with high precision. The patient's head is moved in the focus point using very precise robotics. Stereotactic CT, MRI, PET, magnetoencephalography, or cerebral angiography are used for target determination, depending on the indication.

PROCEDURE

- The Gamma Knife consists of 192 cobalt fixed sources, arranged in 5 concentric rings.
- To achieve irradiation of selected target volume, the radiation emitted by the cobalt sources is aimed to a common focal point by a primary collimator.
- The procedure starts with giving local anesthesia to the patient—peribulbar block and hooking the muscle so as to fix the globe for the procedure.
- A rigid metal frame (Fig. 3) is placed on the patient and attached to the skull at 4 points with pins (Fig. 4).
- A high-resolution MRI scan and planning CT scan are obtained to provide orientation and localization of the target in 3 dimensions.
- Treatment planning is done in relation to spherical points on the Gamma Knife planning system.
- The patient then is brought to the treatment room; the target is immobilized by attaching the frame to the treatment table, and radiation beams are delivered, converging on the target.

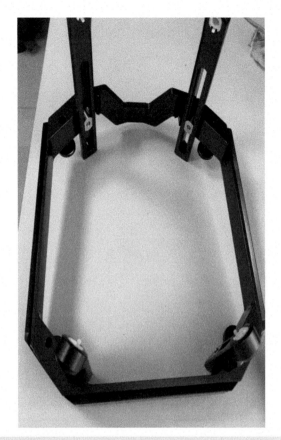

Fig. 3. Gamma Knife frame.

ADVANTAGES OF GAMMA KNIFE

Gamma Knife radiosurgery, initially developed for the treatment of intracranial lesions, has shown promising results in the treatment of uveal melanoma in terms of local tumor control. The primary advantage of Gamma Knife radiosurgery is preservation of the globe, with complete or relative sparing of the visual function. Gamma Knife radiosurgery also serves as a precious resource in cases where brachytherapy is contraindicated, such as large tumors (>15 mm in diameter or 10 mm in height) or lesions within 2 mm from the optic disc [4].

A significant advantage of the Gamma Knife over other available radiosurgical systems is the ability to create conformal and irregular dose plans using multiple target points. Highly conformal and selective radiosurgery is crucial to maintain low side-effect rates by tailoring the effect to the irregular 3D geometry of the target volume. In addition, the Gamma Knife has high selectivity, meaning that the radiation dose falls off outside of the target very steeply, thereby reducing the risk of injury to adjacent structures.

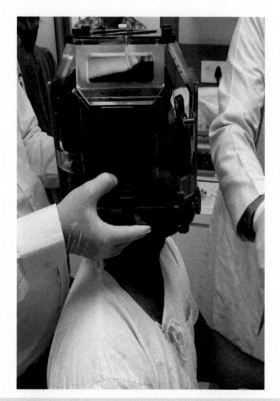

Fig. 4. Frame fixation for Gamma Knife.

CLINICAL OUTCOMES

Gamma Knife radiosurgery has shown promising results in the treatment of intraocular uveal melanoma in terms of local tumor control.

Mazzini and colleagues [10] retrospectively analyzed data from records of 48 patients (48 eyes) treated with Gamma Knife (n = 18) or Ruthenium-106 brachytherapy (n = 30) for uveal melanoma. Patients' demographics and tumor characteristics at diagnosis were recorded. Follow-up data were collected regarding local tumor control, treatment complications, enucleation need, metastases occurrence, and survival status. The median follow-up period was 33.7 months in the Gamma Knife group and 26.2 months in the brachytherapy group. The mean tumor thickness, the largest basal diameter, and the tumor volume were significantly higher in the Gamma Knife group as compared with the brachytherapy group. The local tumor control rate was 100% in the brachytherapy group and 77.8% in the Gamma Knife group. In the Gamma Knife group, 6 patients were enucleated, whereas no patient treated with brachytherapy underwent enucleation. The overall survival rate was 96.7% in the brachytherapy group and 94.44% in the Gamma Knife group. Secondary glaucoma occurred in 10 patients after Gamma Knife and in 1 patient after brachytherapy. However, it may be noted that larger lesions were treated with Gamma Knife, whereas smaller tumors were selected for brachytherapy.

Parker and colleagues [11] did a systematic review and meta-analysis to aggregate the clinical outcomes of patients with uveal melanomas or intraocular metastases treated primarily with Gamma Knife radiosurgery. Local tumor control and tumor regression were extracted as the primary outcomes and analyzed. A total of 840 of 898 patients from 19 studies had local control, and 378 of 478 patients from 16 studies experienced tumor regression.

Thus, Gamma Knife radiosurgery has been found to be an efficacious primary method of treating uveal melanomas and intraocular metastases, with reliable tumor control rates. However, further research is needed in terms of longer follow-up of patients and larger sample size to validate the results in terms of their efficacy.

RADIATION DOSE

Parker and colleagues [11] conducted a systematic review and meta-analysis, which revealed that the average marginal tumor dose for treatment of uveal melanoma ranged from 16 Gy to 59 Gy, with an aggregated median tumor dose of 32 Gy. A linear dose reduction has been tried in Gamma Knife radiosurgery treatments over time to minimize radiation-induced complications. Their review identified that although the average peripheral radiation dose for uveal tumors was 32 Gy, doses as low as 16 Gy have been used with no adverse effect on tumor control. These findings indicate the necessity for additional studies to evaluate lower radiation doses (10–20 Gy) in Gamma Knife radiosurgery treatment for efficacy in achieving local control, and their potential to reduce the incidence of ocular complications, as compared with conventional dosing regimens.

COMPLICATIONS

Although Gamma Knife radiosurgery has yielded promising results in terms of local tumor control, it is not free of complications. Modorati and colleagues [4] conducted a single-center, retrospective, observational study, including all patients with uveal melanoma treated at their institute over a 15-year period. Clinical records of 194 patients were reviewed. Anterior segment complications included a new-onset cataract or a significant worsening of previously known lens opacification (Table 2). Other anterior segment complications included neovascular glaucoma, corneal pannus, and blood in the anterior chamber.

The most frequent posterior segment complication was radiation retinopathy, presenting as peripheral capillary nonperfusion, epiretinal neovascularization, or vascular occlusion. Radiation maculopathy, featuring either macular ischemia/atrophy or intraretinal edema and exudation, also was observed [4]. Optic neuropathy has been documented ranging from acute papillopathy with disc edema and hemorrhages to pale optic disc atrophy. Vitreous hemorrhage is another reported complication [4].

Table 2
Complications following Gamma Knife radiosurgery for uveal melanoma

Complication	Rate (percentage)	Median interval (mo)
Cataract	41.2	18
Neovascular glaucoma	27.3	28.4
Radiation retinopathy	34.5	23.9
Optic neuropathy	18.6	14.9
Radiation maculopathy	11.4	13.7
Vitreous hemorrhage	14.4	26.8
Phthisis bulbi	7.7	53.3
Hyphema	0.5	43.1
Melting	0.5	52.1

Adapted from Modorati GM, Dagan R, Mikkelsen LH, Andreasen S, Ferlito A, Bandello F. Gamma Knife Radiosurgery for Uveal Melanoma: A Retrospective Review of Clinical Complications in a Tertiary Referral Center. Ocul Oncol Pathol. 2020;6(2):115-122.

FUTURE AVENUES

Gamma Knife SRS has yielded positive results in terms of local tumor control. However, only limited studies are currently available to evaluate the results, particularly prospective studies designed to compare results of Gamma Knife with other existing methods of treatment for uveal melanoma to validate its efficacy over other modalities. The complications associated with the use of Gamma Knife SRS need to be studied further to render information on the practicalities of use of this therapy in terms of patient acceptance and long-term visual prognosis. The complications can be studied further in terms of methods that can be used to reduce their severity in order to obtain better clinical outcomes.

CLINICS CARE POINTS

- Stereotactic radiosurgery involves the use of a single high dose of radiation directed to the region of interest in order to obliterate the lesion. Gamma Knife is one of the established methods of stereotactic radiosurgery.
- The primary advantage of Gamma Knife for uveal melanoma is preservation of the globe, with complete or relative sparing of the visual function. It also serves as a precious resource in cases where brachytherapy is contraindicated.
- Although reported to be an efficacious primary method for treating uveal melanomas and intraocular metastases, it is not free of complications.
- Anterior segment complications include a new-onset cataract, neovascular glaucoma, corneal pannus, and blood in the anterior chamber.
- The most frequent posterior segment complication is radiation retinopathy; others include optic neuropathy, maculopathy, and vitreous hemorrhage.

- Gamma Knife stereotactic radiosurgery has yielded positive results in terms of local tumor control. That said, more research is needed to validate its outcomes over other current methods of treatment.

DISCLOSURE

The authors have nothing to disclose. The authors have no commercial or financial conflicts of interest and do not have any funding sources.

References

[1] Spagnolo F, Caltabiano G, Queirolo P. Uveal Melanoma. Cancer Treatment Review 2012;38:P549–53.

[2] Damato B. Progress in the management of patients with uveal melanoma. The 2012 Ashton Lecture. Eye 2012;26(9):1157–72.

[3] Collaborative Ocular Melanoma Study Group. Design and methods of a clinical trial for a rare condition: the Collaborative Ocular Melanoma Study. COMS Report No. 3. Control Clin Trials 1993;14:362–91.

[4] Modorati GM, Dagan R, Mikkelsen LH, et al. Gamma Knife Radiosurgery for Uveal Melanoma: A Retrospective Review of Clinical Complications in a Tertiary Referral Centre. Ocular Oncology Pathology 2020;6:115–22.

[5] Collaborative Ocular Melanoma Study Group. Factors Predictive of Growth and Treatment of Small Choroidal Melanoma. Group, Collaborative Ocular Melanoma Study. Arch Ophthalmology 1997;115(12):1537–44.

[6] Collaborative Ocular Melanoma Study Group. Collaborative Ocular Melanoma Study- Randomized trial of I 125 Brachytherapy for Medium Choroidal Melanoma. Group, Collaborative Ocular Melanoma Study. American Journal Of Ophthalmology 2001;108: 348–66.

[7] Collaborative Ocular Melanoma Study Group. The Collaborative Ocular Melanoma Study Randomized Trial of Pre-enucleation Radiation of Large Choroidal Melanoma: Initial Mortality Findings COMS Report 10. group, Collaborative ocular melanoma study. American Journal Of Ophthalmology 1998;125(6):779–96.

[8] Fanous A, Prasad D, Mathieu D, et al. Intracranial stereotactic radiosurgery. J Neurosurg Sci 2019;63:61–82.

[9] Asgari S, Banaee N, Nedaie H. Comparison of full width at half maximum and penumbra of different Gamma Knife models. J Cancer Res Therapeut 2018;14:260–6.

[10] Mazzini C, Pierreti G, Vicini G, et al. Clinical outcomes and secondary glaucoma after gamma-knife radiosurgery and Ruthenium-106 brachytherapy for uveal melanoma: a single institution experience. Melanoma Res 2021;31(1):38–48.

[11] Parker T, Rigney G, Kallos J, et al. Gamma knife radiosurgery for uveal melanomas and metastases: a systematic review and meta-analysis. Lancet Oncol 2020;21:1526–36.

Advances in Ophthalmology and Optometry 8 (2023) 101–110

ADVANCES IN OPHTHALMOLOGY AND OPTOMETRY

The Pathology of Orbital Mucormycosis

Roshmi Gupta, MD[a],*, Shruthi Mysore Krishna, MD[b],
Ajay Krishnamurthy, MD[c]

[a]Ophthalmic Plastic Surgery, Orbital Disease and Ocular Oncology, Trustwell Hospital, Chandrika Towers, 5 JC Road, Sudhama Nagar, Bangalore, Karnataka 560002, India; [b]Center for Ocular Pathology and Education, Narayana Nethralaya, Narayana Health City, 258/A Bommasandra, Electronic City, Bangalore, Karnataka 560099, India; [c]Ophthalmic Plastic Surgery, Orbital Disease and Ocular Oncology, Narayana Nethralaya, Narayana Health City, 258/A Bommasandra, Electronic City, Bangalore, Karnataka 560099, India

Keywords
- Orbital mucormycosis • Pathogenesis of mucormycosis
- Mucormycosis and role of iron and diabetes • COVID-19 and mucormycosis

Key points
- Mucormycosis in humans is an opportunistic infection, invading where the host defenses fail.
- Mucorales fungi have specific virulence mechanisms allowing angioinvasion, a key step in the infection.
- The complex interaction between fungal virulence factors and host factors determines the clinical manifestation and the management strategy.

Mucormycosis is an invasive fungal disease, caused by fungi of the class of zygomycetes and the order of mucorales. These fungi are ubiquitous thermotolerant saprobes. The leading pathogens among this group are species of the genera *Rhizopus*, *Rhizomucor*, *Lichtheimia*, *Mucor*, and *Cunninghamella*. *Rhizopus oryzae* is the most common organism isolated from patients with mucormycosis and is responsible for more than 70% of all cases of mucormycosis [1].

The incidence of mucormycosis varies across geographic regions, ranging from 0.43 to 6.3 per million population per year across Europe and North

*Corresponding author. *E-mail address:* roshmi_gupta@yahoo.com

https://doi.org/10.1016/j.yaoo.2023.03.007
2452-1760/23/© 2023 Elsevier Inc. All rights reserved.

America, to 140 per million population per year in India [2]. However, multiple reports point to increasing incidence of the disease over the years [2].The recent COVID-19 pandemic saw an unprecedented surge in mucormycosis, particularly in India, where the official reported number of COVID-associated mucormycosis cases on December 3, 2021 was a staggering 51,000 [3].

Mucormycosis is known to affect different parts of the body. Rhino-orbital-cerebral mucormycosis (ROCM) is the commonest followed by cutaneous and pulmonary mucormycosis [4].

Generally, the incidence of ROCM is more in patients with uncontrolled diabetes mellitus, followed by malignancy, organ transplant, and deferoxamine therapy [5]. Mucormycosis primarily is a disease seen in elderly, with hospitalization rates of 7.2 per million population [6]. Men are affected twice as often as women [6]. Usually reported as unilateral disease, cases which are complicated by COVID-19 have reported bilateral involvement [7]. The largest series of ROCM, during the COVID-19 pandemic, reported 2826 cases [8]. No difference occurred in the presentation of ROCM associated with COVID-19 and others, albeit there was a rapid progression and increased incidence, and high mortality rate [7–10].

ROCM patients can present with fever, orbital, and facial pain similar to painful orbital apex syndrome, orbital/facial edema, loss of vision due to optic neuropathy or vascular occlusion, ptosis, proptosis, and nasal block. Less common presentations are proptosis, nasal discharge and nasal eschar, diplopia, headache, orbital and facial discoloration, toothache, loose teeth, epistaxis, and facial deviation [8,10,11].

In the pediatric population, the most common causes for development of mucormycosis are hematopoietic malignancy, post-organ transplant, and stem cell transplant. Sino-orbital mucormycosis accounts for only 15% of infections, whereas gastrointestinal, pulmonary, and cutaneous infections comprise the rest [12].

PATHOGENESIS
Fungal factors
The mucorales causing orbital mucormycosis enter the body through inhalation (other routes are ingestion, implantation in injured skin, and by contaminated needles) (Fig. 1). The spores of the mucorales species are 3 to 11 micron in size. Most of the spores are trapped in the paranasal sinuses, and a small proportion reaches the lungs. Where the epithelium is compromised, the fungal spores attach to the extracellular protein matrices, specifically to laminin and type IV collagen [13].

The spores form germlings, the hyphae, which are the invasive form of the fungus. The hyphae have a fungal ligand, spore coating protein (CotH), which bind to the glucose receptor protein (GRP78) on the host endothelial cells [14]. The CotH is to be found only on the mucorales fungi, and the species that have a larger number of CotH cause disease more often [14]. The hyphae enter the host endothelial cells by endocytosis, and the binding of the CotH to GRP78 activates the platelet-derived growth factor pathway.

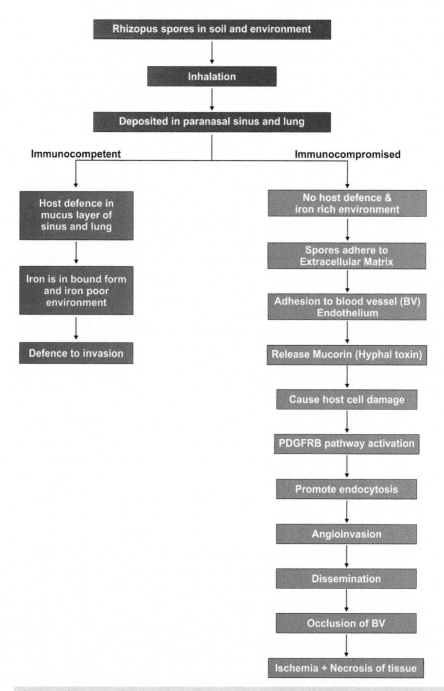

Fig. 1. Pathogenesis of rhino-orbito-cerebal mucormycosis (ROCM). PDGRFB, Platelet derived growth factor receptor beta.

The phagocytosis of the fungus damages the host cells. The angioinvasion is a key feature of invasive mucormycosis. The invasion of the blood vessels allows hematogenous dissemination of the pathogen. The hyphae themselves can block the blood vessels; the platelets are activated and adhere to the hyphae, forming clots. Although the adhesion of the platelets limits the hematogenous dissemination, it also contributes to the occlusion of the vessels. The thrombosis and occlusion of the blood vessels lead to tissue necrosis [15].

The role of iron in mucormycosis

Iron is essential for the growth of the mucorales fungi. Although the intrinsic siderophores of the fungi are not very efficient, they can acquire iron by several mechanisms [15,16].

The fungi can acquire iron from heme. Acidosis in diabetes impairs the ability of transferrin to chelate iron, thus making more iron available to the pathogen. In patients who are on treatment with deferoxamine, the drug acts as a xeno-siderophore after binding the host iron and makes the iron available to the fungi [15,16].

THE ROLE OF DIABETES IN MUCORMYCOSIS

Hyperglycemia inhibits the binding of iron to transferrin, lactoferrin, and ferritin, thus making more free iron available for the pathogen to use. In particular, in diabetic acidosis, the ketone body beta hydroxy butyrate (BHB) prevents transferrin from chelating iron [13].

The presence of BHB directly increases the expression of CotH and GRP78, allowing invasion of the cells by the fungal hyphae. In addition, diabetes impairs the chemotaxis of phagocytic cells, weakening the host defense [14].

Other virulence factors in mucormycosis

The mucorales fungi secrete lytic enzymes and mucoricin, a ricin-like toxin. The toxin is heat stable and remains active even after the death of the fungus. It causes apoptosis and necrosis in the host cells [17].

The fungi also develop Mendelian and epigenetic resistance to antifungals, including voriconazole [16]. Some studies have shown that the use of voriconazole increases the virulence of the fungi, although the exact mechanism is not understood [16].

Host defense factors

The host defense factors include macrophages, neutrophils, platelets, and various cytokines and chemokines. The first line of defense, the tissue macrophages, phagocytoses the spores. The hyphae (growing from the spores that escape phagocytosis) attract neutrophils, which damage the hyphae by oxidative toxicity. The neutrophils also secrete pro-inflammatory cytokines (tumor necrosis factor [TNF α], interferon [INF γ], and interleukin [IL-6]) to attract more inflammatory cells. Activated platelets secrete cytokines and chemokines causing inflammation and damaging the fungi. The platelets aggregate and adhere to the hyphae, preventing further hematogenous spread. However, the platelet aggregation also contributes to thrombosis of the vessels and tissue necrosis [13,16].

The natural killer cells (NK cells) are cytotoxic lymphocytes that secrete TNF α, INF γ, and other chemokines and directly damage the fungal hyphae [13]. A recent paper also attributed the peculiar susceptibility of COVID-19 patient toward mucormycosis to the inadequacy of NK cells in these patients [18].

LABORATORY DIAGNOSIS OF RHINO-ORBITAL-CEREBRAL MUCORMYCOSIS: SAMPLE COLLECTION AND TRANSPORT

1. Tissue scrapings from the involved area (necrotic tissue) are collected using a sterile swab and transported immediately to the microbiology laboratory at room temperature to prevent drying artifacts.
2. Tissue punch biopsy for histopathological examination is sent in 10% neutral-buffered formalin.
3. Frozen section is used for rapid intraoperative infected margin clearance status in cases of radical surgical excision of infected tissue. The sample is sent in normal saline and transported immediately to the histopathology laboratory.
4. Tissue for molecular analysis: Fresh tissue to be sent in phosphate-buffered saline for PCR or formalin-fixed tissue blocks are sent for PCR.

LABORATORY DIAGNOSIS OF MUCORMYCOSIS: MICROBIOLOGY

Potassium hydroxide (KOH) mount examined under light microscope shows branching hyphae with beaded spherical spores. On culture, the mucorales are fast growers in room temperature on Sabouraud Dextrose Agar (SDA) media. They form cotton candy like colonies, which initially are white and then quickly turn gray (Fig. 2).

LABORATORY DIAGNOSIS OF MUCORMYCOSIS: PATHOLOGY

Tissue biopsy or wide excision specimens are the gold standard for demonstration of mucor species. Special stains used for examination of suspected fungal infection are Periodic Acid–Schiff (PAS) and Gomori Methenamine Silver (GMS). Light microscopy shows broad pauci-septate fungal filaments with ribbon like hyphae displaying branching at 90° (Figs. 3 and 4). Angioinvasion (Fig. 5), optic nerve invasion (Fig. 6), and host tissue response can be noted in the tissue sections.

CLINICO-PATHOLOGIC CORRELATION IN ORBITAL MUCORMYCOSIS

The comparatively larger size of the spores of mucorales traps them in the paranasal sinuses, and the sinuses often are involved in the beginning of the infection. The angioinvasion and perineural invasion allows the dissemination of the disease, including the invasion into the orbits. Thrombosis and tissue necrosis are responsible for much of the morbidity from the orbital mucormycosis,

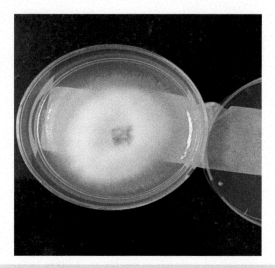

Fig. 2. SDA culture plate showing white cotton candy like mucor colonies.

and the central retinal artery occlusion and ophthalmic artery occlusion are responsible for the loss of vision in many of the patients. The fungi are sequestered in necrotic tissue, and antifungal medication cannot reach the pathogen due to the lack of blood supply. Thus, surgical debridement has to be used in conjunction with systemic antifungal therapy. In addition, voriconazole is to be avoided for treatment of mucormycosis. Local injection of amphotericin B has been seen to be effective in some patients [19,20].

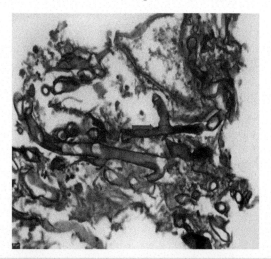

Fig. 3. Microphotograph showing broad pauciseptate fungal hyphal filaments with irregular branching at 90° shown by red arrow (PAS stain 400x).

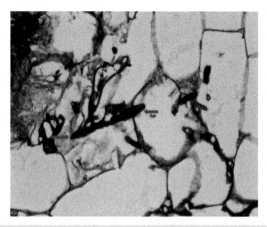

Fig. 4. Microphotograph showing broad blackish-brown fungal hyphal filaments with irregular branching shown by red arrows (GMS stain 400x).

As the primary defense against mucormycosis comes from the monocytes, macrophages, and neutrophils, conditions that cause cytopenia (leukemia, immuno suppression post-organ transplant, or chemotherapy) also are risk factors for contracting mucormycosis. Human immunedeficiency viruses (HIV) seropositivty is not implicated as a risk factors for mucormycosis [13]. Diabetes can decrease the chemotaxis of phagocytic cells, thus increasing the risk of mucormycosis [16]. Myeloproliferative disorders or frequent blood transfusion may increase the susceptibility by increasing the iron load. Diabetes and use of deferoxamine can, in addition, increase the iron available to the fungi, increasing the risk of the disease.

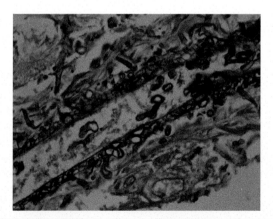

Fig. 5. Microphotograph showing mucor angioinvasion, fungal filaments are seen in the blood vessel lumen shown by red arrows (PAS stain 400x).

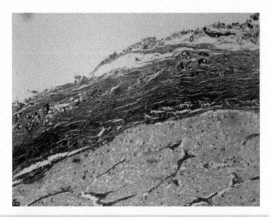

Fig. 6. Microphotograph showing optic nerve invasion of mucor species shown by red arrows (PAS stain 100x).

COVID-19 and orbital mucormycosis

The recent COVID-19 pandemic, caused by the virus SARS-CoV-2, saw an unprecedented number of patients with mucormycosis coinfection [3]. The vast majority of the patients suffered from ROCM. ROCM was more common in patients with moderate to severe COVID infection and progressed rapidly [7–9,21]. ROCM presented with the duration of symptoms of 5 to 6 days, presenting at an average 15 days after the SARS-CoV-2 infection [8,9,21]. Elevated blood sugar levels (irrespective of pre-COVID diabetes status), use of systemic glucocorticoids, and use of IL-6 inhibitors were seen to increase the risk of coinfection with ROCM in COVID-19 patients [8,9,21].

The SARS-CoV-2 virus directly damages pancreatic beta cells and causes new onset diabetes in COVID positive patients [22,23]. SARS-CoV-2 also breaks down hemoglobin, increasing the serum ferritin and makes iron available to the fungi [24]. Systemic glucocorticoids were used widely in moderate to severe SARS-CoV-2 infection; glucocorticoids impaired glucose tolerance as well as interfered with the host defense mechanisms. IL-6 inhibitor tocilizumab, used in severe SARS-CoV-2 infection, suppressed the host defences [25]. Thus, the nature of SARS-CoV-2 infection, the pathogenesis of mucorales infection, and the treatment modalities used for COVID-19 infection, all contributed to the high incidence of the disease.

Orbital mucormycosis, once considered a rare disease, is on the rise. It is difficult to treat and is responsible for extensive loss of function and high mortality. In recent years, we have arrived at a better understanding of the action of the fungi, the host defense, and the complex interactions between the two. In the future, the understanding of the pathology of mucormycosis may help to develop more effective treatments for a devastating disease.

CLINICS CARE POINTS

- Any one examination in microbiology or histopathology, showing pauci septate hyphae, is sufficient to prove the presence of mucormycosis, and treatment should be initiated.
- A strict correction of diabetes and serum iron levels is an essential part of management of rhino-orbito-cerebral mucormycosis (ROCM).
- Treatment of ROCM is by using the appropriate antifungal (amphotericin B, not voriconazole) in combination with surgical debridement of the affected tissue.

DISCLOSURE

The authors have no financial disclosure.

References

[1] Ribes JA, Vanover-Sams CL, Baker DJ. Zygomycetes in human disease. Clin Microbiol Rev 2000;13(2):236–301.

[2] Prakash H, Chakrabarti A. Global Epidemiology of Mucormycosis. J Fungi (Basel) 2019;5(1):26.

[3] https://www.ndtv.com/india-news/51-775-cases-of-mucormycosis-black-fungus-reported-in-india-till-november-29-health-minister-26358. Accessed on 19 February 2023.

[4] Jeong W, Keighley C, Wolfe R, et al. The epidemiology and clinical manifestations of mucormycosis: a systematic review and meta-analysis of case reports. Clin Microbiol Infect 2019;25(1):26–34.

[5] Roden M.M., Zaoutis T.E., Buchanan W.L., et al., Epidemiology and outcome of zygomycosis: a review of 929 reported cases, Clin Infect Dis, **41** (5), 2005, 634-653.

[6] Neofytos D, Treadway S, Ostrander D, et al. Epidemiology, outcomes, and mortality predictors of invasive mold infections among transplant recipients: a 10-year, single-center experience. Transpl Infect Dis 2013 Jun;15(3):233–42.

[7] Fouad YA, Abdelaziz TT, Askoura A, et al. Spike in Rhino-Orbital-Cerebral Mucormycosis Cases Presenting to a Tertiary Care Center During the COVID-19 Pandemic. Front Med 2021;8:645270.

[8] Sen M, Honavar SG, Bansal R, et al. Epidemiology, clinical profile, management, and outcome of COVID-19-associated rhino-orbital-cerebral mucormycosis in 2826 patients in India - Collaborative OPAI-IJO Study on Mucormycosis in COVID-19 (COSMIC), Report 1. Indian J Ophthalmol 2021 Jul;69(7):1670–92.

[9] Al-Tawfiq JA, Alhumaid S, Alshukairi AN, et al. COVID-19 and mucormycosis superinfection: the perfect storm. Infection 2021 Oct;49(5):833–53.

[10] Thurtell MJ, Chiu AL, Goold LA, et al. Neuro-ophthalmology of invasive fungal sinusitis: 14 consecutive patients and a review of the literature. Clin Experiment Ophthalmol 2013;41(6):567–76.

[11] Yohai RA, Bullock JD, Aziz AA, et al. Survival factors in rhino-orbital-cerebral mucormycosis. Surv Ophthalmol 1994;39(1):3–22.

[12] Pana ZD, Seidel D, Skiada A, et al. net and/or FungiScope™ Registries*. Invasive mucormycosis in children: an epidemiologic study in European and non-European countries based on two registries. BMC Infect Dis 2016 Nov 10;16(1):667.

[13] Challa Sundaram. Mucormycosis: Pathogenesis and pathology. Current Fungal Infection Reports 2019;13:11–20.

[14] Baldin C, Ibrahim AS. Molecular mechanisms of mucormycosis-The bitter and the sweet. PLoS Pathog 2017;13(8):e1006408.

[15] Sachdev SS, Chettiankandy TJ, Sardar MA, et al. A comprehensive review of pathogenesis of mucormycosis with implications of COVID-19: Indian perspective. Journal of Global Oral Health 2021;4(2):116–22.

[16] Ibrahim AS, Spellberg B, Walsh TJ, et al. Pathogenesis of mucormycosis. Clin Infect Dis 2012;54(Suppl 1):S16–22.

[17] Soliman SS, Baldin C, Gu Y, et al. Mucoricin is a ricin-like toxin that is critical for the pathogenesis of mucormycosis. Nature microbiology 2021;6(3):313–26.

[18] Gorimanipalli B., Padmanabhan Nair A., Shetty R., et al., Immune profile in patients with COVID-19 associated rhino-orbital-cerebral mucormycosis. ARVO Annual meeting, held in May 1-4 2022, Denver, USA, May 11-12 2022, Virtual. ARVO Annual Meeting Abstract, June 2022.

[19] Rizvi SWA, Khan S, Shahbaz M, et al. Long-term outcomes of transcutaneous retrobulbar amphotericin B in COVID-19-associated mucormycosis. Indian J Ophthalmol 2023;71(2):452–6.

[20] Shakrawal J, Sharma V, Goyal A, et al. Outcomes of transcutaneous retrobulbar Amphotericin B (TRAMB) as an adjuvant therapy for rhino-orbital-cerebral mucormycosis (ROCM) following COVID-19. Int Ophthalmol 2022;1–8; https://doi.org/10.1007/s10792-022-02591-0, Epub ahead of print.

[21] Vasanthapuram VH, Gupta R, Adulkar N, et al. A fungal epidemic amidst a viral pandemic: Risk factors for development of COVID-19 associated rhino-orbital-cerebral mucormycosis in India. Orbit 2023;42(1):30–41.

[22] Hayden MR. An immediate and long-term complication of COVID-19 may be type 2 diabetes mellitus: the central role of β-cell dysfunction, apoptosis and exploration of possible mechanisms. Cells 2020;9:2475.

[23] Müller JA, Groß R, Conzelmann C, et al. SARS-CoV-2 infects and replicates in cells of the human endocrine and exocrine pancreas. Nat Metab 2021;3:149–65.

[24] Habib HM, Ibrahim S, Zaim A, et al. The role of iron in the pathogenesis of COVID-19 and possible treatment with lactoferrin and other iron chelators. Biomed Pharmacother 2021;136:111228.

[25] Song G, Liang G, Liu W. Fungal co-infections associated with global COVID-19 pandemic: a clinical and diagnostic perspective from China. Mycopathologia 2020;185:599–606.

ELSEVIER
MOSBY

Advances in Ophthalmology and Optometry 8 (2023) 111–122

ADVANCES IN OPHTHALMOLOGY AND OPTOMETRY

Applications of Artificial Intelligence in Ocular Oncology

Bhavna Chawla, MD[a],[*], Kusumitha B. Ganesh, MD[a]

[a]Ocular Oncology Service, RP Centre for Ophthalmic Sciences, All India Institute of Medical Sciences, New Delhi, India

Keywords
- Artificial intelligence • Machine learning • Deep learning algorithms
- Artificial neural networks (ANN) • Retinoblastoma • Choroidal nevus
- Choroidal melanoma • OSSN

Key points
- Artificial intelligence (AI) is the simulation of human intelligence by a software/ machine. Machine learning and deep learning are the subsets within AI.
- AI may aid ophthalmologists in accurate prediction and diagnosis of retinoblastoma.
- Clinical database combined with AI technology can be helpful in stratifying patients with uveal melanoma and in predicting survival, thus aiding follow-up and therapy
- In the future, AI has the potential to likely transform current disease diagnostic patterns and generate a significant clinical impact on the management of ocular tumors.
- However, it is important to recognize that AI provides the most effective results only when augmented by the skilled human workforce.

INTRODUCTION

Ocular oncology is a specialty in ophthalmology that deals with the diagnosis and treatment of all tumors that occur in or around the eye–tumors of the eyelid, conjunctiva, intraocular structures, and the orbit. The most common intraocular malignancies are retinoblastoma in the pediatric age group and malignant melanoma in adults. Left untreated, both are highly aggressive and life-threatening malignancies. Conjunctival tumors, such as squamous

*Corresponding author. E-mail address: bhavna2424@hotmail.com

https://doi.org/10.1016/j.yaoo.2023.02.002
2452-1760/23/© 2023 Elsevier Inc. All rights reserved.

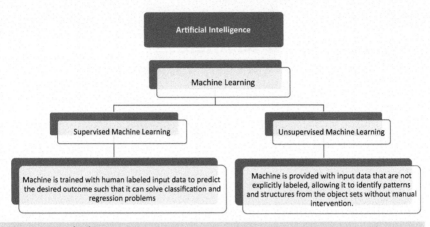

Fig. 1. AI and subtypes.

cell carcinoma, melanoma, and conjunctival lymphoma, are the most common ocular surface malignancies. These often are diagnosed late leading to loss of vision, life, and cosmetic disfigurement. As a result, there is a great need for a system that assists experts in the early detection of ocular tumors, especially malignant ones, through the use of data sets (fundus photographs, radiographs, clinical images, histopathologic images, and bio makers).

Artificial intelligence (AI) has been shown to play a significant role in the analysis of breast histopathology and detection of skin cancer and lung cancer [1–3]. The use of AI to screen and diagnose ophthalmic diseases, such as diabetic retinopathy, age-related macular degeneration, glaucoma, retinopathy of prematurity, age-related or congenital cataract, and retinal vein occlusions, inspired the of evaluation of how AI can be applied to ocular tumors [4].

OVERVIEW OF ARTIFICIAL INTELLIGENCE

AI has emerged as a major frontier in computer science research that deals with the development of algorithms that simulate human intelligence. The term "artificial intelligence" was first used by John McCarthy at Dartmouth Conference in 1956. Machine learning (ML) is a subfield of AI that allows computers to learn from a set of data and subsequently make predictions; these processes can be classified as supervised and unsupervised learning (Figs. 1 and 2).

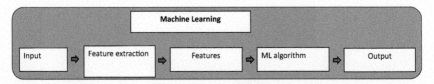

Fig. 2. Steps for development of ML algorithms.

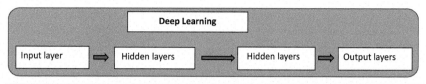

Fig. 3. Steps for development of DL algorithms.

Deep learning (DL) is a subfield of ML characterized by multilayered artificial neural networks. It enables analysis of multiple layers of data simultaneously. The DL system has significant success in the application of pattern recognition, image processing, and speech recognition. DL algorithms are known as "black boxes," as these networks generate features (comprehensive and discriminative) of high dimension to be accessible for human interpretation (Fig. 3).

The steps for developing an AI model are preprocessing of image data, training, validating, and testing the model and finally evaluation of performance of the trained model (Fig. 4). Data preprocessing is necessary to increase the prediction efficiency of the AI model. Noise reduction of data can enhance the quality of data and optimize the learning process. Health care affordability, quality, and accessibility can be amplified using this technology [5].

ROLE OF ARTIFICIAL INTELLIGENCE IN RETINOBLASTOMA

Retinoblastoma is the most common primary intraocular malignancy in childhood, affecting 1 per 16,000 to 18,000 live births worldwide. Durai and colleagues [6] have used DL techniques for early detection and diagnosis of

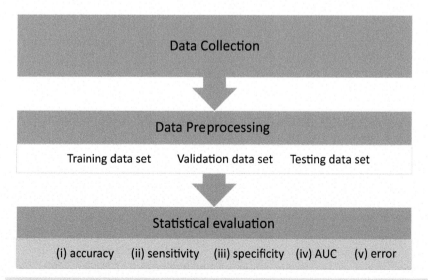

Fig. 4. Steps for developing an AI model.

retinoblastoma. The proposed methodology consists of 3 phases: preprocessing, segmentation, and classification. Initially, the fundus images were preprocessed using the Liner Predictive Decision based Median Filter to remove the noise introduced in the image owing to illumination. The preprocessed images were segmented using the 2.75-D Convolutional Neural Network to distinguish the foreground tumor cells from the background. The segmented tumor cells were classified, and the malignancy was classified into different stages and further grouped. The suggested system had an accuracy of up to 99.82%, a sensitivity of 98.96%, and a specificity of 99.32%.The investigators concluded that the proposed model could reduce the workload of the ophthalmologist by examining and detecting retinoblastoma at the early stage [6].

With advanced screening techniques and multidisciplinary management, most patients with retinoblastoma achieve life salvage, globe salvage, and even useful vision. Following local control and successful overall survival of retinoblastoma, long-term surveillance of survivors and screening for the offspring and relatives of retinoblastoma survivors is a challenge, thus leading to additional disease burden on the health care, socioeconomic, and psychological aspects. Furthermore, in most developing countries, only experienced ophthalmologists at tertiary eye centers can perform examination under anaesthesia (EUAs). Thus, this unbalanced distribution of health care resources may delay the diagnosis and proper management during the referral process. The application of DL techniques was proposed as a reliable and low-cost method for screening and diagnosing retinoblastoma [6].

Zhang and colleagues [7] developed a DL algorithm called Deep Learning Assistant for Retinoblastoma (DLA-RB), which aimed to assist in the fundus surveillance after local control and provide referral advice. It also provided an automatic surveillance of the contralateral eye of retinoblastoma patients and the offspring of retinoblastoma survivors.

In this study, 36,623 images from 713 patients were retrospectively collected and included for DLA-RB development, with 19,045 (52.0%), 2918 (8.0%), and 14,660 (40.0%) images being normal, stable, and active retinoblastoma tumors, respectively. ResNet-50 convolutional neural network with 5-fold cross-validation was used to establish DLA-RB. It achieved an area under the curve (AUC) of 0.9982 in the development data set. Furthermore, 139 eyes of 103 patients were included for prospective validation, and 69 eyes were clinically diagnosed with retinoblastoma. Thus, DLA-RB could accurately identify active retinoblastoma tumors and distinguish them from stable retinoblastoma with AUC, sensitivity, and specificity of 0.991, 0.979, and 1.000, respectively [7].

Also, they observed that compared with competent ophthalmologists, the DLA-RB reached superior sensitivity yet inferior specificity in differentiating active retinoblastoma from stable retinoblastoma. Of all 4 misclassified cases, 3 cases were false-positive, whereas only 1 case was false-negative. Thus, the DLA-RB–based diagnosis mode may be a cost-effective option in both retinoblastoma diagnosis and active lesion identification process. The investigators suggested that, in the future, DLA-RB can incorporate telemedicine programs to reduce diagnostic and follow-up burden and to maximize the use of limited health care resources in multidisciplinary management [7].

APPLICATION OF ARTIFICIAL INTELLIGENCE IN UVEAL TUMORS

Role of artificial intelligence in choroidal nevus

Choroidal nevus is a benign melanocytic tumor, often discovered incidentally on ophthalmic examination. These lesions generally are well circumscribed and pigmented. The overall prevalence of choroidal nevus in the adult population ranges from 5% to 25%. This benign tumor carries risks for vision loss, especially if it is located near the foveola, and risks for transformation into melanoma. Several features allow clinical identification of choroidal nevus and differentiation from melanoma. Based on clinical features, choroidal nevus can be divided into low risk and high risk (see Fig. 3) for future growth into melanoma [8] (Fig. 5).

Recently, Shields and colleagues [9] have described how AI technology can be applied to develop a novel noninvasive diagnostic method for the identification and determination of risk factors for malignant transformation in patients with choroidal nevus. ML is an AI technique that is capable of designing and training software algorithms from human-labeled data sets (fundus photographs). These supervised ML models are eventually capable of identifying choroidal nevi from fundus photographs. Similarly, a different supervised ML model can be trained

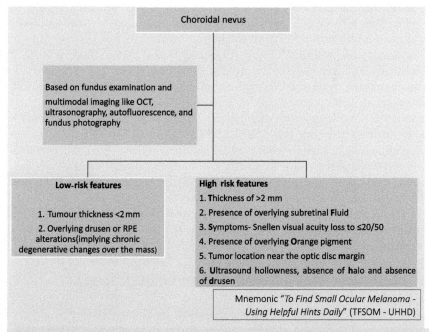

Fig. 5. Low-risk and high-risk choroidal nevus. OCT, optical coherence tomography; RPE retinal pigment epithelium.

using a separate data set labeled as low risk or high risk based on high-risk clinical features. In this regard, DL algorithms hold the potential to find novel or unexpected computational features that might predict nevus at risk of malignant transformation [9]. However, the investigators cautioned that some of the challenges and limitations that must be taken into consideration in these AI models include a lack of homogeneity in the training data set, using 2-dimensional images that lack stereoscopic characteristics, and black boxes within the algorithm. Nevertheless, despite all these challenges, the investigators suggested that AI-based screening for choroidal nevi and factors that may indicate melanoma transformation will enhance the detection and early treatment of melanoma within the eye, thereby improving life expectancy [9].

Role of artificial intelligence in choroidal melanoma

Uveal melanoma (UM) is the most common primary intraocular malignancy in adults, which can affect any part of the uvea (iris, ciliary body, and choroid). In 95% to 98% of cases, UM occurs in the choroid and ciliary body, whereas only 2% occur in the iris.

In recent years, numerous studies have been conducted by collecting large clinical databases that include preclinical data and histopathologic and genetic information, coupled with AI-based strategies (Table 1) to develop robust artificial neural network-based systems to confidently predict patient survival and stratify patients with UM for follow-up and therapy [10–17]. As a result, it is possible that patients with UM around the world will eventually be able to benefit from a model of UM patient prognostication that is widely accepted and used. A few tools developed along these lines include the Liverpool Uveal Melanoma Prognosticator Online (LUMPO) and the Prediction of Risk of Metastasis in Uveal Melanoma (PRiMeUM). LUMPO is a bioinformatic tool developed by assembling clinical, histologic, and genetic data from UK patients with UM. It may be possible to determine the risk of metastases and to estimate the time of survival of individual patients with UM using LUMPO, which is available online [18]. PRiMeUM is a Web-based tool designed for the prognostication of patients with UM in the United States. A reliable personalized metastatic risk assessment is made incorporating clinical features (age, sex, tumor location, largest basal diameter (LBD), and tumor thickness (TT)) and detailed information on chromosomal analysis (chromosome 1p, 3, 6p, 6q, 8p, and 8q status) at 48 months after initial diagnosis. Although both the tools were capable of determining the metastatic risk, neither could predict accurately when the metastasis will develop [19].

ROLE OF ARTIFICIAL INTELLIGENCE IN OCULAR SURFACE SQUAMOUS NEOPLASIA

Ocular surface squamous neoplasia (OSSN) is a broad term encompassing premalignant and malignant changes of the corneal and conjunctival epithelium. The term OSSN includes mild, moderate, and severe dysplasia, squamous cell carcinoma in situ, and invasive squamous cell carcinoma. The gold-standard

Table 1
Application of artificial intelligence in uveal melanoma

Study, year	Study topic	Biosample type	Biomarker studied	Statistical/AI/bioinformatics methods used	Conclusion
Johansson et al [11], 2010	Disease progression, disease prognosis	Tissue	Enzyme-iNOS (inducible nitric oxide synthase)	Supervised regression: Cox proportional hazards regression	iNOS predicts disease-specific survival and disease progression, but not an independent prognostic factor
Ehlers et al [14], 2005	Disease prognosis	Tissue	Protein-Nbs1 gene	1. Supervised regression: logistics regression 2. Supervised: PCA and SVM	Nbs1 is a strong predictor of UM survival and may be used to guide clinical management
Heppt et al [13], 2017	Disease prognosis, disease treatment	Serum	Cytokine, serum products: LDH, CRP, REC	Supervised regression: multivariate Cox regression	Blood markers predict survival in metastatic UM treated with immune checkpoint blockade Normal serum levels of LDH and CRP and a high REC may help to identify patients with better prognosis
Lorenzo et al [17], 2018	Disease prognosis	Blood	Protein: LDH, GGT	1. Supervised regression: logistic regression 2. Supervised ML: decision tree analysis	It demonstrated the bimodal survival pattern and developed a decision tree to facilitate clinical decision making and to counsel patients about the course of disease

(continued on next page)

Table 1
(continued)

Study, year	Study topic	Biosample type	Biomarker studied	Statistical/AI/bioinformatics methods used	Conclusion
Nicholas et al [10], 2018	Disease prognosis, disease treatment	Serum	Serum products: Absolute neutrophil count, LDH, alkaline phosphatase; neutrophil lymphocyte ratio	Supervised regression: multivariate logistic regression	They assessed the prognostic factors for overall survival and developed a novel prognostic model that included patient age, LDH levels, and Eastern Cooperative Oncology Group score
Indini et al [12], 2019	Disease prognosis, disease treatment	Tissue, blood	Cells, protein: NLR, LDH	Unsupervised ML: ANN	They found that ANN can successfully predict the prognosis of patients with melanoma treated with anti-PD1, using easily available patients' and disease's characteristics
Sun et al [16], 2019	Disease prognosis	Tissue	Protein: BAP1	Unsupervised ML: hierarchical neural network	DL model provided an accurate and reproducible method for the prediction of BAP1 expression in UM
Zhang et al [15], 2020	Disease prognosis	Tissue	Immune cells, stromal cells, chemokines	Supervised regression: multivariable Cox regression and Kaplan-Meier survival curves bioinformatics: GO and KEGG	This study showed the effectiveness of DL technology for predicting nBAP1 expression in UM only on the basis of H&E sections

investigation for the diagnosis and management of OSSN is mainly histologic examination, but it may be associated with problems like incomplete excision of lesions or removal of excessive nonneoplastic tissue.

Impression cytology, in vivo confocal microscopy, and anterior segment optical coherence tomography are the other low- to noninvasive investigations used to detect OSSN. However, these techniques are operator dependent and associated with some limitations. Habibalahi and colleagues [20] have recently used autofluorescence multispectral imaging (AFMI) technology to identify OSSN by its specific spectral signature and to differentiate it from normal (nonneoplastic) tissue.

AFMI technology excites eye tissue using a safe level of light in a number of narrow spectral bands (±5 nm) [21]. Tissue autofluorescence in several spectral ranges is captured, thus creating autofluorescent spectral signatures of different types of ocular tissue. AFMI also helps to distinguish between different types of tissue by recognizing chemical tissue composition based on fluorescence spectral signatures of cell-native compounds. Cancerous cells are, in general, highly glycolytic, producing a large proportion of energy from the fermentation of glucose into lactate regardless of oxygen availability, resulting in changes in the concentration and ratios of fluorophores compared with healthy cells, thus making it possible to extract spectral signatures for OSSN [22,23].

In one study, Swarm intelligence, a branch of AI, was used to find the optimized spectral signature of OSSN [21]. This study demonstrated the use of AI and AFMI technology in detecting optimized spectral signature and boundaries of OSSN. Pterygium is a benign, proliferative disorder of the ocular surface, and approximately 10% of cases can coexist with OSSN. Also, the clinical symptoms and appearance of OSSN and pterygium often have similarities, which makes definitive diagnosis challenging at times and results in inappropriate or delayed treatment. Habibalahi and colleagues [21] extended their research by application of multispectral analysis of autofluorescence in combination with AI to characterize and differentiate normal, OSSN, and pterygium cases. Spectral images were processed and then analyzed using the Support Vector Machine algorithm (SVM), which is a supervised learning algorithm, and a new classification framework called fused classification was used to minimize interpatient variability. The SVM classifier performance to distinguish pterygium from OSSN was AUC = 0.94, and in classifying OSSN versus normal and pterygium versus normal, it was AUC = 0.98 and 0.88, respectively. This algorithm also created false color maps for fluorophore analysis and boundary detection. The investigators observed that the margins identified by AI technology were in close agreement with expert evaluation on hematoxylin and eosin sections [21]. The investigators thus concluded that AFMI along with DL technology presents a novel diagnostic tool in clinical management of OSSN, which is noninvasive in nature, inexpensive, time efficient, and user-friendly [21].

POTENTIAL LIMITATIONS OF ARTIFICIAL INTELLIGENCE IN THE FIELD OF OCULAR ONCOLOGY
- There is limited availability of large data of various ocular tumors.

- It requires equally skilled manpower to capture clear and coherent images to be fed as input images.
- The "Black Box" mode of learning inside a neural network or ML algorithm remains unclear, despite familiar inputs and outputs; complete transparency is needed for taking accountability for treatment decisions for patients.
- Several medicolegal issues need to be addressed in relation to the application of AI in the field of ocular oncology.

FUTURE

The use of AI in ocular oncology augments diagnostic imaging, which may be used in real-time in telemedicine screening programs. The DLA-RB with a telemedicine domain has the potential to identify active retinoblastoma tumors and provide fundus surveillance after local control, as well as referral advice. In the future, AI applications could contribute greatly to the support of patients in remote areas by sharing expert knowledge and limited resources. Similarly, several studies have led to the development of robust DL algorithms for detecting the risk of developing choroidal melanoma from nevus, assessing metastatic risk, and prognosticating patients with UM based on clinical, histologic, and genetic markers. Despite this, a need still exists for a unifying and optimized model. The advantages of the use of AI in ophthalmology far outweigh its limitations. However, one should remember that AI provides the most effective results only when augmented by the skilled human workforce. In the future, AI will likely transform current disease diagnostic patterns and generate a significant clinical impact, despite ethical, regulatory, and legal issues.

CLINICS CARE POINTS

- Artificial intelligence is becoming increasingly relevant in the field of ocular oncology.
- Deep learning algorithms are being developed to detect and diagnose retinoblastoma early and to provide long-term follow-up for patients.
- Research is underway to develop a unified and optimized model for predicting prognosis of uveal melanoma.
- A novel and real-time diagnostic tool is being developed using artificial intelligence and autofluorescence multispectral imaging technology for ocular surface squamous neoplasia.
- Early results are promising, and artificial intelligence–based tools are likely to play a key role in the clinical practice of ocular oncology in the future.

DISCLOSURE

The authors have nothing to disclose. The authors have no commercial or financial conflicts of interest. The authors do not have any funding sources.

References

[1] Bejnordi BE, Zuidhof G, Balkenhol M, et al. Context-aware stacked convolutional neural networks for classification of breast carcinomas in whole-slide histopathology images. J Med Imaging 2017;4(04):1.

[2] Esteva A, Kuprel B, Novoa RA, et al. Dermatologist-level classification of skin cancer with deep neural networks. Nature 2017;542(7639):115–8.

[3] van Ginneken B. Fifty years of computer analysis in chest imaging: rule-based, machine learning, deep learning. Radiol Phys Technol 2017;10(1):23–32.

[4] Lu W, Tong Y, Yu Y, et al. Applications of Artificial Intelligence in Ophthalmology: General Overview. J Ophthalmol 2018;2018:1–15.

[5] Grewal PS, Oloumi F, Rubin U, et al. Deep learning in ophthalmology: a review. Can J Ophthalmol 2018;53(4):309–13.

[6] Durai CAD, Jebaseeli TJ, Alelyani S, et al. Early Prediction and Diagnosis of Retinoblastoma Using Deep Learning Techniques. 2021 [cited 2022 Dec 9]; Available at: https://arxiv.org/abs/2103.07622.

[7] Zhang R, Dong L, Li R, et al. Automatic Retinoblastoma Screening and Surveillance Using Deep Learning [Internet]. Ophthalmology 2022 [cited 2022 Dec 9]. Available at: http://medrxiv.org/lookup/doi/10.1101/2022.08.23.22279103.

[8] Shields CL, Furuta M, Berman EL, et al. Choroidal nevus transformation into melanoma: analysis of 2514 consecutive cases. Arch Ophthalmol 2009;127(8):981–7, doi: 10.1001/archophthalmol.2009.151 PMID: 19667334.

[9] Shields CL, Lally SE, Dalvin LA, et al. White Paper on Ophthalmic Imaging for Choroidal Nevus Identification and Transformation into Melanoma. Transl Vis Sci Technol 2021;10(2):24.

[10] Nicholas MN, Khoja L, Atenafu EG, et al. Prognostic factors for first-line therapy and overall survival of metastatic uveal melanoma: The Princess Margaret Cancer Centre experience. Melanoma Res 2018;28(6):571–7.

[11] Johansson CC, Mougiakakos D, Trocme E, et al. Expression and prognostic significance of iNOS in uveal melanoma. Int J Cancer 2010;126(11):2682–9.

[12] Indini A, Di Guardo L, Cimminiello C, et al. Artificial Intelligence Estimates the Importance of Baseline Factors in Predicting Response to Anti-PD1 in Metastatic Melanoma. Am J Clin Oncol 2019;42(8):643–8.

[13] Heppt MV, Heinzerling L, Kähler KC, et al. Prognostic factors and outcomes in metastatic uveal melanoma treated with programmed cell death-1 or combined PD-1/cytotoxic T-lymphocyte antigen-4 inhibition. Eur J Cancer 2017;82:56–65.

[14] Ehlers JP, Harbour JW. NBS1 Expression as a Prognostic Marker in Uveal Melanoma. Clin Cancer Res 2005;11(5):1849–53.

[15] Zhang H, Kalirai H, Acha-Sagredo A, et al. Piloting a deep learning model for predicting nuclear BAP1 immunohistochemical expression of uveal melanoma from hematoxylin-and-eosin sections. Transl Vis Sci Technol 2020;9(2):50.

[16] Sun M, Zhou W, Qi X, et al. Prediction of BAP1 Expression in Uveal Melanoma Using Densely-Connected Deep Classification Networks. Cancers 2019;11(10):1579.

[17] Lorenzo D, Ochoa M, Piulats JM, et al. Prognostic Factors and Decision Tree for Long-Term Survival in Metastatic Uveal Melanoma. Cancer Res Treat 2018;50(4):1130–9.

[18] DeParis SW, Taktak A, Eleuteri A, et al. External Validation of the Liverpool Uveal Melanoma Prognosticator Online. Investig Opthalmology Vis Sci 2016;57(14):6116.

[19] Predicting Mortality from Choroidal Melanoma. Investig Opthalmology Vis Sci 2020;61(4):35.

[20] Habibalahi A, Bala C, Allende A, et al. Novel automated non invasive detection of ocular surface squamous neoplasia using multispectral autofluorescence imaging. Ocul Surf 2019;17(3):540–50.

[21] Habibalahi A, Allende A, Bala C, et al. Optimized Autofluorescence Spectral Signature for Non-Invasive Diagnostics of Ocular Surface Squamous Neoplasia (OSSN). IEEE Access 2019;7:141343–51.

[22] Stringari C, Edwards RA, Pate KT, et al. Metabolic trajectory of cellular differentiation in small intestine by Phasor Fluorescence Lifetime Microscopy of NADH. Sci Rep 2012;2(1): 568.

[23] Skala MC, Riching KM, Gendron-Fitzpatrick A, et al. *In vivo* multiphoton microscopy of NADH and FAD redox states, fluorescence lifetimes, and cellular morphology in precancerous epithelia. Proc Natl Acad Sci 2007;104(49):19494–9.

Cataract & Refractive Surgery

Advances in Ophthalmology and Optometry 8 (2023) 123–138

ADVANCES IN OPHTHALMOLOGY AND OPTOMETRY

Corneal Pathology and Cataract Surgery Considerations

Natalie Cheung, MD, MS[a,b,*], Philip Shands, MD[a,b],
Ashraf Ahmad, MD[c,1], Daniel Daroszewski, MD[d,2],
Shelley Jelineo, MD[e,3]

[a]Corneal and External Diseases, Ophthalmology, Surgical Services, Louis Stokes Cleveland VA
Medical Center, 10701 East Boulevard, Cleveland, OH 44106, USA; [b]Case Western Reserve
University School of Medicine, Cleveland, OH, USA; [c]Cornea, Cataract and Refractive Surgery,
Harvard Eye Associates, Laguna Hills, CA, USA; [d]Cornea, Northeast Ohio Eye Surgeons, Stow,
OH, USA; [e]Case Western Reserve University/University Hospitals, 11100 Euclid Avenue,
Cleveland, OH, USA

Keywords

• Cataract surgery • Fuchs endothelial corneal dystrophy
• Epithelial basement membrane dystrophy • Radial keratotomy
• Corneal transplant • Contact lens • Keratoconus • Pterygium

Key points

- Superficial keratotomy is recommended before cataract surgery in eyes that have diffuse and central epithelial basement membrane dystrophy causing central irregular corneal astigmatism.

- Performing sequential pterygium excision before cataract surgery in eyes that have significant corneal astigmatism yields the most predictable refractive outcomes.

- Using newer IOL formulas that account for posterior corneal curvature and total keratometry can improve refractive outcomes postoperatively in eyes with keratoconus. Avoid astigmatism-correcting IOLs and consider aiming for near vision in patients with KCN that plan to use contact lens postoperatively.

Continued

[1]Present address: 11304 Ansel, Irvine, CA 92618.
[2]Present address: 425 Literary Road, Apartment 414, Cleveland, OH 44113.
[3]Present address: 11100 Euclid Avenue. Cleveland. OH.

*Corresponding author. Corneal and External Diseases, Ophthalmology, Surgical Services, Louis Stokes Cleveland VA Medical Center, 10701 East Boulevard, Cleveland, OH 44106.
E-mail address: natalie.cheung@va.gov

https://doi.org/10.1016/j.yaoo.2023.02.007
2452-1760/23/Published by Elsevier Inc.

Continued

- Stabilization of keratometry readings, corneal maps, and refraction must be achieved before obtaining preoperative cataract surgery measurements in contact lens users to ensure accurate IOL calculations.
- Adjustments in IOL target is needed to counteract the expected hyperopic shift in cases of combined cataract surgery and partial-thickness cornea transplant and cataract surgery in patients with RK.

INTRODUCTION

Cataract surgery remains one of the most common surgical procedures to restore vision around the world. As the aging population continues to rise, the demand for cataract surgery also is projected to climb. Patient expectations on specular independence after surgery continue to grow as the technology for cataract surgery, intraocular lens (IOL) calculations, and intraocular implants is improved and honed. Various corneal pathologies can affect visual outcomes after cataract surgery, which need to be taken under careful consideration for each patient undergoing cataract surgery.

This review focuses on cataract surgery considerations in patients that have concurrent epithelial basement membrane dystrophy (EBMD), pterygium, keratoconus (KCN), contact lens use, Fuchs endothelial corneal dystrophy (FECD), penetrating keratoplasty (PKP), or radial keratotomy (RK).

EPITHELIAL BASEMENT MEMBRANE DYSTROPHY

EBMD, also known as map-dot-fingerprint dystrophy, refers to a corneal epithelial disease that may result in recurrent corneal erosions, irregular corneal astigmatism, and decreased vision. It has been observed to have an autosomal-dominant inheritance pattern, but is commonly sporadic, leading some to consider it a degeneration rather than a dystrophy. On examination, the hallmark of EBMD is negative staining patterns when viewed under cobalt blue light after installation of fluorescein (Fig. 1) [1].

Most patients with EBMD are asymptomatic and do not require treatment or further intervention. However, for patients undergoing cataract surgery in the setting of EBMD, certain considerations need to be taken depending on the extent and severity of the EBMD. If the EBMD is mild and/or peripherally located, no further action needs to be taken especially if the central corneal maps appear regular. However, if the EBMD is more diffuse, central, or encroaching on the visual axis, and causing central irregular astigmatism on corneal imaging, it is recommended that a superficial keratectomy (SK) be done before cataract surgery. This corrects any irregularities in the surface epithelium, improves keratometry readings, and ultimately achieves better visual outcomes after cataract surgery.

Once an SK has been done, an adequate amount of time needs to be given to allow the corneal surface to stabilize. It can take up to 6 to 8 weeks for keratometry readings and topography or tomography to demonstrate stability. Therefore, it is advisable to repeat serial topography or tomography and IOL measurements at least 1 month after SK before proceeding with cataract surgery [2,3].

PTERYGIUM

Pterygium is a benign, wing-shaped lesion extending from the conjunctival limbus onto the cornea, usually in the interpalpebral zones at the 3- and/or 9-o'clock positions. This growth typically is associated with long-term UV light exposure. Pterygia can vary in size, but the larger the growth, the higher likelihood it causes significant corneal astigmatism or affects the vision if they extend into the visual axis. In patients who also have a visually significant cataract, the surgeon must decide whether to perform simultaneous pterygium excision and cataract surgery or sequential surgery. Sequential surgery is preferred if the goal is the best refractive result. However, simultaneous surgery is beneficial in certain situations by offering a single operation and fewer postoperative visits (Fig. 2).

Pterygia can cause corneal flattening and induce astigmatism, which can alter keratometric (K) readings used for IOL power calculations. One study showed that large pterygia (>2.40 mm or 5.45 mm^2 area) tended to have more of an impact on IOL power, and because typically corneal steepening occurs after pterygium excision, IOL power should be decreased by 0.50 diopter (D) [4]. A prospective study of 70 eyes comparing simultaneous with sequential pterygium excision and cataract surgery found the refractive results were more predictable in the group with sequential surgery [5]. Studies have shown no change in mean corneal power between 1 month and 3 months postoperatively after pterygium excision [6]. Therefore, waiting 1 month after pterygium excision before cataract extraction in sequential cases is adequate (Figs. 3 and 4).

In summary, performing pterygium excision, repeating IOL power calculations 1 month after excision, followed by cataract extraction, yields the most predictable refractive outcomes. However, in certain situations where

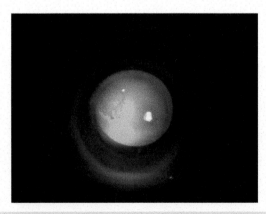

Fig. 1. Slit lamp photograph of epithelial basement membrane dystrophy with negative staining with fluorescein under cobalt blue light.

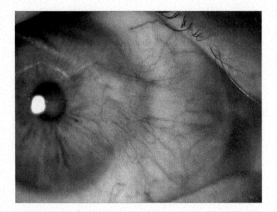

Fig. 2. Slit lamp photograph of large nasal pterygium.

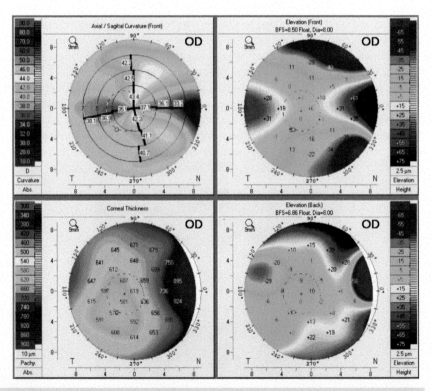

Fig. 3. Tomography of nasal pterygium pre-excision with nasal flattening and steepening 90° away.

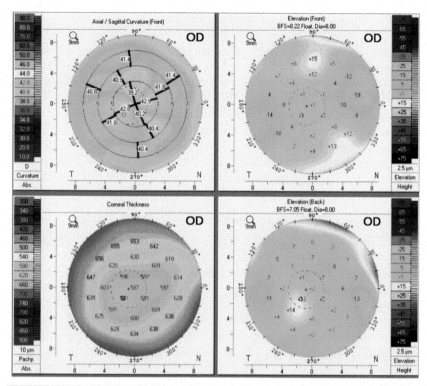

Fig. 4. Tomography of nasal pterygium post-excision with significantly less corneal astigmatism.

simultaneous surgery is preferred, decreasing the IOL power by about 0.5 D may be necessary to avoid a myopic surprise.

KERATOCONUS

In eyes with KCN, establishing stability of the disease process is crucial before proceeding with any surgical intervention. Typically, progression of KCN is most notable through puberty and young adulthood. However, KCN can still be diagnosed in patients of cataract age [7]. These patients may benefit from procedures, such as corneal cross-linking, to halt progression and achieve stability before moving forward with cataract surgery. In patients who currently wear contact lenses, such as scleral or rigid gas permeable (RGP) lenses, a discussion about whether the patient plans to continue wearing those lenses postoperatively is paramount. These lenses help create an optically smooth surface and minimize significant corneal astigmatism. Therefore, astigmatism-correcting IOLs should not be used in patients who plan to continue to wear contact lens correction postoperatively. However, in patients who are unable to use or intolerant of contact lenses and have stable corneal astigmatism, a discussion about the use of astigmatism-correcting IOLs is beneficial to help correct and reduce the patient's total amount of astigmatism (Fig. 5).

IOL calculations in keratoconic eyes can result in a hyperopic surprise for two reasons. The first is that the corneal power often is overestimated, especially in advanced cases with very steep K readings. The second is that the estimated lens position (ELP) tends to be more posterior than predicted [8]. IOL calculation formulas have become more advanced to better predict refractive outcomes by using newer biometers and keratometers that are able to measure the posterior corneal curvature [9]. KCN-specific formulas using total keratometry values seem to yield the most accurate results [10]. However, despite recent adjustments, there still tends to be a hyperopic refractive result. Thus, many advocate aiming for slight myopia of −0.50 to −0.75 D [11]. If the patient plans to wear contact lenses postoperatively, aiming the patient for near vision is helpful.

The steps of cataract surgery in eyes with KCN do not differ significantly from non-KCN eyes. Special care should be taken if there is difficult visualization as a result of the corneal shape or significant scarring and a deeper anterior chamber is often encountered during the surgery. Additionally, in advanced KCN eyes with thinner and steeper corneas, the surgeon should take care when creating the main incision to avoid premature entry and short tunnel length, which could lead to wound leak. There should be a low threshold to place a corneal suture if there is any doubt on the integrity of the corneal wound.

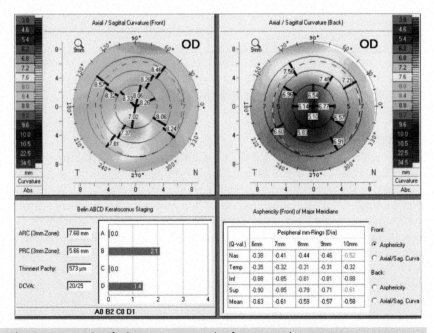

Fig. 5. Tomography of a keratoconic eye with inferior corneal steepening.

The same postoperative risks for routine cataract surgery patients apply to patients with KCN. No studies exist that indicate KCN patients are at a higher risk for complications, such as endophthalmitis or retinal detachment.

CONTACT LENS

Contact lens technology has developed rapidly in recent decades. Although initial studies of polymethyl methacrylate contact lenses were noted to change corneal curvature and cause corneal warpage, subsequent studies of other more modern plastic contact lens materials, including RGPs and soft contact lenses, were noted to cause corneal warpage and thus affect overall corneal curvature [12–14]. Corneal warpage is defined as central irregular corneal astigmatism, loss of radial symmetry, and reversal of the normal pattern of progressive flattening from the center to the periphery [15]. Corneal warpage can significantly affect K measurements and thus affect accuracy of preoperative cataract measurements.

Multiple studies have looked at time to recovery of corneal warpage, often with a focus on refractive stability in the context of refractive surgery. A wide variability seems to occur in RGP users for an average of 5 to 8 weeks with a large standard deviation to achieve refractive stability [16–19]. Some consideration exists that a longer contact lens–free period is needed for those with an extended period of RGP wear [17]. For rigid contact lens users, it is reasonable to be out of contact lenses for at least 4 weeks or for 1 month for every decade of contact lens use.

Soft contact lenses were thought to cause less corneal warpage, and thus an extended contact lens holiday is not necessary as compared with RGPs. However, multiple studies have shown that a longer period may be necessary before obtaining preoperative measurements for cataract surgery for some types of soft contact lenses. A contact lens–free period is recommended for at least 2 weeks but can be up to at least 5 weeks for soft toric contact lenses and 11 weeks for soft extended-wear contact lenses [16,20–23]. Ultimately, stabilization of the corneal maps and refraction out of contact lenses must exist to ensure accurate IOL calculations for cataract surgery.

FUCHS ENDOTHELIAL CORNEAL DYSTROPHY

FECD is an inherited corneal dystrophy that affects corneal endothelial cells. This condition can contribute to glare symptoms and may result in corneal edema, particularly after cataract surgery. Therefore, certain considerations need to be taken when performing cataract surgery on these patients (Fig. 6).

When evaluating patients with FECD and concomitant cataracts, the first decision to be made is performing the cataract extraction alone versus in combination with a partial-thickness corneal endothelial transplant (EK), commonly referred to as a triple procedure. This depends on overall endothelial cell health, density of the cataract, and patient expectations of visual outcomes after surgery. This decision is based on clinical examination findings including severity of corneal guttae, thickening, and preexisting edema and preoperative testing to include pachymetry and endothelial cell count (ECC), which serves

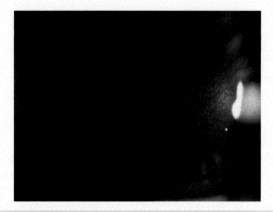

Fig. 6. Slit lamp photograph of corneal guttae in Fuchs endothelial corneal dystrophy.

as surrogate markers for endothelial health. If the clinical examination shows mild to moderate FECD, pachymetry is less than 640 μm, and ECC is more than 1000 cells/mm^2, the likelihood of corneal decompensation after cataract surgery is lower and performing cataract surgery alone is prudent. However, if the clinical examination shows more advanced FECD, pachymetry is greater than 640 μm, and ECC is less than 1000 cells/mm^2, then consideration for combined cataract surgery and EK is warranted [24,25].

The choice of EK in patients with FECD depends on the preexisting additional ocular pathology, vitreous status, and surgeon preference. In patients with no retinal pathology, no prior retinal surgery, and healthy eyes in the setting of FECD, Descemet membrane endothelial keratoplasty (DMEK) is the procedure of choice, giving the best visual outcomes when compared with Descemet stripping endothelial keratoplasty (DSEK). In patients who have a history of incisional glaucoma filtering surgery, retinal surgery, prior vitrectomy, or a unicameral eye, DSEK may be the preferred procedure because of the relative ease of unfolding the graft and achieving attachment. DMEK may be attempted in these patients; however, because of the lack of posterior pressure, crowded or deeper anterior chamber, combined with more difficult fluid dynamics, air/gas bubble management becomes more difficult and unscrolling and positioning of the graft more challenging [26].

Whether planning on cataract surgery alone or in combination with EK, the target refraction for these patients needs to account for the expected hyperopic shift following corneal transplantation. A higher magnitude for hyperopia is expected post-DSEK when compared with DMEK because of the greater amount of tissue addition. Therefore, it is usually recommended to target −1.00 to −1.25 D for DSEK and −0.75 to −1.00 D for DMEK to counteract the expected hyperopic shift [27,28].

Typically, a monofocal lens is recommended for patients with FECD. Multifocal lenses are a relative contraindication in this population because of the risk of decreased contrast sensitivity and visual quality. If patients desire spectacle independence, a thorough preoperative discussion should take place to ensure patient expectations are defined [29].

When performing cataract surgery on these patients, surgeons should take special measures to ensure the best visual outcomes. The first consideration is the creation of a deliberately smaller capsulorrhexis to ensure IOL stability and to avoid unwanted dislocation and decentration of the IOL, especially when performing a triple procedure [30]. Another consideration is using copious dispersive viscoelastic in nontriple cases to protect the cornea endothelium throughout the procedure. One also can use the soft-shell technique, which uses dispersive and cohesive viscoelastic devices to maximize the advantages of both [31].

Most recently, Descemet stripping only has been attempted for patients with milder FECD with symptomatic central guttae. This procedure involves the creation of a 4-mm descemetorhexis without placement of a corneal graft. The belief is that existing healthy peripheral endothelial cells migrate into the central defective area. Strict patient selection is required for this procedure including the primary diagnosis of FECD, central corneal edema, clear peripheral cornea, and peripheral ECC greater than 1000 cells/mm^2. This procedure is done alone or in combination with cataract surgery [32]. Visual recovery is slow and delayed for up to several months after this procedure so careful patient selection and preoperative counseling is needed. Further research is being conducted to better define inclusion and exclusion criteria and factors that contribute to improved and faster visual outcomes.

PENETRATING KERATOPLASTY

Cataract surgery in an eye that has a full-thickness corneal transplant, also known as PKP, requires careful preoperative planning. Some special considerations in these eyes include proper incision placement to not disrupt the graft-host junction, minimizing endothelial cell loss, and accurate preoperative keratometry readings to ensure good refractive outcomes. If there is not enough space between the limbus and graft to place a clear corneal incision for cataract surgery, a more posterior scleral tunnel approach is considered. The same techniques used to minimize endothelial cell loss during cataract surgery, including use of a dispersive viscoelastic and a soft-shell technique for patients with FECD, also are recommended for patients with PKP. Extracapsular cataract surgery technique has shown to cause less endothelial cell damage than phacoemulsification and is considered in certain cases based on overall graft health, ECC, age of graft, density of cataract, and surgeon preference (Fig. 7) [33].

Waiting at least 1 year after PKP surgery to perform preoperative measurements for cataract surgery is ideal. By this time, most or all planned corneal sutures have already been removed and the cornea has had time to take its natural shape. This helps to negate any suture-induced astigmatism, which could lead to increased variability in IOL power prediction [34]. Using an astigmatism-correcting IOL is considered in these patients that have regular

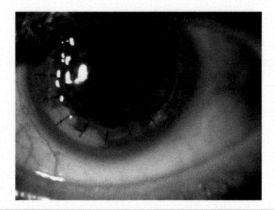

Fig. 7. Slit lamp photograph of penetrating keratoplasty in a patient with paraproteinemic keratopathy from multiple myeloma.

corneal astigmatism, stable K readings, and do not wear contact lenses for best vision [35]. However, in patients who are comfortable wearing contact lenses and plan to continue wearing them postoperatively, a standard monofocal IOL is recommended and a near aim is considered.

In cases where simultaneous cataract surgery and PKP, commonly referred to as the PKP-triple procedure, are performed, additional considerations on what K values are used to calculate the IOL power is needed. At present, there is no good consensus on what K values, IOL formula, or aims to best predict IOL power in these cases [36]. In general, an average keratometry value of between 42.5 and 45 D with a near aim of −1.00 to −2.00 D is used and a larger range of refractive outcomes ± 2 D is expected [36–38]. Sequential cataract surgery after PKP surgery would give a more accurate K reading to better estimate IOL power. However, staged surgery is not without additional risk, because complications can include graft rejection, recurrence of herpetic disease, or late graft failure [39].

When performing simultaneous cataract surgery in these patients, if the surgical view is adequate, phacoemulsification is preferred over open sky cataract extraction to minimize complications from prolonged open sky time. Intravenous mannitol is given to decrease posterior pressure. Core vitrectomy also has been described to relieve posterior pressure [38,40]. Flieringa ring is used for better scleral rigidity and stability. Care is taken to make the capsulorrhexis small enough to cover the IOL optic but large enough to remove the nucleus. Typically, either a one-piece IOL or a three-piece IOL is placed in the capsule or, alternatively, the three-piece IOL is placed in the sulcus space.

RADIAL KERATOTOMY

RK is a refractive procedure that has historically been used to correct myopia with the goal of spectacle independence. RK has largely been supplanted by more advanced techniques, such as laser-assisted in situ keratomileusis, photo-refractive keratectomy, and small incision lenticule extraction, particularly after subsequent studies demonstrated a significant hyperopic shift 2 to 10 years postoperatively after RK [41]. Patients with prior RK undergoing cataract surgery pose certain challenges in the preoperative, surgical, and postoperative periods (Fig. 8).

Patients with RK may demonstrate diurnal fluctuation in vision, which translates to refractive variability and instability [42]. Furthermore, corneal imaging may show similar variations, making IOL selection difficult to estimate. Additionally, standard topography or tomography overestimates central corneal power, which may lead to a hyperopic surprise. Therefore, certain methods are used to estimate effective central corneal power and ELP, to better achieve desired refractive outcomes following cataract surgery. For IOL calculations, several methods are used, typically aiming for -0.50 to -0.75 D in anticipation of a potential hyperopic surprise. The double K formulas use various algorithms (SRK/T, Holladay, or Hoffer Q) to determine ELP by using pre-RK K values and axial length, but also accounts for central corneal power by using post-RK K values. Alternatively, when pre-RK K values and refractions are available, the historical method is used to estimate IOL power. The online American Society of Cataract and Refractive Surgery prior RK IOL calculator, which collects data from more advanced topography or tomography to better estimate the central corneal power, is readily accessible for surgeons to compare various IOL formulas [43].

Recently, several developments in IOL technology have surfaced that may be considered in these patients. Typically, a monofocal lens is recommended for these patients because of the prevalence of irregular astigmatism and highly aberrated corneas. The recently introduced light adjustable lens may be a good option for these patients, because it allows for adjustability of IOL power after implantation [44]. Because this IOL corrects lower-order aberration (ie, sphere and cylinder), it is important to ensure preoperative vision improves with manifest refraction. Adjustments to the IOL power requires demonstration of refractive stability in the postoperative period, which may take 2 to 3 months.

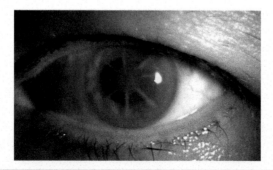

Fig. 8. Slit lamp photograph of an eight-cut radial keratotomy and corneal edema.

Therefore, it is important to manage patient expectations and emphasize the need for prolonged use of UV protective lenses while awaiting adjustment and lock-ins. An additional lens to consider in these patients is the IC-8 Apthera IOL, which uses small aperture technology to provide clear vision across a full range. This lens is set to be available on the market in the coming year [45].

Intraoperative considerations depend on the number of RK cuts in the cornea, because this determines the initial technique for wound creation. For corneas with four to eight cuts, a clear corneal wound is achieved in between cuts as long as care is taken not to bisect any of the cuts to avoid dehiscence and postoperative irregular astigmatism. For corneas with more than eight cuts, a scleral tunnel is the preferred technique, which avoids any complication of intraoperative wound dehiscence and anterior chamber instability [46]. Regardless of whether a clear corneal wound or scleral tunnel is used, most surgeons suture the main incision at the end of the case as a precautionary measure. Additionally, some surgeons use low-flow settings, or lower the bottle height to improve chamber dynamics.

Postoperatively, the main concern for these patients is refractive instability. These patients often have prolonged corneal edema and/or a hyperopic shift that may take 2 to 3 months to resolve before achieving refractive stability [47]. Discussion of postoperative expectations with the patient with RK are paramount before surgery.

SUMMARY

As cataract surgery equipment, techniques, and implant technology continue to advance, visual expectations after cataract surgery also have become more demanding. Many corneal pathologies exist that need to be taken into careful considerations in terms of preoperative, operative, and postoperative care when planning for cataract surgery to ensure the best visual outcomes.

EBMD can not only contribute to glare symptoms but also can cause irregular astigmatism. SK is recommended in patients with diffuse and central EBMD changes to help regulate central corneal astigmatism before cataract surgery. It is advisable to wait at least 1 month after SK before obtaining IOL measurements before proceeding with cataract surgery.

Large pterygium can affect vision by inducing corneal astigmatism or obscuring the visual axis. Sequential pterygium excision followed by cataract surgery is recommended to improve vision and minimize corneal astigmatism for best refractive outcomes. IOL measurements are taken 1 month after pterygium excision. If simultaneous pterygium excision and cataract surgery is performed, decrease the IOL power by 0.5 D to avoid a myopic surprise.

In eyes that have KCN, corneal stability is crucial before proceeding with cataract surgery. Many patients with KCN wear contact lenses for best vision, and it is important to determine contact lens status after cataract surgery. If the patient is to continue contact lens wear after cataract surgery, use a monofocal IOL and consider a near aim. If the patient does not plan on wearing contact lenses after cataract surgery and has stable astigmatism, an astigmatism-correcting IOL is considered. Using a KCN-specific IOL formula that accounts for posterior corneal curvature and total keratometry with an aim of −0.50 to −0.75 D can help prevent a hyperopic surprise.

Contact lens wear causes corneal warpage and can affect keratometric readings. Significant variability occurs in the time it takes for the cornea to recover and show refractive stability. A contact lens–free period of at least 2 weeks for soft contact lens use and at least 4 weeks for soft toric contact lens or hard contact lens is recommended before obtaining IOL measurements. A longer contact lens–free period may be needed for those with extended use.

It is important to determine overall endothelial cell health in patients with concurrent FECD and visually significant cataracts. Cataract surgery is performed safely with a lower risk of corneal decompensation in eyes that have mild to moderate FECD, pachymetry less than 640 μm, and ECC greater than 1000 cells/mm^2. Combined cataract and endothelial keratoplasty should be considered in eyes with more advanced FECD, pachymetry more than 640 μm, and ECC less than 1000 cells/mm^2. In these combined triple cases, target IOL calculations for −1.00 to −1.25 D for DSEK and −0.75 to −1.00 D for DMEK is used to counteract the expected hyperopic shift.

In eyes with prior PKP, IOL measurements are taken a year after surgery as long as all planned suture removal has been completed. In cases where simultaneous PKP and cataract surgery is performed, a larger refractive error is expected. As a general guideline, an average keratometry value of between 42.5 and 45 D with a near aim of −1.00 to −2.00 D is used to calculate IOL power.

RK often causes refractive variability and instability. Newer IOL formulas take into account central corneal power and ELP to counteract a hyperopic surprise.

In all cases of corneal pathology in patients undergoing cataract surgery, it is important to have stable and repeatable corneal and keratometric readings for best IOL power accuracy. Careful preoperative planning, surgical preparation, and counseling on postoperative expectations are crucial to ensure best visual outcomes and to establish realistic expectations.

CLINICS CARE POINTS

- Wait at least 1 month after corneal procedures, such as SK or pterygium excision, before obtaining IOL calculations to allow keratometry readings to stabilize.
- Avoid astigmatism-correcting IOLs and consider aiming for near vision in patients with KCN that plan to use contact lens postoperatively.
- Wound placement and construction for cataract surgery requires more careful planning in patients with KCN, PK, and RK.

• Extra care needs to be taken to protect the corneal endothelium during cataract surgery in patients with FECD or PK.

DISCLOSURE

The authors have nothing to disclose.

References

[1] Stephenson M. When and how to treat EBMD. Review of Ophthalmology. 2019. Available at: https://www.reviewofophthalmology.com/article/when-and-how-to-treat-ebmd.

[2] Yeu E, Hashem O, Sheha H. Treatment of epithelial basement membrane dystrophy to optimize the ocular surface prior to cataract surgery. Clin Ophthalmol 2022;16:785-95.

[3] He X, Huang AS, Jeng BH. Optimizing the ocular surface prior to cataract surgery. Curr Opin Ophthalmol 2022 Jan 1;33(1):9-14.

[4] Koc M, Uzel MM, Aydemir E, et al. Pterygium size and effect on intraocular lens power calculation. J Cataract Refract Surg 2016 Nov;42(11):1620-5.

[5] Joshi RS, Pendke SS, Marewar S. Comparison of intraocular lens power calculation in simultaneous and sequential pterygium and cataract surgery. Rom J Ophthalmol 2021 Apr-Jun;65(2):157-62.

[6] Kim SW, Park S, Im CY, et al. Prediction of mean corneal power change after pterygium excision. Cornea 2014 Feb;33(2):148-53.

[7] Yildiz EH, Diehl GF, Cohen EJ, et al. Demographics of patients older than 50 years with keratoconus. Eye Contact Lens 2009 Nov;35(6):309-11.

[8] Watson MP, Anand S, Bhogal M, et al. Cataract surgery outcome in eyes with keratoconus. Br J Ophthalmol 2014 Mar;98(3):361-4.

[9] Ton Y, Barrett GD, Kleinmann G, et al. Toric intraocular lens power calculation in cataract patients with keratoconus. J Cataract Refract Surg 2021 Nov 1;47(11):1389-97.

[10] Riaz Kamran. Current Practice Patterns for IOL Calculations in Patients with Corneal Disease [Video]. Eversight. 2022. Available at: https://www.youtube.com/watch?v=cTOLhhVOBxM.

[11] Ghiasian L, Abolfathzadeh N, Manafi N, et al. Intraocular lens power calculation in keratoconus: a review of literature. J Curr Ophthalmol 2019 Mar 15;31(2):127-34.

[12] Hartstein J. Corneal warping due to wearing of corneal contact lenses. A report of 12 cases. Am J Ophthalmol 1965;60(6):1103-4.

[13] Levenson DS. Changes in corneal curvature with long-term PMMA contact lens wear. Eye Contact Lens 1983;9(2):121-5.

[14] Asbell PA, Wasserman D. Contact lens–induced corneal warpage. Int Ophthalmol Clin 1991;31(2):121-6.

[15] Wilson SE, Lin DT, Klyce SD, et al. Topographic changes in contact lens-induced corneal warpage. Ophthalmology 1990;97(6):734-44.

[16] Wang X, McCulley JP, Bowman RW, et al. Time to resolution of contact lens-induced corneal warpage prior to refractive surgery. Eye Contact Lens 2002;28(4):169-71.

[17] Tsai PS, Dowidar A, Naseri A, et al. Predicting time to refractive stability after discontinuation of rigid contact lens wear before refractive surgery. J Cataract Refract Surg 2004;30(11):2290-4.

[18] Budak K, Hamed AM, Friedman NJ, et al. Preoperative screening of contact lens wearers before refractive surgery. J Cataract Refract Surg 1999;25(8):1080-6.

[19] Pannu JS, Mutyala S, Pannu D. When to perform LASIK in contact lens wearers. J Cataract Refract Surg 2000;26(3):311-2.

[20] Hashemi H, Firoozabadi MR, Mehravaran S, et al. Corneal stability after discontinued soft contact lens wear. Contact Lens Anterior Eye 2008;31(3):122-5.

[21] Lloyd McKernan A, O'Dwyer V, Simo Mannion L. The influence of soft contact lens wear and two weeks cessation of lens wear on corneal curvature. Contact Lens Anterior Eye 2014;37(1):31–7.

[22] Rayess Y, Arej N, Abdel Massih Y, et al. Influence of soft contact lens material on corneal warpage: prevalence and time to resolution. Can J Ophthalmol 2018;53(2):135–8.

[23] Ng LT, Lee EM, Nguyen AL. Preoperative assessment of corneal and refractive stability in soft contact lens wearing photorefractive candidates. Optom Vis Sci 2007;84(5):401–9.

[24] Seitzman GD, Gottsch JD, Stark WJ. Cataract surgery in patients with Fuchs' corneal dystrophy: expanding recommendations for cataract surgery without simultaneous keratoplasty. Ophthalmology 2005;112(3):441–6.

[25] Kaup S, Pandey SK. Cataract surgery in patients with Fuchs' endothelial corneal dystrophy. Community Eye Health 2019;31(104):86–7.

[26] Price MO, Feng, Matthew MT, et al. Endothelial keratoplasty update 2020. Cornea 2021 Nay 1;40(5):541–7.

[27] Terry MA, Shamie N, Chen ES, et al. Endothelial keratoplasty for Fuchs' dystrophy with cataract: complications and clinical results with the new triple procedure. Ophthalmology 2009;116(4):631–9.

[28] Wacker K, Cavalcante LCB, Baratz KH, et al. Hyperopic trend after cataract surgery in eyes with Fuchs' endothelial corneal dystrophy. Ophthalmology 2018;125(8):1302–4.

[29] Braga-Mele R, Chang D, Dewey S, et al. Multifocal intraocular lenses: relative indications and contraindications for implantation. J Cataract Refract Surg 2014;40(2):313–22.

[30] Ahmad A, Daroszewski D, Cheung N. Cataract surgery in the setting of Fuchs dystrophy. American Academy of Ophthalmology, EyeWiki. 2020. Available at: https://eyewiki.aao.org/Cataract_Surgery_in_the_Setting_of_Fuchs_Dystrophy.

[31] Arshinoff Steve AMD. FRCSC. Dispersive-cohesive viscoelastic soft shell technique. J Cataract Refract Surg 1999;25(2):167–73.

[32] Fernandes DH, Luis ME, Figueiredo R. Descemetorhexis without endothelial keratoplasty. American Academy of Ophthalmology, EyeWiki. 2018. Available at: https://eyewiki.org/Descemetorhexis_Without_Endothelial_Keratoplasty.

[33] Acar BT, Buttanri IB, Sevim MS, et al. Corneal endothelial cell loss in post-penetrating keratoplasty patients after cataract surgery: phacoemulsification versus planned extracapsular cataract extraction. J Cataract Refract Surg 2011 Aug;37(8):1512–6.

[34] Dietrich T, Viestenz A, Langenbucher A, et al. Accuracy of IOL power prediction in cataract surgery after penetrating keratoplasty: retrospective study of 72 eyes. Klin Monbl Augenheilkd 2011 Aug;228(8):698–703.

[35] Srinivasan S, Ting DS, Lyall DA. Implantation of a customized toric intraocular lens for correction of post-keratoplasty astigmatism. Eye 2013 Apr;27(4):531–7.

[36] Flower CW, McLeod SD, McDonnell PJ, et al. Evaluation of intraocular lens power calculation formulas in the triple procedure. J Cataract Refract Surg 1996 Jan-Feb;22(1):116–22.

[37] Gruenauer-Kloevekorn C, Kloevekorn-Norgall K, Duncker GI, et al. Refractive error after triple and non-simultaneous procedures: is the application of a standard constant keratometry value in IOL power calculation advisable? Acta Ophthalmol Scand 2006 Oct;84(5):679–83.

[38] Inoue Y. Corneal Triple Procedure Senin Ophthalmol 2001 Sep;16(3):113–8.

[39] Hsiao CH, Chen JJ, Chen PY, et al. Intraocular lens implantation after penetrating keratoplasty. Cornea 2001 Aug;20(6):580–5.

[40] Oie Y, Nishida K. Triple Procedure: cataract extraction, intraocular lens implantation, and corneal graft. Curr Opin Ophthalmol 2017. Jan;28(1):63–6.

[41] Waring GO, Lynn MJ, McDonnell PJ. Results of the prospective evaluation of radial keratotomy (PERK) study 10 years after surgery. Arch Ophthalmol 1994 Oct;112(10):1298–308.

[42] Rashid ER, Waring GO. Complications of radial and transverse keratotomy. Surv Ophthalmol 1989;34:73–106.

[43] Turnbull A.M.J., Crawford G.J., Barrett G.D., Methods for intraocular lens power calculation in cataract surgery after radial keratotomy, *Ophthalmology*, **127** (1), 2020, 45–51.
[44] Moshirfar M, Duong AA, Shmunes KM, et al. Light adjustable intraocular lens for cataract surgery after radial keratotomy. J Refract Surg 2020;36(12):852–4.
[45] Franco F, Branchetti M, Vicchio L, et al. Implantation of a small aperture intraocular lens in eyes with irregular corneas and higher order aberrations. J Ophthalmic Vis Res 2022 Aug 15;17(3):317–23.
[46] Meduri A, Urso M, Signorino GA, et al. Cataract surgery on post radial keratotomy patients. Int J Ophthalmol 2017 Jul 18;10(7):1168–70.
[47] Stephenson M. Refractive surprises after cataract surgery. Review of Ophthalmology. 2014. Available at: https://www.reviewofophthalmology.com/article/refractive-surprises-after-cataract-surgery.

Advances in Ophthalmology and Optometry 8 (2023) 139–153

ADVANCES IN OPHTHALMOLOGY AND OPTOMETRY

Dropless Cataract Surgery

Anvesh Annadanam, MD, Angela J. Verkade, MD*

Department of Ophthalmology, Kellogg Eye Center, University of Michigan, 1000 Wall Street, Ann Arbor, MI 48105, USA

Keywords

- Postoperative cystoid macular edema • Irvine-gass syndrome
- Intracanalicular steroids • Subconjunctival steroids • Transzonular
- Intracameral steroids

Key points

- Cystoid macular edema (CME), although relatively rare, is an unwanted consequence after cataract surgery. Traditional methods of using postoperative drops as prophylaxis have been more recently replaced by dropless methods to reduce the risk of patient non-compliance.
- Intracanalicular, subconjunctival, and intraocular routes are being utilized to reduce postoperative drop burden. However, few studies exist comparing these dropless methods for CME prophylaxis.
- New devices are rapidly being tested to improve sustained drug delivery for inflammation control.

 Video content accompanies this article at http://www. advancesinophthalmology.com.

INTRODUCTION

Cataract surgery is one of the most commonly performed surgeries in the United States and other developed countries [1]. Similar to many other intraocular surgeries, cataract extraction induces a significant postoperative inflammatory response, primarily concentrated in the anterior segment, but also can have effects on the posterior segment. Cystoid macular edema (CME) is the most common cause of postoperative decreased visual acuity (VA), and usually

*Corresponding author. Department of Ophthalmology and Visual Sciences, University of Michigan, 1000 Wall Street, Ann Arbor, MI 48105. E-mail address: ajverkad@med.umich.edu

https://doi.org/10.1016/j.yaoo.2023.02.008
2452-1760/23/© 2023 Elsevier Inc. All rights reserved.

takes 4 to 8 weeks to develop [2,3]. It may resolve spontaneously, but it also can result in permanent vision loss if untreated. Though this relatively rare condition was initially described decades ago, its pathogenesis is not fully understood [4]. It is thought to be triggered by surgical trauma and disruption of the blood–aqueous barrier leading to diffusion of prostaglandins and other inflammatory mediators. This causes leakage from dilated retinal capillaries leading to intraretinal and subretinal extracellular fluid accumulation.

Prophylaxis of postoperative inflammation and CME has historically been addressed with monotherapy or combination of topical corticosteroid and non-steroidal anti-inflammatory (NSAID) drops. Common corticosteroid drops in use are prednisolone acetate 1%, dexamethasone 0.1%, difluprednate 0.05%, and loteprednol etabonate 0.5%. They exhibit their effect after binding to glucocorticoid receptors causing an alteration in gene expression, resulting in the blockade of various inflammatory cascade mechanisms [5]. NSAIDs work by inhibiting the expression of cyclooxygenase enzymes, thus reducing the intraocular release of pro-inflammatory prostaglandins which cause vasodilation and disruption of the blood–ocular barrier [4]. Common NSAID drops include ketorolac tromethamine 0.5%, bromfenac 0.09%, nepafenac 0.1%, and diclofenac 0.1%, among others. The appropriate treatment regimen is widely debated. Differences in intraocular inflammation reduction between steroids and NSAIDs have not been significant [6–8], but trials have shown a synergistic effect when administered concurrently [9,10].

All of these prophylactic measures require strict patient compliance in drop usage for optimal effect. However, patients often are inconsistent in drop administration in terms of frequency, amount, and duration of treatment. One study described a nearly 40% self-reported non-adherence to the prescribed medication regimen [11], whereas another review reported patient deviation ranged from 5% to 80% [12]. Patients with glaucoma often are instructed to continue their preoperative anti-hypertensive drops, further increasing the drop burden. This unpredictable variability has encouraged the development and utilization of dropless techniques for prophylaxis of postoperative inflammation and CME [13]. This article describes the currently available techniques in dropless cataract surgery ranging from periocular to intraocular methods of administering medication. We also describe novel approaches that are under investigation.

INTRACANALICULAR STEROIDS

In 2018, the United States (US) Food and Drug Administration (FDA) approved a novel method to treat ocular pain following ophthalmic surgery. Dextenza (Ocular Therapeutix, Inc., Bedford, MA), is a sustained-release intracanalicular insert of preservative-free dexamethasone 0.4 mg that is applied directly after cataract surgery and releases the medication over a period of 30 days [14]. In 2019, the device also received approval for the treatment of ocular inflammation after surgery.

Dextenza is composed of dexamethasone conjugated in fluorescein and suspended in a polyethylene glycol (PEG) hydrogel. Measuring 0.5 mm in diameter and 3 mm in length [14], the device is inserted into the vertical canaliculus after the completion of cataract surgery and releases the drug onto the ocular surface as the PEG hydrogel degrades. Insertion instructions can be found on the manufacturer's website [15].

Previous animal studies in dogs have shown the efficacy of the sustained release of intracanalicular dexamethasone to day 28 after insertion [16]. No changes in intraocular pressure (IOP) or ocular or systemic toxicity were noted [17].

The safety of Dextenza was tested in a randomized controlled trial by Walters and colleagues in which patients were randomized to the sustained-release dexamethasone implant or a placebo vehicle inserted into the inferior canaliculus. More patients who received the dexamethasone implant had an absence of intraocular pain (79.3% vs 30%, $P < 0.01$) and an absence of anterior chamber cells (20.7% vs 10%, $P = 0.1495$) at 8 days compared with placebo [18]. A second phase 3 trial confirmed similar results [19].

Few studies exist comparing Dextenza to other methods of CME prophylaxis [20–22]. Larsen and colleagues [21] randomized 20 patients undergoing refractive lens exchange to one eye with the intracanalicular insert and the fellow eye with topical corticosteroid drops. At 4 to 8 weeks postoperatively, no differences occurred in pain, corneal staining, anterior chamber cell and flare, IOP, or VA between the two groups. Similar rates of postoperative breakthrough inflammation were found between the two groups in a different study [22].

Patient response to using intracanalicular dexamethasone has been positive, with the majority preferring it over topical drops in surveys [21,23,24]. Physicians who were surveyed regarding their use of Dextenza thought that using it would improve patient compliance and would prefer it over traditional postoperative drops [25]. They reported feeling comfortable using the device after placing it three times.

Contraindications to the use of Dextenza include an active corneal, conjunctival, or canalicular infection [14]. Side effects of the implant are similar to those of topical steroids, including increased IOP, rebound inflammation, and delayed wound healing. Canalicular obstruction with resulting epiphora has been reported [26].

SUBCONJUNCTIVAL STEROIDS

Subtenon and subconjunctival steroid depots are widely used to treat various ocular inflammatory syndromes [27,28]. Most commonly, betamethasone, dexamethasone, and triamcinolone have been used. When administered subconjunctivally, the drug usually is injected inferior to the limbus underneath the conjunctiva, thus bypassing the conjunctival barrier which limits the bioavailability of topically administered drugs (Video 1) [5]. The medication then directly diffuses through the sclera into the anterior and posterior segments.

In the early 1990s, Corbett and colleagues [29] described the postoperative use of a short-acting subconjunctival betamethasone 2 mg (Betnesol) depot as an adjunctive treatment to topical betamethasone with the goal of controlling the robust inflammatory response in the immediate postoperative period.

Those who received subconjunctival betamethasone, rather than placebo, had significantly less postoperative inflammation, which was more pronounced in patients with pre-existing ocular inflammatory conditions. Of note, the cataract surgery described in their study was either extracapsular extraction or large incision (7 mm) phacoemulsification–techniques that may be more pro-inflammatory than modern methods.

More recently, the goal of perioperative subconjunctival steroids was to obviate the need for topical steroids to decrease the risk of patient non-compliance. One study in the Netherlands divided 200 patients into two groups, with one group receiving postoperative subconjunctival betamethasone 1 mg and the other group receiving topical dexamethasone 0.1% drops three times per day for 4 weeks [1]. Both groups had a similar rate of macular edema on optical coherence tomography (OCT) (7.0% vs 6.0%). No differences occurred in postoperative IOP or VA. Of note, patients with glaucoma were excluded from the study.

Another study in India divided 400 patients into two groups, each receiving either postoperative subconjunctival triamcinolone acetonide 5 mg or topical loteprednol etabonate 0.5% tapered over 5 weeks [30]. Both groups received topical ketorolac tromethamine 0.5% and ofloxacin 0.3% tapered over 3 weeks. Both groups had similar IOP and anterior chamber inflammation scores at each visit over the postoperative follow-up period of 12 weeks. None of the patients in either group had CME. Patients with glaucoma or known steroid responders were excluded from the study.

Lindholm and colleagues [31] compared subconjunctival triamcinolone acetonide 20 mg versus topical dexamethasone and showed a relative postoperative decrease in central retinal thickness in the triamcinolone group than the dexamethasone group. Patients with glaucoma had comparable IOP rise between the two groups, and no steroid response was noted among any patients. In diabetic patients, the addition of subconjunctival triamcinolone acetonide 40 mg to a topical regimen of bromfenac 0.09% and dexamethasone 0.1% resulted in no CME [32].

Overall, a wide variation exists in the type and concentration of subconjunctival corticosteroid used postoperatively. Most studies have reported non-inferiority to conventional topical steroid or NSAID regimens. Benign side effects of subconjunctival hemorrhage and chemosis do exist with this route of administration. It also is possible that some of the medication may leak out of the needle tract through which it is injected, reducing the total amount of drug administered [5]. However, the feared effect of elevated IOP in glaucoma patients receiving subconjunctival steroid depots has not been thoroughly explored, as most studies exclude this population.

INTRACAMERAL MEDICATIONS
Corticosteroids
Steroids also have achieved success when injected intracamerally. Triamcinolone acetonide often is used in the anterior chamber to assist in the visualization

and removal of unwanted vitreous in complicated cases [33]. Given its anti-inflammatory effect, some surgeons routinely use 1 to 2 mg preservative-free triamcinolone alone without postoperative drops as a means to control postoperative inflammation [34,35]. Gungor and colleagues [35] compared the postoperative administration of intracameral triamcinolone 2 mg versus dexamethasone 0.4 mg and found similar control of inflammation, though the postoperative day (POD) 1 IOP was higher in the triamcinolone group. Glaucoma patients were excluded, and CME was not discussed. An earlier study by Chang and colleagues [36] showed that intracameral dexamethasone can safely be administered in glaucoma patients with little concern for IOP elevations postoperatively.

To better control and predict drug elution, anterior segment sustained-release devices have been developed. Dexamethasone can be embedded into a biodegradable polymer with varying ratios of polylactic acid and polyglycolic acid to control the rate of degradation [37].

The first sustained-release biodegradable steroid implant created was Surodex (Oculex Pharmaceuticals, Inc., Sunnyvale, CA). It is a rod-shaped implant that is placed either in the anterior chamber angle or ciliary sulcus, and achieves a sustained release of dexamethasone 60 μg over 7 to 10 days [38]. Previous studies have shown similar or lower levels of anterior chamber cell and flare for Surodex when compared with topical steroid therapy [39–42]. Although it has only completed phase II trials in the United States, Surodex commonly is used in Asia and other countries [43].

Another such implant, called Dexycu (Icon Bioscience, Inc., Sunnyvale, CA), is the first long-acting intracameral product approved by the FDA for the treatment of postoperative inflammation after cataract surgery [44]. In this system, dexamethasone 9% is injected as a 5 μL droplet into the anterior segment after surgery, allowing for 21 days of controlled steroid release. Donnenfeld and Holland found that two different concentrations of intracameral dexamethasone were superior to placebo in anterior chamber clearance of cell and flare on POD 8 [44]. The rate of IOP increase was similar between the three groups, but the treatment groups had a higher proportion of patients with an increase ≥10 mm Hg. Rates of CME were less than 3% in all groups. Another study compared Dexycu against topical prednisolone four times a day for 3 weeks and found similar rates of anterior chamber cell and flare clearing at all-time points [45]. A clinical trial is underway to compare Dexycu + topical antibiotics + NSAIDs against standard topical steroids, antibiotics, and NSAIDs [46]. This method is not truly dropless; however, the burden of topical steroids would be eliminated. In this trial, the medication was injected intracapsular at the optic-haptic junction. Iris atrophy has been reported as a potential complication of Dexycu administration [47]. A potential exists of the medication spherule migrating to the anterior chamber to cause focal corneal edema; therefore, various injection locations have been attempted including the ciliary sulcus and intracapsular optic–haptic junction [48].

Phenylephrine and ketorolac

In 2014, the FDA approved Omidria (Rayner Surgical, Inc., West Sussex, United Kingdom), a drug consisting of a combination of phenylephrine 1% and ketorolac 0.3%, for the prevention of intraoperative miosis and postoperative pain [49]. It is added to the irrigating solution to provide continuous intraoperative administration. The phenylephrine component maintains mydriasis and ketorolac works to continuously block the inflammatory cascade.

Visco and colleagues [49] compared the effect of Omidria versus postoperative topical loteprednol 0.5% on CME, iritis, pain, and photophobia after cataract surgery. All patients received topical bromfenac 0.07% postoperatively for 10 weeks. The Omidria group was found to have a lower rate of CME (0.52% vs 1.47%), breakthrough iritis, and pain. Of note, patients who were at higher risk of CME, such as those with retinal vein occlusion, vitreomacular traction, and epiretinal membrane were excluded from the study. Though the use of Omidria seems to eliminate the necessity of topical steroid drops, no studies have been conducted comparing the use of Omidria against no drops at all. The issues of patient compliance remain. In addition, there is a variable cost burden to the patient or ophthalmology practice for the utilization of this commercial drug.

TRANSZONULAR MEDICATIONS

In an effort to further simplify cataract surgery protocols, pharmacologic prophylaxis for endophthalmitis and inflammation have been combined into single compounded drug formulations. Rather than intracamerally, antibiotic or antibiotic-steroid combination medications may be injected transzonularly into the anterior vitreous at the end of cataract surgery (Fig. 1). It is thought

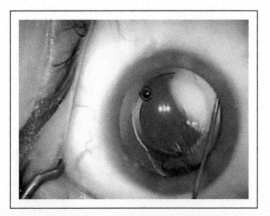

Fig. 1. Surgical view of a transzonular intravitreal injection of a compounded triamcinolone–moxifloxacin–vancomycin formulation. (*From* Tyson SL, Bailey R, Roman JS, Zhan T, Hark LA, Haller JA. Clinical outcomes after injection of a compounded pharmaceutical for prophylaxis after cataract surgery. *Curr Opin Ophthalmol.* 2017;28(1):73-80.)

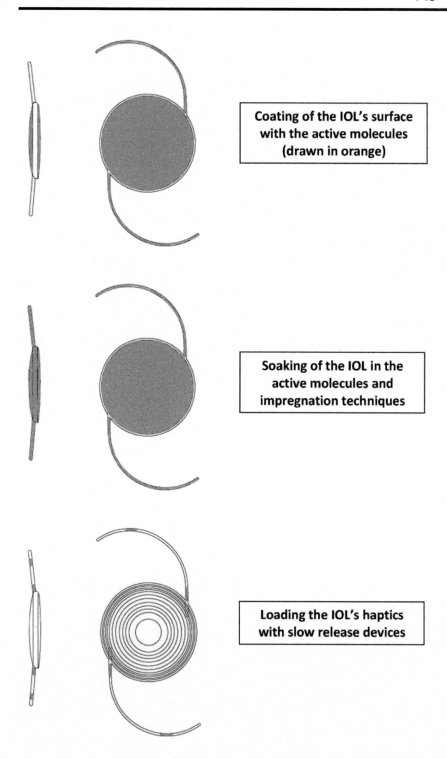

Coating of the IOL's surface with the active molecules (drawn in orange)

Soaking of the IOL in the active molecules and impregnation techniques

Loading the IOL's haptics with slow release devices

that medication is cleared less quickly in the vitreous than in the anterior chamber [50].

One medication, Tri-Moxi-Vanc (Imprimis Pharmaceuticals, Carlsbad, CA), consists of triamcinolone acetonide 3 mg, moxifloxacin 0.2 mg, and vancomycin 2 mg. It has been shown to have similar rates of rebound inflammation, IOP spikes, and CME when compared with topical regimens [50,51]. However, the risk of hemorrhagic occlusive retinal vasculitis (HORV) with intraocular vancomycin use has been well reported, resulting in a statement by the FDA against the usage of this medication [52,53]. Tri-Moxi-Vanc is no longer available on the Imprimis Pharmaceuticals website.

A formulation without vancomycin, called Tri-Moxi, also is available from the same company. Patients who received Tri-Moxi plus topical NSAIDs had lower levels of anterior chamber inflammation at day 1, week 1, and month 1 postoperatively when compared with patients receiving standard topical therapy for steroids plus NSAIDs [54]. In that study, Tri-Moxi was instilled through a pars-plana injection rather than through the anterior chamber. The difference in rates of CME and IOP increases was not statistically significant. In contrast, a smaller study found higher rates of breakthrough inflammation in the Tri-Moxi group when compared with the topical steroid group [55]. In this study, however, patients were not given NSAID drops in either group, suggesting that NSAID use may be a confounding variable. Interestingly, HORV recently has been reported with the use of Tri-Moxi in two patients [56].

The only commercially available combination medication formula containing an NSAID for postoperative use is Dex-Moxi-Ketor (Imprimis Pharmaceuticals, Carlsbad, CA), consisting of dexamethasone 0.1%, moxifloxacin 0.05%, and ketorolac 0.04%. Kuriakose and colleagues compared patients on topical steroids, Tri-Moxi, or Dex-Moxi-Ketor. All patients received topical NSAIDs postoperatively. Their study showed similar rates of anterior chamber inflammation, corneal edema, CME, and endophthalmitis between all groups. The Tri-Moxi group had higher IOP at postoperative month 1 compared with Dex-Moxi-Ketor (15.64 vs 14.16), which may not be clinically significant to patients without glaucoma.

OTHER APPROACHES
Drug-loaded intraocular lenses
Drug-coated intraocular lenses (IOL) were described more than 25 years ago as a method for sustained intraocular delivery of medications, however, no commercially available product utilizing this system exists. One of the first studies showed that rabbit eyes with indomethacin-coated IOLs had lower rates

Fig. 2. Methods for intraocular lens drug delivery. (*From* Mylona I, Tsinopoulos I. A Critical Appraisal of New Developments in Intraocular Lens Modifications and Drug Delivery Systems for the Prevention of Cataract Surgery Complications. *Pharmaceuticals (Basel)*. 2020;13(12):448. Published 2020 Dec 8.)

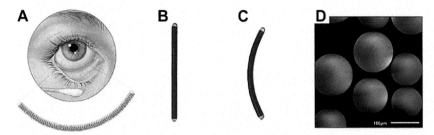

Fig. 3. (A) Location of the ocular coil in the inferior conjunctival fornix. (B) Photograph of a straight ocular coil and (C) a curved ocular coil. (D) Scanning electron microscopic photograph of the microsphere filling of the ocular coil (SEI, 1 kV, 220 × magnification). (*From* Bertens CJF, Dunker SL, Dias AJAA, van den Biggelaar FJHM, Nuijts RMMA, Gijs M. Safety and Comfort of an Innovative Drug Delivery Device in Healthy Subjects. *Transl Vis Sci Technol.* 2020;9(13):35. Published 2020 Dec 18.)

of posterior capsular opacification than eyes with control non-coated IOLs [57]. More recent research has discussed the efficacy of loading IOLs with antibiotics or steroids to help prevent endophthalmitis and control inflammation [58–61].

Several methods are used to modify IOLs as drug delivery systems: coating, soaking, or attaching slow-release drug reservoirs to the optic or haptic (Fig. 2) [61,62]. Prior methods for drug incorporation have been extensively reviewed elsewhere [61]. Several practical issues with the creation of IOL drug delivery systems include maintaining the optical clarity and foldability of the IOL. Essentially, the widely accepted physical and biomechanical properties of modern IOLs would need to remain undisturbed or improved before the adoption of drug-loaded IOLs into clinical practice. It is unclear what obstacles are preventing the translation of this research into patient care.

Novel devices

New approaches to dropless surgery continue to be created. One group has developed a stainless steel-coated ocular coil that can be filled with a drug-eluting matrix (Fig. 3). This coil could be inserted into the inferior conjunctival fornix for sustained release of medication. However, there may be issues regarding comfort, retention, and conjunctival injection [63]. Another group has studied ketorolac-loaded silica particles in vitro drug release assays and in vivo subconjunctival injections in guinea pig eyes, but research still is in its preliminary stages [64]. Finally, temperature-sensitive hydrogels loaded with dexamethasone and moxifloxacin are being investigated to provide sustained drug delivery when injected intracamerally [65]. It remains to be seen whether these preliminarily assessed devices can be commercialized and used in routine surgical practice.

SUMMARY

Cataract surgery has become a safe and well-tolerated procedure to establish ideal visual outcomes. Historically, unwanted postoperative side effects such as inflammation and CME, which could be visually debilitating, were treated with varying combinations of topical steroids and NSAIDs. These methods require strict patient compliance and may be financially burdensome. In this review, we discussed the available devices and methods in the burgeoning field of dropless cataract surgery.

The closer the route of administration is to the intraocular space, the higher the efficacy as well as side effects of the medication will be. It has been well-studied that the combination of NSAID and steroids is the optimal regimen for the treatment of CME. Dropless formulations of steroids are a good start but do not completely avoid drops in the cases of rebound inflammation in which adjunct topical steroids are needed, or if the addition of topical NSAIDs is necessary for the treatment of CME.

In addition, many of the studies discussed have compared the use of an injectable drug along with fewer topical drops versus the standard regimen of only topical drops. Therefore, they are not truly "dropless" cataract surgery. Future studies may be needed to assess the safety of medications or drug delivery devices without the use of additional drops. However, any reduction in drop burden is likely to be advantageous to the patient to improve compliance.

Many studies employing the use of periocular or intraocular medications excluded glaucoma patients given the fear of IOP spikes with the use of non-modifiable steroid doses once injected. It has been shown that formulations with steroids may potentially increase IOP at later time points when compared with formulations with steroids and NSAIDs or topical regimens, suggesting that they may be best avoided in patients with glaucoma or a history of steroid-induced IOP spikes. In cases of uncontrolled IOP, it may be possible to excise the subconjunctival steroid. However, methods such as Dextenza or intraocular steroids may need to be surgically removed or washed out, respectively, in case of any unwanted complications [26]. Patients with pre-existing diabetic retinopathy or epiretinal membrane are at higher risk of developing CME, but this population has also been minimally studied using dropless methods.

The risk of toxic anterior segment syndrome exists with any compounded formulation due to dilution errors [66]. Given the known low rate of endophthalmitis with the advent of intraocular antibiotics during surgery, many of the studies referenced in this article were not powered to detect statistically significant differences in endophthalmitis rates between the various regimens and products compared.

In addition to patient compliance, the high out-of-pocket cost and insurance coverage issues may discourage or prevent patients from obtaining the necessary topical therapy [13]. Although it is unclear the extent of cost savings for the overall health care system when utilizing dropless methods, the cost burden may shift to the clinician's practice to pay for the extra intraoperative devices and medications.

Overall, intracanalicular steroids, subconjunctival steroids, and transzonular formulations have each been compared against standard topical therapy with similar outcomes in terms of inflammation and CME. However, no studies compare each of the dropless methods. The decision to utilize a particular approach is based primarily on patient selection, clinician comfort, availability of method, and insurance reimbursement.

CLINICS CARE POINTS

- Consider dropless methods for inflammation prophylaxis in most cataract surgery patients, especially those with difficulty administering drops or high preexisting drop burden.
- Patients with severe glaucoma may experience postoperative IOP spikes after surgery if dropless steroid formulations are used. These patients may benefit from topical steroids, which can be titrated as needed.
- Protocols and training for compounded medications should be established by each practice before use to decrease the risk of medication dilution errors.

DISCLOSURE

The authors have nothing to disclose.

SUPPLEMENTARY DATA

Supplementary data related to this article can be found online at https://doi.org/10.1016/j.yaoo.2023.02.008.

References

[1] Dieleman M, Wubbels RJ, van Kooten-Noordzij M, et al. Single perioperative subconjunctival steroid depot versus postoperative steroid eyedrops to prevent intraocular inflammation and macular edema after cataract surgery. J Cataract Refract Surg 2011;37(9):1589–97.

[2] Gulkilik G, Kocabora S, Taskapili M, et al. Cystoid macular edema after phacoemulsification: risk factors and effect on visual acuity. Can J Ophthalmol 2006;41(6):699–703.

[3] Rotsos T. Cystoid macular edema. Clin Ophthalmol 2008;919; https://doi.org/10.2147/OPTH.S4033.

[4] Russo A, Costagliola C, Delcassi L, et al. Topical nonsteroidal anti-inflammatory drugs for macular edema. Mediators Inflamm 2013;2013:1–11.

[5] Gaballa SA, Kompella UB, Elgarhy O, et al. Corticosteroids in ophthalmology: drug delivery innovations, pharmacology, clinical applications, and future perspectives. Drug Deliv Transl Res 2021;11(3):866–93.

[6] Missotten L, Richard C, Trinquand C. Topical 0.1% indomethacin solution versus topical 0.1% dexamethasone solution in the prevention of inflammation after cataract surgery. Ophthalmologica 2001;215(1):43–50.

[7] Simone JN, Pendelton RA, Jenkins JE. Comparison of the efficacy and safety of ketorolac tromethamine 0.5% and prednisolone acetate 1% after cataract surgery. J Cataract Refract Surg 1999;25(5):699–704.

[8] Flach AJ, Kraff MC, Sanders DR, et al. The quantitative effect of 0.5% ketorolac tromethamine solution and 0.1% dexamethasone sodium phosphate solution on postsurgical blood-aqueous barrier. Arch Ophthalmol 1988;106(4):480–3.

[9] Erichsen JH, Holm LM, Forslund Jacobsen M, et al. Prednisolone and ketorolac vs ketorolac monotherapy or sub-tenon prophylaxis for macular thickening in cataract surgery. JAMA Ophthalmol 2021;139(10):1062.

[10] Heier JS, Topping TM, Baumann W, et al. Ketorolac versus prednisolone versus combination therapy in the treatment of acute pseudophakic cystoid macular edema. Ophthalmology 2000;107(11):2034–8.

[11] Vandenbroeck S, De Geest S, Dobbels F, et al. Prevalence and correlates of self-reported nonadherence with eye drop treatment. J Glaucoma 2011;20(7):414–21.

[12] Olthoff C, Schouten J, Vandeborne B, et al. Noncompliance with ocular hypotensive treatment in patients with glaucoma or ocular hypertensionan evidence-based review. Ophthalmology 2005;112(6):953–61.e7.

[13] Liegner J, Grzybowski A, Galloway M, et al. Dropless cataract surgery: an overview. Curr Pharm Des 2017;23(4):558–64; https://doi.org/10.2174/1381612822666161129 150628.

[14] Ocular Therapeutix. Dextenza (dexamethasone ophthalmic insert) [package insert]. U.S. Food and Drug Administration website. https://www.accessdata.fda.gov/drugsatfda_-docs/label/2019/208742s001lbl.pdf. Revised June 2019. Accessed November 2022.

[15] Handling of Dextenza. Ocular Therapeutix Inc. 2022. Available at: https://www.dextenza.com/insertion-and-storage/. Accessed November 13, 2022.

[16] Blizzard C, Desai A, Driscoll A. Pharmacokinetic studies of sustained-release depot of dexamethasone in beagle dogs. J Ocul Pharmacol Ther 2016;32(9):595–600.

[17] Driscoll A, Blizzard C. Toxicity and pharmacokinetics of sustained-release dexamethasone in beagle dogs. Adv Ther 2016;33(1):58–67.

[18] Walters T, Endl M, Elmer TR, et al. Sustained-release dexamethasone for the treatment of ocular inflammation and pain after cataract surgery. J Cataract Refract Surg 2015;41(10): 2049–59.

[19] Walters T, Bafna S. Efficacy and safety of sustained release dexamethasone for the treatment of ocular pain and inflammation after cataract surgery: results from two phase 3 studies. J Clin Exp Ophthalmol 2016;7(4); https://doi.org/10.4172/2155-9570.1000572.

[20] Jackson KJ, Akrobetu D, Guduru A, et al. Intracanalicular dexamethasone insert or topical prednisolone following istent and hydrus surgery for glaucoma. J Glaucoma 2022;31(8): 694–9.

[21] Larsen J, Whitt T, Parker B, et al. a randomized, controlled, prospective study of the effectiveness and safety of an intracanalicular dexamethasone ophthalmic insert (0.4 mg) for the treatment of post-operative inflammation in patients undergoing refractive lens exchange (RLE). Clin Ophthalmol 2021;15:2211–7.

[22] Lu AQ, Rizk M, O'Rourke T, et al. Safety and efficacy of topical versus intracanalicular corticosteroids for the prevention of postoperative inflammation after cataract surgery. J Cataract Refract Surg 2022; https://doi.org/10.1097/j.jcrs.0000000000000963.

[23] Gira J, Sampson R, Silverstein S, et al. Evaluating the patient experience after implantation of a 0.4 mg sustained release dexamethasone intracanalicular insert (Dextenza™): results of a qualitative survey. Patient Prefer Adherence 2017;11:487–94.

[24] Ibach MJ, Shafer BM, Wallin DD, et al. The effectiveness and safety of dextenza 0.4 mg for the treatment of postoperative inflammation and pain in patients after photorefractive keratectomy: the RESTORE trial. J Refract Surg 2021;37(9):590–4.

[25] Matossian C, Stephens JD, Rhee MK, et al. Early real-world physician experience with an intracanalicular dexamethasone insert. Clin Ophthalmol 2022;16:2429–40.

[26] Williams KJ, Blieden LS, Koch DD, et al. Intractable epiphora with the dexamethasone ophthalmic insert. J Cataract Refract Surg 2021; https://doi.org/10.1097/j.jcrs.00000 00000000665.

[27] HELM CJ, HOLLAND GN. The effects of posterior subtenon injection of triamcinolone acetonide in patients with intermediate uveitis. Am J Ophthalmol 1995;120(1):55–64.

[28] Zamir E, Read RW, Smith RE, et al. A prospective evaluation of subconjunctival injection of triamcinolone acetonide for resistant anterior scleritis. Ophthalmology 2002;109(4): 798–805.

[29] Corbett MC, Hingorani M, Boulton JE, et al. Subconjunctival betamethasone is of benefit after cataract surgery. Eye 1993;7(6):744–8.

[30] Reddy JK, Chaitanya V, Shah N, et al. Safety & efficacy of single subconjunctival triamcinolone 5 mg depot vs topical loteprednol post cataract surgery: less drop cataract surgery. Int J Ophthalmol 2019;12(5):774–8.

[31] Lindholm J, Taipale C, Ylinen P, et al. Perioperative subconjunctival triamcinolone acetonide injection for prevention of inflammation and macular oedema after cataract surgery. Acta Ophthalmol 2020;98(1):36–42.

[32] Wielders LHP, Schouten JSAG, Winkens B, et al. Randomized controlled European multicenter trial on the prevention of cystoid macular edema after cataract surgery in diabetics: ESCRS PREMED Study Report 2. J Cataract Refract Surg 2018;44(7):836–47.

[33] Yamakiri K, Uchino E, Kimura K, et al. Intracameral triamcinolone helps to visualize and remove the vitreous body in anterior chamber in cataract surgery. Am J Ophthalmol 2004;138(4):650–2.

[34] Karalezli A, Borazan M, Akova YA. Intracameral triamcinolone acetonide to control postoperative inflammation following cataract surgery with phacoemulsification. Acta Ophthalmol 2008;86(2):183–7.

[35] Gungor S, Bulam B, Akman A, et al. Comparison of intracameral dexamethasone and intracameral triamcinolone acetonide injection at the end of phacoemulsification surgery. Indian J Ophthalmol 2014;62(8):861.

[36] Chang DTW, Herceg MC, Bilonick RA, et al. Intracameral dexamethasone reduces inflammation on the first postoperative day after cataract surgery in eyes with and without glaucoma. Clin Ophthalmol 2009;345; https://doi.org/10.2147/OPTH.S5730.

[37] Shah TJ, Conway MD, Peyman GA. Intracameral dexamethasone injection in the treatment of cataract surgery induced inflammation: design, development, and place in therapy. Clin Ophthalmol 2018;12:2223–35.

[38] Lee SS, Hughes P, Ross AD, et al. Biodegradable implants for sustained drug release in the eye. Pharm Res (N Y) 2010;27(10):2043–53.

[39] Tan D. Randomized clinical trial of surodex steroid drug delivery system for cataract surgery anterior versus posterior placement of two surodex in the eye. Ophthalmology 2001;108(12):2172–81.

[40] Chang DF, Garcia IH, Hunkeler JD, et al. Phase II results of an intraocular steroid delivery system for cataract surgery. Ophthalmology 1999;106(6):1172–7.

[41] Tan DT, Chee S-P, Lim L, et al. Randomized clinical trial of a new dexamethasone delivery system (surodex) for treatment of post-cataract surgery inflammation11The authors have no financial interest in this or competing products or in Surodex or Oculex Pharmaceuticals, Inc. Ophthalmology 1999;106(2):223–31.

[42] Wadood AC, Armbrecht AM, Aspinall PA, et al. Safety and efficacy of a dexamethasone anterior segment drug delivery system in patients after phacoemulsification. J Cataract Refract Surg 2004;30(4):761–8.

[43] Wang J, Jiang A, Joshi M, et al. Drug delivery implants in the treatment of vitreous inflammation. Mediators Inflamm 2013;2013:1–8.

[44] Donnenfeld E, Holland E. Dexamethasone intracameral drug-delivery suspension for inflammation associated with cataract surgery. Ophthalmology 2018;125(6):799–806.

[45] Donnenfeld E. Study to Evaluate the Safety for the Treatment of Inflammation Associated With Cataract Surgery. Clinicaltrials.gov. 2018. Available at: https://clinicaltrials.gov/ct2/show/study/NCT02547623. Accessed October 23, 2022.

[46] Weinstock RJ. A Prospective study of the efficacy of intracameral dexamethasone (dexycu™) compared to standard of care treatment for post-cataract surgical pain and anterior

chamber inflammation. Clinicaltrials.gov. 2021. Available at: https://clinicaltrials.gov/ct2/show/NCT04781335. Accessed October 16, 2022.

[47] Bergman Z, Thompson R, Malouf A, et al. Iris atrophy after administration of intracameral dexycu in routine cataract surgery: a case series. Eye Contact Lens Sci Clin Pract 2022;48(4):185–7.

[48] McCabe C, Desai P, Nijm L, et al. Real-world experience with intracapsular administration of dexamethasone intraocular suspension 9% for control of postoperative inflammation. Clin Ophthalmol 2022;16:1985–92.

[49] Visco DM, Bedi R. Effect of intracameral phenylephrine 1.0%–ketorolac 0.3% on postoperative cystoid macular edema, iritis, pain, and photophobia after cataract surgery. J Cataract Refract Surg 2020;46(6):867–72.

[50] Potvin R, Fisher B. Transzonular vitreous injection vs a single drop compounded topical pharmaceutical regimen after cataract surgery. Clin Ophthalmol 2016;10:1297–303.

[51] Tyson SL, Bailey R, Roman JS, et al. Clinical outcomes after injection of a compounded pharmaceutical for prophylaxis after cataract surgery. Curr Opin Ophthalmol 2017;28(1):73–80.

[52] Witkin AJ, Chang DF, Jumper JM, et al. Vancomycin-associated hemorrhagic occlusive retinal vasculitis. Ophthalmology 2017;124(5):583–95.

[53] A case of hemorrhagic occlusive retinal vasculitis (HORV) following intraocular injections of a compounded triamcinolone, moxifloxacin, and vancomycin formulation. U.S. Food & Drug Administration. 2017. Available at: https://www.fda.gov/drugs/human-drug-compounding/case-hemorrhagic-occlusive-retinal-vasculitis-horv-following-intraocular-injections-compounded. Accessed October 23, 2022.

[54] Nassiri S, Hwang FS, Kim J, et al. Comparative analysis of intravitreal triamcinolone acetonide–moxifloxacin versus standard perioperative eyedrops in cataract surgery. J Cataract Refract Surg 2019;45(6):760–5.

[55] Singhal R, Luo A, O'Rourke T, et al. Transzonular triamcinolone–moxifloxacin versus topical drops for the prophylaxis of postoperative inflammation after cataract surgery. J Ocul Pharmacol Ther 2019;35(10):565–70.

[56] Pan WW, Miller AR, Young BK, et al. Hemorrhagic occlusive retinal vasculitis associated with triamcinolone-moxifloxacin use during uncomplicated cataract surgery. JAMA Ophthalmol 2022; https://doi.org/10.1001/jamaophthalmol.2022.4697.

[57] Nishi O, Nishi K, Yamada Y, et al. Effect of indomethacin-coated posterior chamber intraocular lenses on postoperative inflammation and posterior capsule opacification. J Cataract Refract Surg 1995;21(5):574–8.

[58] Liu Y-C, Wong TT, Mehta JS. Intraocular lens as a drug delivery reservoir. Curr Opin Ophthalmol 2013;24(1):53–9.

[59] Tsuchiya Y, Kobayakawa S, Tsuji A, et al. Preventive effect against post-cataract endophthalmitis: drug delivery intraocular lens versus intracameral antibiotics. Curr Eye Res 2008;33(10):868–75.

[60] Kleinmann G, Apple DJ, Chew J, et al. Hydrophilic acrylic intraocular lens as a drug-delivery system for fourth-generation fluoroquinolones. J Cataract Refract Surg 2006;32(10):1717–21.

[61] Mylona I, Tsinopoulos I. A critical appraisal of new developments in intraocular lens modifications and drug delivery systems for the prevention of cataract surgery complications. Pharmaceuticals 2020;13(12):448.

[62] Filipe HP, Bozukova D, Pimenta A, et al. Moxifloxacin-loaded acrylic intraocular lenses: in vitro and in vivo performance. J Cataract Refract Surg 2019;45(12):1808–17.

[63] Bertens CJF, Dunker SL, Dias AJAA, et al. Safety and comfort of an innovative drug delivery device in healthy subjects. Transl Vis Sci Technol 2020;9(13):35.

[64] Sun Y, Huffman K, Freeman WR, et al. Single subconjunctival injection formulation using sol-gel mesoporous silica as a controlled release system for drop-free post-cataract surgery care. J Cataract Refract Surg 2020;46(11):1548–53.

[65] Yan T, Ma Z, Liu J, et al. Thermoresponsive GenisteinNLC-dexamethasone-moxifloxacin multi drug delivery system in lens capsule bag to prevent complications after cataract surgery. Sci Rep 2021;11(1):181.

[66] Kuriakose RK, Cho S, Nassiri S, et al. Comparative outcomes of standard perioperative eye drops, intravitreal triamcinolone acetonide-moxifloxacin, and intracameral dexamethasone-moxifloxacin-ketorolac in cataract surgery. J Ophthalmol 2022;2022:1–8; https://doi.org/10.1155/2022/4857696, Figus M.

Advances in Ophthalmology and Optometry 8 (2023) 155–164

ADVANCES IN OPHTHALMOLOGY AND OPTOMETRY

Three-Dimensional Heads-Up Cataract Surgery

Eileen L. Mayro, MD*, Rachel A.F. Wozniak, MD, PhD

Flaum Eye Institute, University of Rochester Medical Center, 601 Elmwood Avenue, Box 659, Rochester, NY 14642, USA

Keywords
- Three-dimensional visualization system • Heads-up cataract surgery • Ergonomics
- Educational value • Depth perception

Key points
- Heads-up cataract surgery involves the surgeon viewing the surgical field on a three-dimensional display screen rather than through the oculars of a traditional microscope.
- Advantages of heads-up cataract surgery over traditional cataract surgery include improved ergonomics, superior educational value, and better depth perception.
- Integrating artificial intelligence algorithms into heads-up visualization systems has the potential to improve intraoperative decision-making.

INTRODUCTION

Heads-up surgery refers to a surgical field that is viewed through a pair of three-dimensional (3D) polarized glasses on a specialized 3D display screen rather than through a traditional binocular viewing microscope. A heads-up display was first conceived in the field of military aviation during World War II with the hope of keeping military pilots' eyes on the sky as opposed to on the control panel [1]. During the next 50 years, this technology has improved immensely and now has been adapted to the surgical field in efforts to improve visualization and surgeon ergonomics. The first eye surgery performed using heads-up visualization was a cataract surgery in 2009 [2]. Since then, 3D display systems have rapidly been adopted in a wide range of ophthalmic surgeries including cataract, vitreoretinal, cornea [3,4], strabismus

*Corresponding author. E-mail address: Eileen_Mayro@urmc.rochester.edu

https://doi.org/10.1016/j.yaoo.2023.02.009
2452-1760/23/© 2023 Elsevier Inc. All rights reserved.

[5], and minimally invasive glaucoma [6] procedures. This article offers an overview of heads-up cataract surgery and reviews its advantages and disadvantages as well as the future directions of this innovative technology.

SIGNIFICANCE
Overview
The 3D heads-up system consists of 1 or 2 cameras, a central processing unit, a display monitor, and 3D polarized glasses. The camera(s) is attached to a traditional ophthalmic operating microscope, which captures the individual field of view from each ocular. Images are then transmitted to the central processing unit, which organizes and recreates the entire operating field on the display monitor. To achieve 3D viewing, right-eye images are presented in odd-numbered rows that are polarized in one direction and left-eye images are presented in even numbered rows that are polarized in the opposite direction. The viewer wears passive polarized 3D glasses in which the right eye polarization filter is in the same direction as the odd-numbered rows and the left eye polarization filter is in the same direction as even-numbered rows (Fig. 1). As a result, when looking at the display screen, the observer achieves a stereoscopic view, such that the image appears 3D [7].

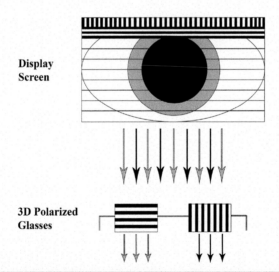

Fig. 1. Passive polarized 3D glasses are worn when observing the display screen. The right eyeglass lens is vertically polarized. The left eyeglass lens is horizontally polarized. Odd-numbered rows of the display screen are vertically polarized. Even-numbered rows of the display screen are horizontally polarized. Images from the vertically polarized odd-numbered rows go through the vertically polarized right eyeglass lens to reach the right eye (*black arrows*). Images from the horizontally polarized even-numbered rows go through the horizontally polarized left eyeglass lens to reach the left eye (*gray arrows*).

Advantages

Ergonomics

Heads-up surgery offers a solution to one of the most common problems experienced by ophthalmologists: musculoskeletal pain. Similar to other surgical specialties, ophthalmology has higher rates of musculoskeletal pain then nonsurgical specialties [8]. Performing slit-lamp biomicroscopy and indirect ophthalmoscopy in the office setting as well as using a surgical microscope in the operating room requires specific postures that can be physically demanding. Bending and twisting motions, repetitive tasks, and awkward positions contribute to the development of pain [9]. In fact, the prevalence of neck and back pain in eye doctors ranged from 51.8% to 81% in studies from the Northeastern United States [10], the United Kingdom [11], India [12], Saudi Arabia [13], and Germany [14]. Unfortunately, decreased productivity is an important consequence of work-related pain. In a survey of 127 United States ophthalmologists, Schechet and colleagues [8] found that 14% of ophthalmologists decided to retire early, 3% reduced operating room time and clinic hours, 2% planned to change careers, and 1% stopped operating due to work-related pain.

Heads-up surgery has the potential to decrease surgeons' musculoskeletal pain as ophthalmic surgeons can adopt a more comfortable, neutral posture. This is particularly important for cataract surgery given that one study found that anterior segment surgeons have a higher proportion of baseline pain than posterior segment surgeons (76% compared with 62.2%, respectively) [15]. Although it is not entirely clear why anterior segment surgeons reported worse pain, the caseload of high-volume cataract surgeons may be a contributor. In the study by Weinstock and colleagues, [15] 84% of anterior segment surgeons endorsed improved posture and comfort as well as reduced severity or frequency of pain when operating using a heads-up display rather than with a conventional surgical microscope.

Educational value

A 3D heads-up display allows for an enhanced view of the surgical field by all surgical team members, including surgical technicians and nurses. This can promote improved teamwork and coordination, as well as improve the trainee educational experience [16]. In fact, both nurses and residents reported that heads-up cataract surgery had increased educational value [17] and medical students reported better depth of field and visibility with heads-up visualization when viewing femtosecond laser-assisted cataract surgery [18]. This improved vantage point led trainees to report improved detail understanding, knowledge retention, and educational value associated with a heads-up approach [18]. Surgeons agree that heads-up display systems are valuable educational tools. In one study of 12 surgeons, 83% thought that heads-up cataract surgery had greater teaching potential than traditional cataract surgery [19].

Heads-up surgical systems also may improve mentor–trainee communication during cataract surgery. Eckardt and colleagues [20] conducted a study in which a trainee was guided through cataract surgery exclusively using the heads-up approach. Utilizing a Bluetooth earpiece to hear verbal feedback, the trainee performed cataract surgery while the mentor was positioned approximately 2 meters from the trainee [20]. The mentor was close enough to observe every detail of the procedure on the display screen, yet far enough from the surgical field such that comments were not audible to the patient. This allowed the mentor to instruct freely and openly explain concepts and approach without disrupting the patient experience, which is an important advantage given that most cataract surgeries are performed under local anesthesia. Although this study only included one participant, it demonstrates the educational potential associated with heads-up surgical systems.

Visualization
Heads-up systems may be associated with better visualization of the surgical field than traditional microscopes due to superior depth perception and image quality. In 2 studies, cataract surgeons reported they had better depth perception with heads-up visualization systems than with traditional microscopes [17,21]. In a study by Wang and colleagues, 65 cataract surgeons rated their satisfaction with the depth perception of a heads-up display system and a traditional microscope on a scale of 1 through 10. The ratings for depth perception were 9.40 ± 0.81 and 6.51 ± 1.5, respectively [18]. Del Turco and colleagues [19] found that surgeons reported 3D heads-up systems had higher image quality than traditional microscopes. Surgeons also reported better image resolution with heads-up displays in a study by Bawankule and colleagues [17].

Retinal phototoxicity
Retinal phototoxicity, or damage to retinal pigment epithelial cells and photoreceptors due to prolonged exposure to light [22], is a rare phenomenon during cataract surgery that is more common in longer cases more than 100 minutes but has been seen in cases less than 30 minutes [23]. Heads-up display systems require lower light illumination than traditional microscopes but produce brighter images—23 times brighter according to Matsumoto and colleagues [24]. In one study, Rosenberg and colleagues found that on average 50% less light illumination was used in 3D heads-up cataract surgery than in cataract surgery under a traditional microscope. In some cases, 75% less light illumination was used in the 3D heads-up group than in the traditional microscope group [25]. In this single-surgeon series of 35 patients, Rosenberg and colleagues [25] also found that heads-up cataract surgery may be associated with faster postoperative recovery—50% more patients who underwent heads-up cataract surgery had a postoperative day one visual acuity that was within 2 lines of their postoperative month one visual acuity than patients in the traditional cataract surgery group. Differences in macular light exposure may contribute to early visual acuity recovery following surgery.

Eyestrain
Unlike with traditional cataract surgery, surgeons utilizing heads-up visualization systems do not need to utilize near vision and, as a result, may experience

less asthenopia [26]. In traditional cataract surgery, viewing a magnified field at a close distance often induces accommodation and resultant eye strain, particularly for presbyopic surgeons. In contrast, higher magnification without eyestrain is possible with heads-up cataract surgery because the image is at a distance from the viewer [27].

Operative fluency and case duration
Heads-up visualization systems may improve operative fluency and decrease time required to complete cataract surgery. A recent study by Berquet and colleagues [28] demonstrated that those surgeons operating with heads-up displays significantly shortened their surgical times by 5 minutes on average (16.44 ± 4.36 vs 21.44 ± 7.50 minutes; $P = .007$). Although Berquet and colleagues [28] found that heads-up cataract surgery was shorter than traditional cataract surgery under a microscope, other studies [27,29] found that surgery using the 2 techniques took a similar amount of time.

Surgical complications and visual outcomes
With regards to operative and postoperative complications, most published reports have not identified any difference in the complication rates between heads-up and traditional cataract surgery [18,27–30]. A small, single-surgeon study reported a 3-fold higher rate of unplanned vitrectomy during cataract surgery utilizing a standard microscope versus a 3D heads-up display [2], perhaps due to superior visualization of the posterior capsule with the heads-up system. However, all other studies have found no difference in the rate of posterior capsule rupture between heads-up and traditional cataract surgery.

With regards to postoperative corneal edema, a study by Qian and colleagues [29] found no difference in corneal endothelial cell density between the 2 groups at 1 month. However, Sandali and colleagues [31] did report reduced corneal edema in the 3D heads-up group compared with the traditional microscope group (postoperative central corneal thickness of 17.3 μm $\pm$ 3.2 and 44.0 μm $\pm$ 9.3, respectively). Again, the authors thought the reduced cornea edema may be secondary to improved depth perception with heads-up display systems [31]. Importantly, despite potential small differences in surgical complication rates, across all currently published studies, no differences occurred in final visual acuity between patients who underwent heads-up versus those who underwent traditional cataract surgery [17,18,29].

Integrated technology
The 3D heads up display system also provides the ability to display data or other ophthalmic imaging next to or overlaid onto the surgical field on the display monitor. For example, split screens can show optical coherence tomography images [32], preoperative data obtained from the slit lamp, or phacoemulsification parameters. In addition, data, or enhanced imagery such as incision markings or toric intraocular lens axes, can be overlaid on top of the surgical field on the display screen. These integrated displays can improve surgical technique by providing comprehensive and real-time patient data during surgery.

Disadvantages
Learning curve
Ophthalmologists may not want to consider learning a new way to operate, given the time and training that went into mastering surgery under a conventional microscope. Ophthalmologists most willing to utilize a heads-up visualization system were between 11 and 20 years in clinical practice [21]. Bin Helayel and colleagues postulated 2 likely reasons for this: (1) a level of comfort in trying new technologies given an increased level of experience and (2) musculoskeletal pain from previous years of practice that predisposes a willingness to try a new way of operating that may be associated with less pain.

With regards to adopting heads-up cataract surgery, certain steps may be associated with a steeper learning curve than others. Bawankule and colleagues [17] conducted a study in which surgeons rated the ease of completing steps with a traditional microscope versus with a 3D heads-up display system during a learning phase and after the learning phase (postlearning phase).

Surgeons reported feeling equally comfortable entering the anterior chamber in the microscope group and the heads-up group. However, surgeons reported performing the capsulorrhexis and phacoemulsification fragmentation were easier with the traditional microscope than with the heads-up display in the postlearning phase. Given that capsulorrhexis and phacoemulsification fragmentation typically are the most challenging steps of cataract surgery, a longer learning phase may be required to improve physician comfort in completing those specific steps with 3D visualization. Of note, surgeons found that irrigation and aspiration as well as intraocular lens insertion were easier with the 3D heads-up display than with the traditional microscope [17].

Overall, surgeons reported feeling comfortable and efficient in performing heads-up cataract surgery after 3 to 4 cases [28]. However, approximately 20 cases were required until surgeons could perform as quickly as the predetermined average time for cataract surgery [33].

Crosstalk
A key drawback of 3D visualization systems is the possibility of crosstalk on the display screen [34]. Three-dimensional display screens consist of an organic light-emitting diode (OLED) panel and micropolarizer film. Right-eye images are present in odd-numbered rows and left-eye images are present in even number rows. When the viewer looks at the 3D display using passive polarized 3D glasses, there should be perfect overlap of the micropolarizer and display rows leading to each eye only seeing its respective image. However, if the viewer is not at the correct angle and distance from the display screen, row misalignment results in crosstalk and separate eye images may overlap causing blurring. Importantly, the optimal position of the viewer with respect to the display screen is not universal and is different for each display screen model. A study evaluating the NGENUITY 3D Visualization System with 3 different display screen models found that different optimal distances occurred for each type of screen ranging from 1.25 to 1.8 meters. A viewer's optimal position with

respect to the display screen should be calculated before a case in order to reduce crosstalk [7].

Cost

There is a high cost associated with heads-up visualization systems. Currently 2 commercially available systems exist: (1) NGENUITY 3D Visualization System (Fort Worth, TX) and (2) ZEISS ARTEVO 800 Digital Microscope (Dublin, CA). These systems generally retail for US$50,000 to US$100,000. In addition to a high upfront cost, there are additional costs associated with heads-up visualization systems including machine maintenance and upgrades.

Image latency

The ZEISS ARTEVO 800 Digital Microscope and NGENUITY 3D Visualization System were found to have a 50-millisecond and 80-millisecond image latency, respectively [35]. Although most surgeons did not find the delay particularly noticeable [29], the time delay may be more apparent in anterior segment surgery than in posterior segment surgery due to more rapid surgical steps.

Visual comfort

Viewing a 3D display screen has the potential to cause visual discomfort as well as motion sickness [36]. Although in a recent survey of 73 cataract surgeons, Berquet and colleagues [28] found no overall difference in visual comfort between heads-up and traditional cataract surgery, a small subset of surgeons experienced temporary visual discomfort for the first 10 to 15 cases before they adjusted to the heads-up visualization system. It is thought that this time-limited phenomenon is more likely to affect surgeons with exophoria [37]. Additionally, surgeons who never wore spectacles previously reported some discomfort wearing glasses [28].

Future avenues

The 2 major disadvantages of 3D heads-up visualization systems, cost and crosstalk, should be further explored and addressed. With regards to cost, given the high price tag of 3D heads-up display systems, a cost–benefit analysis of heads-up cataract surgery and surgical outcomes, physician pain, and trainee learning would lead to a better understanding of how these systems could be integrated into clinical practice. With regards to crosstalk, improved polarization designs could decrease this phenomenon. For example, current heads-up display systems use linear polarization, in which each eye is polarized in a different direction (eg, the right eye may be vertically polarized, whereas the left eye is horizontally polarized). Linear polarization is subject to crosstalk at different head positions causing overlap of right and left eye images, leading to blurring. Circular polarization minimizes crosstalk at different head positions allowing an observer to tilt their head, to adopt the most comfortable posture, without visual consequences. An example of circular polarization is a clockwise orientation for right-eye images and a counterclockwise orientation for left-eye image with corresponding passive polarized glasses.

In the future, heads-up visualization systems could incorporate artificial intelligence (AI) algorithms with intraoperative data to make cataract surgery safer and more effective. Intraoperative patient head drift and eye movements are significant challenges during cataract surgery [38]. AI could alert the surgeon of the patient position change and adjust the surgical view on the display screen so that the middle of the surgical field always is in the center of the screen. AI could include mapping of intraocular architecture [39] and trigger an alert if the surgeon is in danger of a complication, such as posterior capsule rupture or iris prolapse. Improved intraoperative decision-making may be possible with artificial intelligence algorithms on heads-up 3D displays. In addition, the incorporation of vocal commands into heads-up visualization systems could make surgical cases faster and improve patient outcomes. For example, a surgeon could seamlessly turn on the intraoperative aberrometry display with a voice command, thereby avoiding an additional foot or hand movement during surgery.

SUMMARY
Although heads-up cataract surgery has only existed for about 10 years, great strides have been made with respect to heads-up visualization systems. Numerous advantages exist to these systems, including ergonomics, educational value, and depth perception. In the future, the integration of other technologies and artificial intelligence algorithms into heads-up display systems has the potential to make cataract surgery even safer and more effective.

CLINICS CARE POINTS

- Surgeons with preexisting musculoskeletal pain may want to consider performing cataract surgery with a heads-up display to improve their positioning and comfort.
- Before performing heads-up cataract surgery, a surgeon should calculate their optimal distance from the display screen to prevent crosstalk and image blurring.
- Surgeons performing heads-up cataract surgery should take advantage of the system's ability to display data and imaging next to or on top of the surgical field.

FINANCIAL DISCLOSURES
The authors received no specific funding for this study. The authors' employer, Flaum Eye Institute, has received a Research to Prevent Blindness, United States Departmental Unrestricted Grant.

References
[1] Johnson J. The past and future of the head-up display, the original augmented reality. Intelligencer. Available at: https://nymag.com/intelligencer/2019/01/the-past-and-future-of-the-head-up-display.html. 2019. Accessed December 15, 2022.

[2] Weinstock, RJ. First clinical use of on-screen 3-D image guidance templates during small-incision cataract surgery. Paper presented at: The American Society of Cataract and Refractive Surgery Annual Meeting; April 12, 2010; Boston, MA.

[3] Panthier C, Courtin R, Moran S, et al. Heads-up descemet membrane endothelial keratoplasty surgery: feasibility, surgical duration, complication rates, and comparison with a conventional microscope. Cornea 2021;40(4):415–9.

[4] Galvis V, Berrospi RD, Arias JD, et al. Heads up Descemet membrane endothelial keratoplasty performed using a 3D visualization system. J Surg Case Rep 2017;2017(11):rjx231.

[5] Hamasaki I, Shibata K, Shimizu T, et al. Lights-out surgery for strabismus using a heads-up 3D vision system. Acta Med Okayama 2019;73(3):229–33.

[6] Ohno H. Utility of three-dimensional heads-up surgery in cataract and minimally invasive glaucoma surgeries. Clin Ophthalmol 2019;13:2071–3.

[7] Tsuboi K, Shiraki Y, Ishida Y, et al. Optimal display positions for heads-up surgery to minimize crosstalk. Transl Vis Sci Technol 2020;9(13):28.

[8] Schechet SA, DeVience E, DeVience S, et al. Survey of musculoskeletal disorders among US ophthalmologists. Digit J Ophthalmol 2021;26(4):36–45.

[9] Kitzmann AS, Fethke NB, Baratz KH, et al. A survey study of musculoskeletal disorders among eye care physicians compared with family medicine physicians. Ophthalmology 2012;119(2):213–20.

[10] Dhimitri KC, McGwin G Jr, McNeal SF, et al. Symptoms of musculoskeletal disorders in ophthalmologists. Am J Ophthalmol 2005;139(1):179–81.

[11] Hyer JN, Lee RM, Chowdhury HR, et al. National survey of back & neck pain amongst consultant ophthalmologists in the United Kingdom. Int Ophthalmol 2015;35(6):769–75.

[12] Venkatesh R, Kumar S. Back pain in ophthalmology: National survey of Indian ophthalmologists. Indian J Ophthalmol 2017;65(8):678–82.

[13] Al-Marwani Al-Juhani M, Khandekar R, Al-Harby M, et al. Neck and upper back pain among eye care professionals. Occup Med (Lond) 2015;65(9):753–7.

[14] Bertelmann T, Heutelbeck A, Bopp S, et al. Prevalence of back pain among german ophthalmologists. Ophthalmic Res 2021;64(6):974–82.

[15] Weinstock RJ, Ainslie-Garcia MH, Ferko NC, et al. Comparative assessment of ergonomic experience with heads-up display and conventional surgical microscope in the operating room. Clin Ophthalmol 2021;15:347–56.

[16] Agranat JS, Miller JB, Douglas VP, et al. The scope of three-dimensional digital visualization systems in vitreoretinal surgery. Clin Ophthalmol 2019;13:2093–6.

[17] Bawankule PK, Narnaware SH, Chakraborty M, et al. Digitally assisted three-dimensional surgery - Beyond vitreous. Indian J Ophthalmol 2021;69(7):1793–800.

[18] Wang K, Song F, Zhang L, et al. Three-dimensional heads-up cataract surgery using femtosecond laser: efficiency, efficacy, safety, and medical education-a randomized clinical trial. Transl Vis Sci Technol 2021;10(9):4.

[19] Del Turco C, D'Amico Ricci G, Dal Vecchio M, et al. Heads-up 3D eye surgery: Safety outcomes and technological review after 2 years of day-to-day use. Eur J Ophthalmol 2021;32(2):1–7.

[20] Eckardt C, Ahdab K, Eckert T. Use of mobile phones during heads-up surgery-a new way of teaching cataract and vitreoretinal surgery. Retina 2019;39(Suppl 1):S191–3.

[21] Helayel HB, Al-Mazidi S, AlAkeely A. Can the three-dimensional heads-up display improve ergonomics, surgical performance, and ophthalmology training compared to conventional microscopy? Clin Ophthalmol 2021;15:679–86.

[22] Tso MO, Woodford BJ. Effect of photic injury on the retinal tissues. Ophthalmology 1983;90(8):952–63.

[23] Kleinmann G, Hoffman P, Schechtman E, et al. Microscope-induced retinal phototoxicity in cataract surgery of short duration. Ophthalmology 2002;109(2):334–8.

[24] Matsumoto CS, Shibuya M, Makita J, et al. Heads-up 3D surgery under low light intensity conditions: new high-sensitivity HD camera for ophthalmological microscopes. J Ophthalmol 2019;2019:5013463.

[25] Rosenberg ED, Nuzbrokh Y, Sippel KC. Efficacy of 3D digital visualization in minimizing coaxial illumination and phototoxic potential in cataract surgery: pilot study. J Cataract Refract Surg 2021;47(3):291–6.

[26] Kumar A, Hasan N, Kakkar P, et al. Comparison of clinical outcomes between "heads-up" 3D viewing system and conventional microscope in macular hole surgeries: A pilot study. Indian J Ophthalmol 2018;66(12):1816–9.

[27] Weinstock RJ, Diakonis VF, Schwartz AJ, et al. Heads-up cataract surgery: complication rates, surgical duration, and comparison with traditional microscopes. J Refract Surg 2019;35(5):318–22.

[28] Berquet F, Henry A, Barbe C, et al. Comparing heads-up versus binocular microscope visualization systems in anterior and posterior segment surgeries: a retrospective study. Ophthalmologica 2020;243(5):347–54.

[29] Qian Z, Wang H, Fan H, et al. Three-dimensional digital visualization of phacoemulsification and intraocular lens implantation. Indian J Ophthalmol 2019;67(3):341–3.

[30] Bedar MS, Kellner U. Digital 3D "heads-up" cataract surgery: safety profile and comparison with the conventional microscope system. Klin Monbl Augenheilkd 2022;239(8):991–5.

[31] Sandali O, El Sanharawi M, Tahiri Joutei Hassani R, et al. Early corneal pachymetry maps after cataract surgery and influence of 3D digital visualization system in minimizing corneal oedema. Acta Ophthalmol 2022;100(5):e1088–94.

[32] Kelkar JA, Kelkar AS, Bolisetty M. Initial experience with three-dimensional heads-up display system for cataract surgery - A comparative study. Indian J Ophthalmol 2021;69(9):2304–9.

[33] Velasque L, Dominguez M, Fourmaux E, et al. Heads-up learning curve. Poster presented at: European Society of Retina Specialists; June 9, 2019; Paris, FR.

[34] Shibata TS Y, Kamei M. Clinical utility of stereoscopic 3D displays in heads-up surgery. SID Symp Dig Tech Papers 2018;49:1327–30.

[35] Kaur M, Titiyal JS. Three-dimensional heads up display in anterior segment surgeries- Expanding frontiers in the COVID-19 era. Indian J Ophthalmol 2020;68(11):2338–40.

[36] Ong CW, Tan MCJ, Lam M, et al. Applications of extended reality in ophthalmology: systematic review. J Med Internet Res 2021;23(8):e24152.

[37] Kim SH, Suh YW, Song JS, et al. Clinical research on the ophthalmic factors affecting 3D asthenopia. J Pediatr Ophthalmol Strabismus 2012;49(4):248–53.

[38] Brogan K, Dawar B, Lockington D, et al. Intraoperative head drift and eye movement: two under addressed challenges during cataract surgery. Eye 2018;32(6):1111–6.

[39] Muecke TP, Casson RJ. Three-dimensional heads-up display in cataract surgery: a review. Asia Pac J Ophthalmol (Phila) 2022;11(6):549–53.

Vitreoretinal Disease

Advances in Ophthalmology and Optometry 8 (2023) 165–178

ADVANCES IN OPHTHALMOLOGY AND OPTOMETRY

Evolution and Advances in Wet Age-Related Macular Degeneration Treatments

Samantha Goldburg, MD[a], George Jiao, MD[a],
Ronni M. Lieberman, MD[b],*

[a]Department of Ophthalmology, Northwell Health Eye Institute, 600 Northern Boulevard, Suite 214, Great Neck, NY 11021, USA; [b]Department of Ophthalmology, Mount Sinai Health Systems, New York, NY, USA

Keywords
- Macular degeneration • Choroidal neovascularization
- Vascular endothelial growth factor • Port delivery system

Key points
- Macular degeneration is a chronic progressive disease and a leading cause of vision loss with several known validated treatments.
- Current treatments for neovascular age-related macular degeneration include anti-vascular endothelial growth factor (VEGF) therapy and, less frequently, laser photocoagulation, photodynamic therapy, and surgical management.
- Treatment with intravitreal anti-VEGF requires frequent injections and visits to the clinic, which can lead to patient nonadherence.
- Newer trials investigating port delivery systems, gene therapy, complement inhibition, and stem cell therapy have the potential to change the scope of macular degeneration treatment by offering equally effective treatment, but reducing the number of clinic visits required.

INTRODUCTION

Age-related macular degeneration (AMD) is the leading cause of irreversible blindness in developed countries, affecting 10% of the population more than age 65 years and 25% of those more than 75 years [1]. The global prevalence of AMD is predicted to increase from 196 million people in 2020 to 288 million

*Corresponding author. 82-68 164th Street Pavilion, 452, Jamaica, NY 11432. *E-mail address:* LIEBERMR@nychhc.org

https://doi.org/10.1016/j.yaoo.2023.02.010

by 2040 [2]. In the United States, an estimated 11 million people suffer from dry-AMD, whereas 1.5 million have wet-AMD, an advanced stage with neovascularization [3]. Risk factors include older age, cigarette smoking, family history, hypertension, cardiovascular disease, nutrient deficiency, and visible light exposure [4,5]. AMD is a degenerative disease of the retina that leads to significant central vision loss. Large, confluent, or soft drusen concentrated within the macula are hallmarks of AMD. Cumulative oxidative injury leads to the loss of photoreceptors and accumulation of lipofuscin granules in the retinal pigmented epithelium (RPE) [6]. The neovascular form of AMD is characterized by the presence of vascular endothelial growth factors (VEGFs), leading to vessels formation from the choroid and disruption Bruch's membrane. This can lead to various clinical manifestations such as subretinal and intraretinal fluid, RPE detachments, or subretinal and sub-RPE hemorrhages, resulting in hypertrophic fibrovascular scar formation and permanent vision loss [7]. Given its high prevalence and devastating complications, neovascular AMD treatment has been the target of research across the world for potential therapeutic agents and methods (Fig. 1).

Thermal laser photocoagulation, photodynamic therapy, and radiation therapy

The earliest treatments for neovascular AMD involved using thermal laser photocoagulation to seal leaking vessels outside the fovea. The Macular Photocoagulation Study (MPS) from the 1980s showed that patients with extrafoveal and juxtafoveal classic choroidal neovascularization (CNV) from AMD had better long-term visual prognosis with photocoagulation compared with those without treatment [8,9]. Patients with subfoveal neovascular lesions with classic

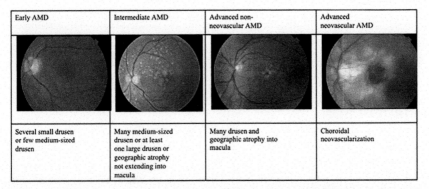

Early AMD	Intermediate AMD	Advanced non-neovascular AMD	Advanced neovascular AMD
Several small drusen or few medium-sized drusen	Many medium-sized drusen or at least one large drusen or geographic atrophy not extending into macula	Many drusen and geographic atrophy into macula	Choroidal neovascularization

Fig. 1. Fundus photos and classes of early, intermediate, advanced AMD and neovascular AMD. (Reprinted with permission from Elsevier. The Lancet, November 2008; 372(9652): 1835-1845 and Stringham JM, Hammond BR, Nolan JM, et al. The utility of using customized heterochromatic flicker photometry (cHFP) to measure macular pigment in patients with age-related macular degeneration. *Exp Eye Res.* 2008;87(5):445-453.)

CNV, well-demarcated boundaries, and equal or smaller than 3.5 disc areas treated with photocoagulation were associated with better visual acuity than untreated eyes at 48 months [10]. Laser photocoagulation does not address the underlying issue of neovascularization [11]. The high recurrence rate, coupled with the strict eligibility criteria of the MPS trials and modern therapies, has made thermal laser photocoagulation fall out of favor.

Photodynamic therapy (PDT) emerged in the 1990s for predominantly classic CNV. Intravenously injected verteporfin accumulates in neovascular membranes and releases reactive oxygen species when irradiated with laser light at 689 nm, leading to destruction of the choroidal neovascular endothelium [12]. The treatment of age-related macular degeneration with photodynamic therapy study and the visudyne in photodynamic therapy trials demonstrated that patients with greater than 50% of classic CNV were less likely to lose more than three lines of vision when treated with PDT compared with patients who received placebo [13,14]. Although it demonstrated some efficacy in preventing vision loss, verteporfin rarely improved vision in patients with AMD. PDT has been largely relegated to management of polypoidal choroidal vasculopathy and central serous chorioretinopathy as per the EVEREST trial [15] and may be used as an adjunct to anti-VEGF treatments [16].

Radiation therapy has been tried in wet AMD, including brachytherapy, external beam radiotherapy, and stereotactic radiotherapy. It was hypothesized that as radiation preferentially targets rapidly dividing cells, and that cumulative doses up to 25 Gy rarely cause damage to healthy retina or optic nerve, radiotherapy may be effective in targeting endothelial cells in CNV to halt the progression of neovascularization. However, studies have not shown a clear benefit in using radiotherapy to treat neovascular AMD and may even be harmful with certain techniques such as epimacular brachytherapy [17]. Currently, the Stereotactic Radiotherapy for Wet AMD trial is evaluating the effect of using radiotherapy in conjunction with anti-VEGF therapy [18] with the aim to reduce the need for regular injections.

Submacular surgery, macular translocation surgery, and pneumatic submacular hemorrhage displacement

Submacular surgery to remove fibrovascular tissue and blood has been tried in patients with subfoveal neovascular AMD. The Submacular Surgery Trials evaluated whether surgical removal of CNV with associated hemorrhage in neovascular AMD can stabilize or improve vision compared with observation and the effect on patients' reception of health- and vision-related "quality of life," as measured by the Medical Outcome Survey Short Form-36 (MOS SF-36), the Hospital Anxiety and Depression Scale, and the National Eye Institute Visual Function Questionnaire (NEI VFQ-25). The authors found that submacular surgery did not increase chance of stable or improved vision, reduce risk of severe vision loss, and had no effect on subjective quality-of-life measures in patients with large hemorrhages from subfoveal neovascular AMD lesions [19,20]. In patients with untreated, new CNV due to AMD, submacular surgery did not improve or preserve vision compared with observation [21]. Although quality-of-life outcomes were improved in this subset of patients [22], the investigators could not recommend the intervention due to suboptimal visual outcomes. Future studies on submacular surgery noted high-quality evidence of no benefit in preventing visual loss, with an increased risk of retinal detachments and need for cataract surgery in patients who underwent submacular surgery [23].

Macular translocation surgery, the detachment of macula from the RPE by subretinal infusion of fluid followed by macular translocation, was demonstrated to improve visual acuity for at least 5 years with both full macular translocation and limited macular translocation [24,25]. However, these studies are limited in generalizability and in a high rate of vision-threatening complications such as CNV recurrence, proliferative vitreoretinopathy, and foveal RPE atrophy [24]. Despite these limitations, future research for RPE and stem cell transplantations should be encouraged, as the neurosensory retina has proven to be able to survive and function for at least 5 years when translocated to areas of healthy RPE.

Intravitreal air and gas and subretinal tissue plasminogen activator injection for pneumatic displacement of submacular hemorrhage have been attempted and demonstrated some efficacy in improving short-term visual acuity [26,27]. No general consensus or guidelines have been achieved for the use of these techniques, as the underlying cause of CNV is not addressed.

Anti-vascular endothelial growth factor treatments

The development of anti-VEGF agents revolutionized the treatment of neovascular AMD in the 2000s. VEGF is a potent angiogenic protein that stimulates vascular endothelial cell growth and hyperpermeability of blood vessels [28]. This growth factor, especially the subgroup A isoform 165, plays a major role in the development of CNV when overexpressed in the RPE. Anti-VEGF agents prevent VEGF from binding to cell surfaces. Several major clinical trials have demonstrated continued efficacy of anti-VEGF injections and superiority over previously used treatment modalities.

The first of these agents, pegaptanib (Macugen, Eyetech Pharmaceuticals, Palm Beach Gardens, FL, USA), received FDA approval in 2004. Pegaptanib is a pegylated single strand of nucleic acid that specifically binds to the 165 isoform of VEGF and works as an antagonist when injected intravitreally. The VEGF Inhibition Study in Ocular Neovascularization trial demonstrated that patients who received 0.3 mg of pegaptanib every 6 weeks were protected from a visual acuity loss of greater than 15 letters at higher proportion compared with those who received sham injections at 1 year [29]. The rate of visual decline also was lower in the treated group. However, both the 0.3 mg treated group and the placebo group continued to experience vision loss, and the second year of treatment was proven to be less effective than the first year.

Ranibizumab (Lucentis, Genentech, Inc, San Francisco, CA) is a recombinant humanized immunoglobulin G (IgG)1 monoclonal antibody fragment that binds to the receptor-binding site on all isoforms of VEGF-A [30]. The

Minimally Classic/Occult Trial of the Anti-VEGF Antibody Ranibizumab in the Treatment of Neovascular AMD (MARINA) and the Anti-VEGF Antibody for the Treatment of Predominantly Classic Choroidal Neovascularization in AMD (ANCHOR) trials independently evaluated the efficacy and safety of 0.3 and 0.5 mg of intravitreal ranibizumab. The primary end point for both trials was proportion of patients who lost fewer than 15 letters from baseline at 12 months. The MARINA study demonstrated successful prevention of vision loss and significant improvement in visual acuity over 24 monthly intravitreal injections with both 0.3 and 0.5 mg injections, in patients with minimally classic or occult CNV compared with sham injections [31]. The ANCHOR study compared monthly 0.3 and 0.5 mg intravitreal injections and sham PDT therapy to sham injections and PDT therapy, in predominantly classic CNV. Again, intravitreal injection with ranibizumab achieved significant improvement in visual acuity and prevented vision loss in a greater proportion of patients compared with treatment with verteporfin PDT [16].

Bevacizumab (Avastin, Genentech, Inc, San Francisco, CA), such as ranibizumab, also is a recombinant humanized monoclonal IgG1 antibody. Unlike ranibizumab, which is a fragment of the antibody, bevacizumab is the complete IgG molecule and also binds to all isoforms of VEGF [32]. Bevacizumab is FDA-approved for the treatment of metastatic colorectal cancer, lung cancer, and breast cancer, and despite its wide use in ophthalmology, is not FDA-approved for ophthalmic use. Initially administered systemically in the Systemic Avastin for Neovascular AMD trial, bevacizumab increased visual acuity and decreased central retinal thickness in all 15 patients in the trial [33]. Further studies on intravitreal bevacizumab demonstrated comparable efficacy to ranibizumab, longer duration of action, and lower cost for patients, which prompted National Institute of Health (NIH)-supported noninferiority clinical trials to evaluate the efficacy and safety of bevacizumab compared with ranibizumab. The Comparison of AMD Treatment Trials (CATT) randomly assigned patients into four groups: ranibizumab or bevacizumab, on an as-needed regiment (PRN) or monthly basis. At 1 year, bevacizumab and ranibizumab had similar therapeutic benefits when administered on the same schedule [34]. Ranibizumab given PRN had an equivalent effect on vision to ranibizumab administered monthly. The 2-year CATT results showed ranibizumab and bevacizumab had similar effects on visual acuity, and treatment on a monthly basis resulted in a slight improvement in visual acuity compared with PRN dosing in both agents [35]. A 5-year follow-up was completed with 71% of the original patients. Although half of the eyes had visual acuity greater than 20/40, the vision gained during the first 2-years of CATT were not maintained at 5 years, decreasing by three letters compared with baseline and by 11 letters compared with 2-year follow-up [36]. High variability in individual treatments between years 2 and 5 limits any conclusive statements regarding effects of different drugs, safety profiles, and dosing regimens.

Aflibercept (Eylea, Regeneron Pharmaceuticals, Inc, Tarrytown, NY) is a soluble decoy molecule, consisting of an IgG backbone fused to extracellular VEGF receptor sequence, binding to VEGF-A and VEGF-B, as well as placental growth factor with higher affinity than the natural VEGF receptors [37]. This "VEGF-trap" binds to both sides of the VEGF dimer and prevents subsequent activation of native VEGF receptors. The VEGF Trap-Eye: Investigation of Efficacy and Safety in Wet AMD 1 and 2 studies randomized patients into four treatment groups: 0.5 mg aflibercept monthly, 2 mg aflibercept monthly, 2 mg aflibercept every 2 months after 3 initial monthly injections, or 0.5 mg ranibizumab monthly. The primary end point in both studies was the percentage of patients who lost fewer than 15 letters at 52 weeks. All aflibercept regimens demonstrated noninferiority to monthly ranibizumab injections, including the group treated with 2 mg aflibercept every 2 months after 3 initial monthly doses [38]. At 2 years, mean letter increase was 7.9 in the monthly ranibizumab group and 7.6 in the 2 mg aflibercept every 2 months group [38]. Anatomic response was strong at 2 years as well, as the decrease in central retinal thickness was maintained from year 1 to year 2 across all treatment groups.

Brolucizumab (Beovu, Novartis, Basel, Switzerland) is a single-chain variable fragment (scFv) that was developed by grafting complementarity-determining regions of a novel anti-VEGF-A antibody to a human scFv scaffold, which is the smallest functional unit of an antibody [39]. Because brolucizumab lacks the Fc region, it has a smaller molecular weight [40], allowing for higher molar dosing and more rapid and evenly distributed tissue penetration [41]. It binds VEGF-A in a 2:1 ratio and has a significantly higher binding affinity to VEGF-A isoforms compared with bevacizumab [40]. HAWK [42] and HARRIER [43] are two phase 3 trials comparing brolucizumab with aflibercept to treat neovascular AMD [39]. A total of 1817 patients with untreated active CNV due to AMD were randomized to brolucizumab 3 mg (HAWK only), brolucizumab 6 mg, or aflibercept 2 mg. Brolucizumab treated eyes were loaded with 3 monthly injections and then received an injection every 12 weeks, or adjusted to every 8 weeks if disease was still active. Aflibercept-treated eyes received an injection every 8 weeks. At week 48, each brolucizumab arm demonstrated noninferiority to aflibercept in best corrected visual acuity (BCVA) change from baseline. Fifty-six percent of HAWK patients and 51% from HARRIER were maintained on injections every 12 weeks when treated with 6 mg of brolucizumab [39]. At week 16, after identical treatment exposure, fewer eyes treated with 6 mg brolucizumab had disease activity compared with aflibercept-treated eyes. At week 48, brolucizumab was noninferior to aflibercept in visual acuity, and greater than 50% of eyes treated with 6 mg brolucizumab were maintained on injections every 12 weeks. Brolocizumab was generally found to have similar, mild adverse effects compared with aflibercept. More importantly, however, it has been associated with an increased rate of intraocular inflammation, retinal vasculitis, and retinal occlusive events [44]. HAWK and HARRIER reported intraocular inflammation at a rate of 4%, including reports of severe vision loss [39].

Conbercept (Lumitin, Chengdu Kang Hong Biotech Co, Ltd, Sichuan, China) is a fusion protein composed of the extracellular domain 2 of VEGF receptor 1 and extracellular domains 3 and 4 of VEGF receptor 2 combined with the Fc portion of the human immunoglobulin G1. It has a higher affinity to VEGF than ranibizumab and bevacizumab; its affinity is similar to that of aflibercept [41]. One meta-analysis found intravitreal conbercept was noninferior to intravitreal ranibizumab; however, low-quality evidence occurred, and a lack of trials comparing conbercept to other anti-VEGF treatments exists [45]. In a retrospective review of 66 eyes treated with 0.5 mg intravitreal conbercept monthly for 3 months, followed by a PRN protocol, a statistically significant improvement occurred in BCVA as well as central macular thickness at 3 months [46]. Forty-eight patients completed 1 year of follow-up, with BCVA and central macular thickness improving at each follow-up visit (every 3 months). No serious adverse reactions occurred; however, further prospective randomized double-blind trials are needed to confirm the efficacy and safety of conbercept.

Faricimab (Vabysmo, Genentech, San Francisco, CA) is a bi-specific antibody directed against both VEGF and angiopoietin-2. This dual-targeted treatment was dosed up to 4-month intervals and was found to be non-inferior to aflibercept given every 2 months in the first year. In the phase 3 TENAYA [47] and LUCERNE [48] trials, Faricimab dosed up to every 16 weeks resulted in similar visual acuity and anatomical outcomes compared with aflibercept given every 8 weeks [49]. At week 48, more than three-quarters of patients were dosed every 12 weeks or longer. Data up to week 48 show the drug was well tolerated, with low rates of intraocular inflammation and no vasculitis or occlusive retinitis events.

Port delivery system

The ranibizumab port delivery system (PDS; Susvimo, Genentech, San Francisco, CA) includes an ocular implant, a customized formulation of ranibizumab, and four ancillary devices for initial fill, surgical implantation, refill-exchange, and explantation (Fig. 2). This device allows for continuous delivery of ranibizumab into the vitreous over an extended period. It has been approved by the US Food and Drug Administration (FDA) for treatment of neovascular AMD in adults who have previously responded to at least two anti-VEGF injections [50]. Ranibizumab is ideal for PDS given its stability and high solubility. Release rates have been found to remain consistent 6 months after initial fill and first, second, and third refills [50]. The Ladder trial was a Phase 2 multi-center, randomized, treatment-controlled study including 220 patients randomized to PDS with 10, 40, and 100 mg/mL ranibizumab or intravitreal ranibizumab (IVR) 0.5 mg/month [51]. In the 100 mg/mL group, the mean time to first refill (primary endpoint) was 15.8 months. In the 40 and 10 mg/mL groups, the mean time was 13 and 8.7 months, respectively. Archway is a phase 3 open-label, randomized, visual acuity assessor-masked noninferiority and equivalence trial including patients with neovasular age related macular degeneration (nAMD) diagnosed within 9 months of screening, responsive to previous anti-VEGF therapy [52]. Patients were randomized to PDS with

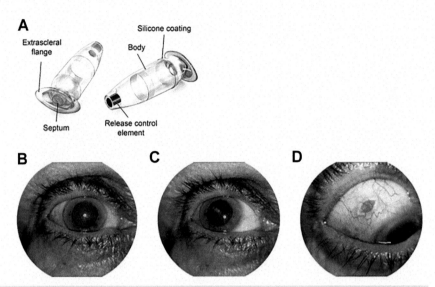

Fig. 2. (A) Port delivery system with ranibizumab implant demonstrating the extrascleral flange that anchors implant in sclera, septum which allows for refills, body of the device, and release control element. (B) Eye in primary position, no visible implant. (C) Eye looking up, device visible in superotemporal quadrant. (D) Eye looking down, device visible in sclera. (*From* Campochiaro PA, Marcus DM, Awh CC, et al. The Port Delivery System with Ranibizumab for Neovascular Age-Related Macular Degeneration: Results from the Randomized Phase 2 Ladder Clinical Trial. Ophthalmology. 2019;126(8):1141-1154.)

ranibizumab 100 mg/mL with fixed 24-week refills or intravitreal ranibizumab 0.5-mg injections every 4 weeks. A total of 418 patients were enrolled. Mean change in BCVA from baseline averaged over 36 and 40 weeks was +0.2 letters in the PDS arm and +0.5 letters in the monthly ranibizumab arm; PDS was non-inferior and equivalent to monthly ranibizumab. 98.4% of patients in the PDS arm did not receive supplemental treatment in the first 24-week interval [52].

Gene therapy delivery
RGX-314 (REGENXBIO Inc, Rockville, MD) is in development as a one-time subretinal injection that includes the NAV AAV8 vector containing a gene encoding an anti-VEGF monoclonal antibody fragment (fab protein) similar to ranibizumab, potentially producing continuous anti-VEGF therapy in the eye [53]. AAVIATE is an open-label trial evaluating the efficacy, safety, and tolerability of suprachoroidal delivery of RGX-314 via the SCS Microinjector. Twenty patients in cohort 1 and 20 patients in cohort 2 were randomized to receive RGX-314 at doses of 2.5 × 1011 and 5 × 1011 genomic copies per eye, respectively, compared with monthly 0.5 mg ranibizumab intravitreal injections. Patients in cohorts 1 and 2 had stable BCVA and central retinal thickness at 6 months and had a greater than 70% reduction in anti-VEGF burden [53]. Twenty-nine percent of patients in cohort 1 and 40% of patients in cohort 2 received no anti-VEGF injections over 6 months after RGX-314 administration. Adverse

events were mild including mild intraocular inflammation in 23% of patients that resolved with topical corticosteroids. The ATMOSPHERE trial is an ongoing Randomized, Partially Masked, Controlled, Phase 2b/3 Clinical Study to Evaluate the Efficacy and Safety of RGX-314 Gene Therapy in Participants With nAMD that started in December 2020 [54]. It will enroll 300 participants with two RGX-314 dose arms versus ranibizumab. The primary endpoint is non-inferiority to ranibizumab based on change from baseline BCVA at 1 year.

Ixoberogene soroparvovec (Ixo-vec, formerly referred to as ADVM-022; AAV.7m8-aflibercept; Adverum Biotechnologies, Inc, Redwood City, CA) is another gene therapy developed for the treatment of nAMD. The phase 1 OPTIC trial showed that using a dose of 2E11 vg a greater than 80% reduction occurred in annual anti-VEGF injection frequency and after a median follow-up of 1.7 years, greater than 50% of patients did not require any supplemental anti-VEGF injections [55]. Aflibercept expression levels were sustained through year 2 after a single injection, and mean BCVA remained stable. Most of the adverse events were mild, and no cases of vasculitis, retinitis, choroiditis, vascular occlusions, or endophthalmitis occurred [55]. LUNA is a Phase 2 trial underway at about 40 sites in the United States and Europe in which subjects are randomized between the 2E11 Ixo-vec dose, a new lower 6E10 dose, and across four prophylactic steroid regimens. Initial data are expected to be reported in 2023 [56].

Stem cells

In 2019, the National Eye Institute launched the first phase 1/IIa clinical trial to test the safety of patient-specific stem cell-based therapy to treat geographic atrophy (GA) in AMD patients. This therapy involves converting patients' blood cells into induced pluripotent stem cells (iPSCs), which are then programmed to become RPE cells [57]. iPSC-derived RPE is grown on a biodegradable scaffold designed to promote integration of cells with the retina, which has been shown to be more effective compared to RPE cells in suspension used in studies using animal models [58]. The patch is positioned between the patient's RPE and photoreceptors. An estimated 20 participants will be enrolled in this clinical trial with at least 14 study visits over 5.5 years. The use of an individual's autologous blood cells is expected to minimize the risk of the body rejecting the implant. Several possible risks exist associated with the use of stem cell-based therapy including oncogenic potential. Preclinical studies using a mouse model showed no tumor growth 7 months after injection of stem cells; however, further long-term safety of cells derived from iPSCs is needed [59].

SUMMARY

Most current treatment options available for AMD have a mechanism aimed at preventing further progression of neovascularization. The gold-standard therapy for neovascular AMD is intravitreal anti-VEGF injections. Several drugs exist in this category that have been developed over the past few decades, as neovascular AMD treatment has been a primary focus of research within the field. These include bevacizumab and aflibercept, which are widely used.

Brolucizumab seemed to be a promising alternative, but data have revealed an increased risk of intraocular inflammation associated with it, making this drug a less desirable option. Faricimab is the first bi-specific antibody directed against both VEGF and angiopoietin-2. This is an exciting new option, given data showing similar visual acuity and anatomical outcomes when dosed every 16 weeks compared with aflibercept given every 8 weeks.

Although these medications have significantly improved visual prognosis in many patients, several downsides exist. Frequent intravitreal injections are costly and inconvenient for patients. Although generally well tolerated, injections can lead to pain and discomfort. These factors can make it difficult for patients to adhere to treatment regimens.

Newer treatment modalities under investigation may help eliminate these limitations. For instance, RGX-314 is a gene therapy administered as a onetime suprachoroidal injection. Early data have shown lasting effects up to 6 months after the injection in many patients.

There also has been a more recent shift in attention and research to treatment for non-neovascular AMD and GA. Although there are not many options available, Pegcetacoplan was approved by the FDA in November 2022 and has been shown to reduce lesion growth. However, data revealed that patients treated with this medication also had an increased rate of conversion to neovascular AMD. This may lead to difficulty in determining the best course of treatment, and possibly increased inconvenience and discomfort for patients if they end up requiring both pegcetacoplan injections as well as anti-VEGF injections.

Stem cells are another area of focus in treating GA in AMD patients. The first clinical trial to test the safety of patient-specific stem cell-based therapy for this purpose is currently underway.

Despite the promise of these newer treatment options including gene therapy and stem cell therapy, the long-term safety and efficacy remains unknown. Moreover, these treatments have tremendous costs. If costs do not change, it could lead to a substantial burden on patients and the health care system. Continued prospective trials are needed to provide us with enough data to make decisions about which treatment will be most beneficial and least harmful to patients moving forward.

CLINICS CARE POINTS

- Physicians should strongly consider treatment with an intravitreal anti-vascular endothelial growth factor (VEGF) medication for patients with neovascular age-related macular degeneration (AMD).
- The choice of anti-VEGF may vary depending on systemic health, lesion type, social circumstances, and cost.
- Faricimab has similar visual acuity and anatomical outcomes when dosed every 16 weeks compared with aflibercept every 8 weeks.

- The ranibizumab port delivery system was approved for patients with neovascular AMD and allows for continuous intravitreal ranibizumab delivery over several months.
- A onetime suprachoroidal injection of RGX-314 may be effective for several months, allowing patients to avoid monthly anti-VEGF injections.
- Stem cell therapy is currently under investigation for the treatment of geographic atrophy in AMD, but more data are needed to determine the safety and efficacy.

DISCLOSURE

The authors have nothing to disclose.

References

[1] Joachim N, Mitchell P, Burlutsky G, et al. The incidence and progression of age-related macular degeneration over 15 years: the blue mountains eye study. Ophthalmology 2015;122(12):2482–9.

[2] Wong WL, Su X, Li X, et al. Global prevalence of age-related macular degeneration and disease burden projection for 2020 and 2040: a systematic review and meta-analysis. Lancet Glob Health 2014;2(2):e106–16.

[3] Chou R, Dana T, Bougatsos C, et al. Screening for impaired visual acuity in older adults: updated evidence report and systematic review for the US preventive services task force. JAMA 2016;315(9):915–33.

[4] Tomany SC, Wang JJ, Van Leeuwen R, et al. Risk factors for incident age-related macular degeneration: pooled findings from 3 continents. Ophthalmology 2004;111(7):1280–7.

[5] Katsi VK, Marketou ME, Vrachatis DA, et al. Essential hypertension in the pathogenesis of age-related macular degeneration: a review of the current evidence. J Hypertens 2015;33(12):2382–8.

[6] Zarbin MA. Current concepts in the pathogenesis of age-related macular degeneration. Arch Ophthalmol 2004;122(4):598–614.

[7] Ferris FL 3rd, Wilkinson CP, Bird A, et al. Clinical classification of age-related macular degeneration. Ophthalmology 2013;120(4):844–51.

[8] Argon laser photocoagulation for senile macular degeneration. Results of a randomized clinical trial. Arch Ophthalmol 1982;100(6):912–8.

[9] Krypton laser photocoagulation for neovascular lesions of age-related macular degeneration. Results of a randomized clinical trial. Macular Photocoagulation Study Group. Arch Ophthalmol 1990;108(6):816–24.

[10] Subfoveal neovascular lesions in age-related macular degeneration: guidelines for evaluation and treatment in the macular photocoagulation study. Arch Ophthalmol 1991;109(9): 1242–57.

[11] Tezel TH, Del Priore LV, Flowers BE, et al. Correlation between scanning laser ophthalmoscope microperimetry and anatomic abnormalities in patients with subfoveal neovascularization. Ophthalmology 1996;103(11):1829–36.

[12] Schlotzer-Schrehardt U, Viestenz A, Naumann GO, et al. Dose-related structural effects of photodynamic therapy on choroidal and retinal structures of human eyes. Graefes Arch Clin Exp Ophthalmol 2002;240(9):748–57.

[13] Blumenkranz MS, Bressler NM, Bressler SB, et al. Verteporfin therapy for subfoveal choroidal neovascularization in age-related macular degeneration: three-year results of an open-label extension of 2 randomized clinical trials–TAP Report no. 5. Arch Ophthalmol 2002;120(10):1307–14.

[14] Blinder KJ, Bradley S, Bressler NM, et al. Effect of lesion size, visual acuity, and lesion composition on visual acuity change with and without verteporfin therapy for choroidal neovascularization secondary to age-related macular degeneration: TAP and VIP report no. 1. Am J Ophthalmol 2003;136(3):407–18.

[15] Koh A, Lai TYY, Takahashi K, et al. Efficacy and safety of ranibizumab with or without verteporfin photodynamic therapy for polypoidal choroidal vasculopathy: a randomized clinical trial. JAMA Ophthalmol 2017;135(11):1206–13.

[16] Potter MJ, Claudio CC, Szabo SM. A randomised trial of bevacizumab and reduced light dose photodynamic therapy in age-related macular degeneration: the VIA study. Br J Ophthalmol 2010;94(2):174–9.

[17] Evans JR, Igwe C, Jackson TL, et al. Radiotherapy for neovascular age-related macular degeneration. Cochrane Database Syst Rev 2020;8(8):CD004004.

[18] Neffendorf JE, Desai R, Wang Y, et al. Stereotactic radiotherapy for wet age-related macular degeneration (STAR): study protocol for a randomised controlled clinical trial. Trials 2016;17(1):560.

[19] Bressler NM, Bressler SB, Childs AL, et al. Surgery for hemorrhagic choroidal neovascular lesions of age-related macular degeneration: ophthalmic findings: SST report no. 13. Ophthalmology 2004;111(11):1993–2006.

[20] Childs AL, Bressler NM, Bass EB, et al. Surgery for hemorrhagic choroidal neovascular lesions of age-related macular degeneration: quality-of-life findings: SST report no. 14. Ophthalmology 2004;111(11):2007–14.

[21] Hawkins BS, Bressler NM, Miskala PH, et al. Surgery for subfoveal choroidal neovascularization in age-related macular degeneration: ophthalmic findings: SST report no. 11. Ophthalmology 2004;111(11):1967–80.

[22] Miskala PH, Bass EB, Bressler NM, et al. Surgery for subfoveal choroidal neovascularization in age-related macular degeneration: quality-of-life findings: SST report no. 12. Ophthalmology 2004;111(11):1981–92.

[23] Giansanti F, Eandi CM, Virgili G. Submacular surgery for choroidal neovascularisation secondary to age-related macular degeneration. Cochrane Database Syst Rev 2009;(2): CD006931.

[24] van Romunde SH, Polito A, Bertazzi L, et al. Long-term results of full macular translocation for choroidal neovascularization in age-related macular degeneration. Ophthalmology 2015;122(7):1366–74.

[25] Oshima H, Iwase T, Ishikawa K, et al. Long-term results after limited macular translocation surgery for wet age-related macular degeneration. PLoS One 2017;12(5):e0177241.

[26] Martel JN, Mahmoud TH. Subretinal pneumatic displacement of subretinal hemorrhage. JAMA Ophthalmol 2013;131(12):1632–5.

[27] Haupert CL, McCuen BW 2nd, Jaffe GJ, et al. Pars plana vitrectomy, subretinal injection of tissue plasminogen activator, and fluid-gas exchange for displacement of thick submacular hemorrhage in age-related macular degeneration. Am J Ophthalmol 2001;131(2): 208–15.

[28] Campochiaro PA. Retinal and choroidal neovascularization. J Cell Physiol 2000;184(3): 301–10.

[29] Gragoudas ES, Adamis AP, Cunningham ET Jr, et al, Group VISiONCT. Pegaptanib for neovascular age-related macular degeneration. N Engl J Med 2004;351(27):2805–16.

[30] Chen Y, Wiesmann C, Fuh G, et al. Selection and analysis of an optimized anti-VEGF antibody: crystal structure of an affinity-matured Fab in complex with antigen. J Mol Biol 1999;293(4):865–81.

[31] Rosenfeld PJ, Brown DM, Heier JS, et al. Ranibizumab for neovascular age-related macular degeneration. N Engl J Med 2006;355(14):1419–31.

[32] Ferrara N. Vascular endothelial growth factor: basic science and clinical progress. Endocr Rev 2004;25(4):581–611.

[33] Michels S, Rosenfeld PJ, Puliafito CA, et al. Systemic bevacizumab (Avastin) therapy for neo-vascular age-related macular degeneration twelve-week results of an uncontrolled open-label clinical study. Ophthalmology 2005;112(6):1035–47.

[34] Group CR, Martin DF, Maguire MG, et al. Ranibizumab and bevacizumab for neovascular age-related macular degeneration. N Engl J Med 2011;364(20):1897–908.

[35] Comparison of Age-related Macular Degeneration Treatments Trials Research G, Martin DF, Maguire MG, Fine SL, et al. Ranibizumab and bevacizumab for treatment of neovascular age-related macular degeneration: two-year results. Ophthalmology 2012;119(7): 1388–98.

[36] Comparison of Age-related Macular Degeneration Treatments Trials Research G, Maguire MG, Martin DF, Ying GS, et al. Five-Year Outcomes with Anti-Vascular Endothelial Growth Factor Treatment of Neovascular Age-Related Macular Degeneration: The Comparison of Age-Related Macular Degeneration Treatments Trials. Ophthalmology 2016;123(8):1751–61.

[37] Papadopoulos N, Martin J, Ruan Q, et al. Binding and neutralization of vascular endothelial growth factor (VEGF) and related ligands by VEGF Trap, ranibizumab and bevacizumab. Angiogenesis 2012;15(2):171–85.

[38] Heier JS, Brown DM, Chong V, et al. Intravitreal aflibercept (VEGF trap-eye) in wet age-related macular degeneration. Ophthalmology 2012;119(12):2537–48.

[39] Dugel PU, Koh A, Ogura Y, et al. HAWK and HARRIER: Phase 3, multicenter, randomized, double-masked trials of brolucizumab for neovascular age-related macular degeneration. Ophthalmology 2020;127(1):72–84.

[40] Tadayoni R, Sararols L, Weissgerber G, et al. Brolucizumab: a newly developed anti-VEGF molecule for the treatment of neovascular age-related macular degeneration. Ophthalmologica 2021;244(2):93–101.

[41] Ahmad ZA, Yeap SK, Ali AM, et al. scFv antibody: principles and clinical application. Clin Dev Immunol 2012;2012:980250.

[42] Alcon R. Efficacy and Safety of RTH258 Versus Aflibercept - Study 1. 2017.

[43] Alcon R. Efficacy and Safety of RTH258 Versus Aflibercept - Study 2. 2017.

[44] Mones J, Srivastava SK, Jaffe GJ, et al. Risk of inflammation, retinal vasculitis, and retinal occlusion-related events with brolucizumab: post hoc review of HAWK and HARRIER. Ophthalmology 2021;128(7):1050–9.

[45] Zhou P, Zheng S, Wang E, et al. Conbercept for treatment of neovascular age-related macular degeneration and visual impairment due to diabetic macular edema or pathologic myopia choroidal neovascularization: a systematic review and meta-analysis. Front Pharmacol 2021;12:696201.

[46] Wu BH, Wang B, Wu HQ, et al. Intravitreal conbercept injection for neovascular age-related macular degeneration. Int J Ophthalmol 2019;12(2):252–7.

[47] Hoffmann-La R. A Study to Evaluate the Efficacy and Safety of Faricimab in Participants with Neovascular Age-Related Macular Degeneration (TENAYA). 2020.

[48] Hoffmann-La R. A Study to Evaluate the Efficacy and Safety of Faricimab in Participants with Neovascular Age-Related Macular Degeneration (LUCERNE). 2020.

[49] London N, Guymer RH, Demetriades A, et al. Faricimab in neovascular age-related macular degeneration: updated week 48 efficacy, safety, and durability in the phase 3 TENAYA and LUCERNE trials. Investigative ophthalmology & Visual Sciences 2022;63(7):252–7.

[50] Ranade SV, Wieland MR, Tam T, et al. The Port Delivery System with ranibizumab: a new paradigm for long-acting retinal drug delivery. Drug Deliv 2022;29(1):1326–34.

[51] Khanani AM, Callanan D, Dreyer R, et al. End-of-study results for the ladder phase 2 trial of the port delivery system with ranibizumab for neovascular age-related macular degeneration. Ophthalmol Retina 2021;5(8):775–87.

[52] Holekamp NM, Campochiaro PA, Chang MA, et al. Archway randomized phase 3 trial of the port delivery system with ranibizumab for neovascular age-related macular degeneration. Ophthalmology 2022;129(3):295–307.

[53] Khanani AM. Suprachoroidal delivery of RGX-314 gene therapy for neovascular AMD: the phase II AAVIATETM study. Investigative ophthalmology & Visual Sciences 2022;63(7): 1152.

[54] Inc R. Pivotal 1 Study of RGX-314 Gene Therapy in Participants With nAMD. 2023.

[55] Busbee B, Boyer DS, Khanani AM, et al. Phase 1 study of intravitreal gene therapy with ADVM-022 for neovascular AMD (OPTIC Trial). Investigative Ophthalmology & Visual Sciences 2021;62(8):352.

[56] Adverum Biotechnologies I, Parexel. Safety and Efficacy of ADVM-022 in Treatment-Experienced Patients With Neovascular Age-related Macular Degeneration LUNA. 2024.

[57] O'Neill HC, Limnios IJ, Barnett NL. Advancing a stem cell therapy for age-related macular degeneration. Curr Stem Cell Res Ther 2020;15(2):89–97.

[58] Sharma R, Khristov V, Rising A, et al. Clinical-grade stem cell-derived retinal pigment epithelium patch rescues retinal degeneration in rodents and pigs. Sci Transl Med 2019;11(475): eaat5580.

[59] Sharma A, Jaganathan BG. Stem cell therapy for retinal degeneration: the evidence to date. Biologics 2021;15:299–306.

Advances in Ophthalmology and Optometry 8 (2023) 179–189

ADVANCES IN OPHTHALMOLOGY AND OPTOMETRY

Advances in Pneumatic Retinopexy

Challenges and Innovations

Ravneet S. Rai, MD[a], Rina Su, MD[a], Samuel Gelnick, MD[a], Ronni M. Lieberman, MD[b],*, Alan Sheyman, MD[b],1

[a]Department of Ophthalmology, Northwell Health Eye Institute, 600 Northern Boulevard, Suite 214, Great Neck, NY 11021, USA; [b]Department of Ophthalmology, Mount Sinai Health Systems, New York, NY, USA

Keywords
- Pneumatic retinopexy • Rhegmatogenous retinal detachment • Gas bubble
- Laser retinopexy • Cryotherapy

Key points
- Pneumatic retinopexy uses injection of a gas bubble along with cryotherapy or laser photocoagulation and patient positioning to repair rhegmatogenous retinal detachments.
- Pneumatic retinopexy classically treats breaks within the superior 8 clock hours; however, expanded indications during the past decades also have been shown to be successful, with no difference in anatomic outcomes and superior visual outcomes as compared with pars plana vitrectomy and scleral buckling.
- New or missed retinal breaks are the most common complications and largest contributions to failure.
- As a procedure performed in the office rather than in an operating room, pneumatic retinopexy allows for increased convenience, decreased morbidity, and improved health, saving costs.

F irst described by George Hilton in 1986 [1], pneumatic retinopexy has become an important technique for repairing select retinal detachments in the office setting. It has since become a well-accepted alternative to

[1]Present address: 82-68 164th Street Pavilion. 452. Jamaica. NY 11432.

*Corresponding author. 82-68 164th Street Pavilion, 452, Jamaica, NY 11432. E-mail address: liebermr@nychhc.org

https://doi.org/10.1016/j.yaoo.2023.02.011
2452-1760/23/© 2023 Elsevier Inc. All rights reserved.

scleral buckling and vitrectomy for repair of select cases of rhegmatogenous retinal detachments, and has been used for expanded indications in the decades since its introduction [2]. Pneumatic retinopexy offers the opportunity to repair rhegmatogenous retinal detachments in the superior 8 clock hours of the fundus at lower cost, with less tissue trauma, and with minimal complications [2].

Pneumatic retinopexy involves 3 steps: injection of a gas bubble to tamponade a superior retinal break, use of laser photocoagulation or cryotherapy to create permanent adhesions between the choroid and retina 360° around the break, and patient positioning after the procedure to keep the bubble tamponade in place. This technique relies on the surface tension of the bubble to retain its shape and prevent its passage into the subretinal space. It also uses the buoyancy of the gas to provide constant upwards pressure on the retina against the eye's wall [3].

The gas bubble must be adequate to cover all breaks. A 60° retinal arc can be covered by a 0.3-cc gas bubble, and a 90° arc requires a 1.2-cc gas bubble [3]. Individual ocular characteristics should be considered, as for instance a myopic eye will require a larger volume of gas to cover the same amount of retinal surface as an emmetropic eye [3]. In the United States, gases used for the procedure are SF6 and C3F8. These gases have the ideal properties for intraocular use in retinopexy: they are inert, they last for an adequate amount of time to allow for the retinopexy scar to form, and they expand to allow for all breaks to be covered [2,4]. The size of the injected SF6 will double between 24 and 36 hours after injection and can last up to 12 days in the eye. C3F8 will quadruple in size by 3 days after injection and lasts around 38 days in the eye [2].

The ideal patient for pneumatic retinopexy is one who is phakic [5–7], has a superior retinal break, and will be compliant with head positioning for up to 16 hours per day after the procedure. Worse operative outcomes in pseudophakic eyes may be due to posterior capsular opacification preventing full examination of the peripheral retina, with resultant failure to identify additional small peripheral breaks [8]. Ideally, patients should have a single break, or multiple breaks confined to 1 clock hour. Cases in which pneumatic retinopexy can be particularly effective include those with retinal breaks located under the superior rectus muscle (which avoids the diplopia created by scleral buckle), recurrent retinal detachment following scleral buckle, and large, irregular breaks difficult to repair with scleral buckle [2,3]. Pneumatic retinopexy is most useful when one is not considering a pars plana vitrectomy (PPV). Pneumatic retinopexy also may be favored over scleral buckling in patients with thin sclera at risk of perforation or those with conjunctival scarring that makes peritomy in scleral buckling difficult [2].

Pneumatic retinopexy commonly is performed in the outpatient office setting, and, depending on the protocol that is used, the procedure may take anywhere from 30 minutes to more than 2 hours (Fig. 1) [9]. As an office-based procedure, it obviates an anesthesiologist, an operating room, and perioperative staff. First, the patient is dilated and examined to identify all retinal

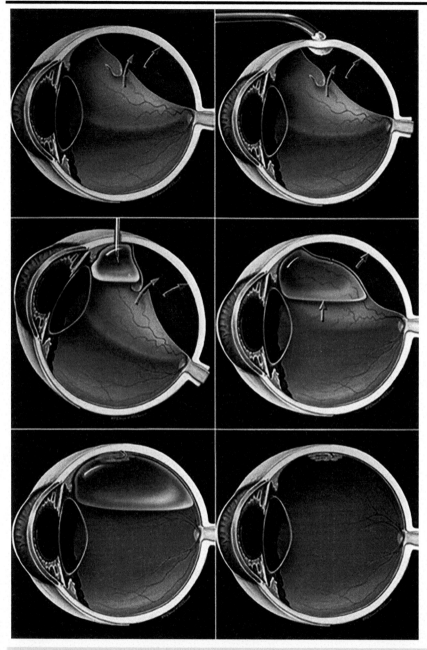

Fig. 1. Top left: Vitreous fluid flows through a retinal break (*green arrow*) causing a rhegmatogenous retinal detachment. Top right: Cryotherapy is used to treat the area of retinal break. Middle left: A gas bubble is injected with a 30-gauge needle through the pars plana. Middle right: The patient's head is repositioned to allow the expanding gas bubble to cover the retinal break and prevent further subretinal vitreous flow through the break. Bottom left: The break is closed and the retina is reattached. Bottom right: The gas bubble is reabsorbed. RPE (*red arrow*). (*From* Hilton GF, Grizzard WS. Pneumatic retinopexy. A two-step outpatient operation without conjunctival incision. Ophthalmology. 1986;93(5):626-641.)

breaks. The peripheral retina is examined with scleral depression to ensure that no breaks are missed [9]. The eye is prepped with an antiseptic solution such as 5% povidone iodine solution and is draped in sterile fashion [9]. A local anesthetic is usually administered subconjunctivally but a retrobulbar or peribulbar block may be used as well.

The gas, usually SF6 or C3F8, is injected into the vitreous using a 30G needle through the pars plana [9]. Retinopexy may be performed via cryotherapy either before injection of the gas, or 1 to 2 days after. Alternatively, laser retinopexy can be performed either on the same day, after the gas has been injected, or 1 to 2 days later [9]. Same day laser may be difficult because the gas may form "fish eggs," and it may be difficult to visualize the retina through them. Waiting a day or two for the gas bubble to coalesce is usually best. In many cases, repeated cryopexy or laser retinopexy can be performed in the days following the procedure [9]. One may need to repeat the laser on multiple, consecutive days.

It is important to monitor the intraocular pressure after the procedure, both immediately and on subsequent visits. Mild-to-moderate increases in intraocular pressure usually are well tolerated; however, patients who are susceptible to glaucoma or have poor arterial perfusion should be treated for elevated pressures. Treatment includes topical or oral hypotensive medications but a paracentesis may be necessary if intraocular pressures are not adequately lowered or evidence exists of central retinal artery nonperfusion [9]. Following the procedure, the patient must keep strict positioning for up to 18 hours per day for 1 week, or half of all hours for 2 weeks [9]. Tamponade of the retina with the gas bubble for this length of time allows for the bond between retina and RPE to reach its maximal strength after retinopexy [10]. Close monitoring of the eye is required to minimize complications [2].

Single operation anatomic success rate for pneumatic retinopexy is around 75%, with final operative anatomic success at 96%, new retinal breaks occurring in 12% and development of proliferative vitreoretinopathy in 5% of patients [2]. Primary pneumatic retinopexy has been compared with primary PPV in repairing rhegmatogenous retinal detachments. Although the single operation anatomic success rate for PPV at 93% was significantly higher than that of pneumatic retinopexy at 81% in a large randomized trial, the final anatomic success rate was similar in the 2 groups at 98.7% and 98.6%, respectively [11].

Since pneumatic retinopexy was first introduced by Dr Hilton, challenges inherent to the technique have been solved by enterprising retinal surgeons. For instance, pneumatic retinopexy creates the risk of iatrogenic macular detachment by pushing extramacular subretinal fluid under the macula [12]. This challenge led to the development of the steamroller technique (Fig. 2). In this modification of pneumatic retinopexy, the patient is positioned facedown for approximately 5 hours immediately after intravitreal gas injection [12]. The buoyant gas bubble immediately pushes some fluid out through the retinal break. After 5 hours, the head is elevated by 30° per hour until the patient is fully upright.

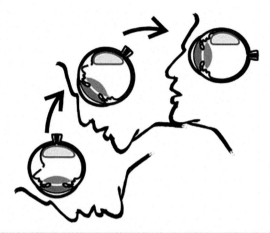

Fig. 2. The steamroller technique where the patient starts in a facedown position after gas bubble injection. Gradual elevation of the head allows for the subretinal fluid to be slowly pushed by the gas bubble from the posterior to superior fundus away from the macula. (*From* Chan CK, Lin SG, Nuthi AS, Salib DM. Pneumatic retinopexy for the repair of retinal detachments: a comprehensive review (1986-2007). Surv Ophthalmol. 2008;53(5):443-478.)

In this way, the gas bubble slowly pushes, or "steamrolls," the subretinal fluid superiorly toward the superior retinal break and away from the macula [12]. At the end of the maneuver, the gas bubble tamponades the superior retinal break against the RPE, allowing for easy subsequent laser [2].

Although pneumatic retinopexy has become a proven technique that has established its place in the retina surgeon's armamentarium, after more than 35 years in use, it remains with its challenges. The surgeon must be meticulous and skilled in detecting all retinal breaks. Inadequate detection can lead to failure of the procedure. Novel or missed breaks constitute one of the most common complications after pneumatic retinopexy [12]. Unlike scleral buckling or PPV, the retinal surgeon performing pneumatic retinopexy does not have the opportunity to examine the retina under anesthesia or, as in the case of PPV, surgically clear any vitreous opacities to provide an unobstructed view to the far peripheral retina [13].

Although pneumatic retinopexy traditionally has been used in cases of small retinal breaks in the superior 8 clock hours, it has also been used in other scenarios as well. Cases in which pneumatic retinopexy have been used, and which had previously thought to be contraindications include eyes with a small amount of vitreous hemorrhage, small proliferative vitreoretinopathy, lattice, degeneration, giant retinal tears, multiple retinal breaks in multiple clock hours, absence of a previously identified break, and even inferior breaks [14]. In a study of 141 eyes with rhegmatogenous retinal detachment, eyes were separated into traditional or nontraditional groups based on their preoperative characteristics. The traditional group had the ideal candidates for pneumatic retinopexy, with a single retinal break or multiple superior breaks within 1 clock hour. The nontraditional group had previously contraindicated characteristics as described above [14]. Anatomic success did not differ between the traditional and nontraditional groups (84.1% vs 74.4%, $P = .16$), and no difference occurred in visual outcome at 6 months. However, anatomic failure was significantly associated with the presence of an inferior retinal break [14].

The difficulty with treating inferior retinal breaks with pneumatic retinopexy is due to the postprocedure patient positioning required, which involves remaining prone with a pillow under the chest to keep the head at a negative angle [15]. An alternative, more comfortable, postprocedure position for inferior retinal breaks has recently been described. Rather than remaining prone on top of a pillow, patients maintained a lateral recumbent position with varying degrees of head tilt. This positioning resulted in a good final result with only mild patient discomfort [15].

Pneumatic retinopexy also has been used as a rescue procedure in cases of unsuccessful scleral buckles and pars plana vitrectomies [12]. After vitrectomy and scleral buckle, rhegmatogenous retinal detachment most commonly recurs due to retinal breaks that were missed during the original procedure, or are novel due to the entry site in vitrectomy [16]. A study of 42 cases of rhegmatogenous retinal detachment that failed primary scleral buckling or vitrectomy, 100% of the scleral buckling group and 90% of the vitrectomy group were successfully reattached with a single pneumatic retinopexy procedure [16]. In these patients who would otherwise have to return to the operating room for a second costly surgery, pneumatic retinopexy offers the opportunity for a quick and inexpensive repair that can be performed in the office at a lower cost and with generally excellent results [16].

As mentioned earlier, the final anatomic success rates between pneumatic retinopexy and other methods of rhegmatogenous retinal detachment repair are similar [11]. Shortly after pneumatic retinopexy was first described by Dr Hilton, a large, randomized, multicenter trial with nearly 200 patients compared anatomic results and final visual outcomes between pneumatic retinopexy and scleral buckling [17]. The patients in this trial had the classic indications for pneumatic retinopexy: retinal breaks less than or equal in size to 1 clock hour, located within the superior two-thirds of the retina, and with minimal or no proliferative vitreoretinopathy [17].

After a minimum of 6 months postoperatively, pneumatic retinopexy was no different than scleral buckling with regard to single-operation success rate, overall success rate, rate of proliferative vitreoretinopathy, and novel retinal breaks [17]. With similar anatomical outcomes to scleral buckling, pneumatic retinopexy had statistically superior postoperative visual acuity and less morbidity [17]. These results held in the same group of patients 2 years after surgery, with similar surgical success rates between pneumatic retinopexy and scleral buckling, and significantly better final visual outcome with pneumatic retinopexy [18].

PPV eventually superseded scleral buckling as the preferred method of rhegmatogenous retinal detachment repair globally [11]. The Pneumatic Retinopexy versus Vitrectomy for the Management of Primary Rhegmatogenous Retinal Detachment Outcomes Randomized Trial (PIVOT) compared 1-year Early Treatment Diabetic Retinopathy Study visual acuity between pneumatic retinopexy and PPV 1 year postoperatively [11]. Inclusion criteria for the trial were again the classic indications for pneumatic retinopexy: retinal break no larger than 1 clock hour, and all breaks in detached retina occurring between the 8:00 and 4:00 sectors. This trial did, however, allow for breaks in any area of attached retina, including the inferior quadrant.

The study included 176 patients. Visual acuity was better in the pneumatic retinopexy group at both 3 and 12 months postoperatively. A composite score measuring visual function outcomes were higher in the pneumatic retinopexy group at 3 and 6 months postoperatively. Pneumatic retinopexy patients had less metamorphopsia at 12 months. No statistically significant difference existed in primary or secondary anatomic success at 12 months [11]. Pneumatic retinopexy offers equivalent, if not superior, postoperative results while simultaneously avoiding morbidity associated with anesthesia and reducing time and financial strain for the patient.

Most cases of failure occur within 1 month of the procedure, and of these failures, most occur within 10 days [19]. Although factors such as poor preoperative visual acuity, pseudophakia/aphakia, and older age contribute to the risk of failure, the greatest predictor is a new or missed break causing redetachment [19]. New retinal breaks may occur due to increased traction from a gas bubble located between the retina and posterior hyaloid face. Approximately three-quarters of new breaks after pneumatic retinopexy are located in the upper two-thirds of the retina and just more than one-half are located within 3 clock hours of the initial break [13].

Reopening of the original break also can occur. This is of concern in pneumatic retinopexy because, unlike in scleral buckling or PPV, no release occurs of vitreoretinal traction in this technique [13]. The strength of the chorioretinal adhesion due to the applied cryopexy or laser retinopexy is solely relied on to counter the force of retinal traction [13].

Fortunately, even in cases of primary pneumatic retinopexy failure, the retinal break can be successfully repaired with another procedure. In a study comparing 42 eyes that underwent PPV after a failed pneumatic retinopexy to 29 eyes that were successfully treated with a single PPV, no difference occurred in anatomical retinal reattachment or visual acuity [20]. It is important to note that in cases of failed pneumatic retinopexy, a repeat pneumatic retinopexy has significantly worse outcomes than rescue with scleral buckle or vitrectomy [21]. Therefore, although pneumatic retinopexy is an excellent rescue technique for failed vitrectomy or scleral buckle, it should not be relied on as a rescue for itself.

Some complications associated with the procedure itself include subretinal trapping of gas, endophthalmitis, macular hole, proliferative vitreoretinopathy, choroidal detachment, and increase in intraocular pressure [2]. These complications generally are infrequent and also can be seen in other techniques used to repair rhegmatogenous retinal detachments [2]. Beyond procedural complications, one negative aspect of pneumatic retinopexy is the postoperative care required. In comparison to scleral buckling and PPV, pneumatic retinopexy places a significant postoperative burden on the patient with strict positioning for most of the day for up to several weeks [9]. The patient also is required to be seen in the office on (potentially) a daily basis and undergo repeated, potentially painful laser treatment.

Given postoperative positioning difficulties and issues with patient compliance, Velez-Montoya and colleagues developed a novel wearable device to monitor head position and provide real-time positioning data. The device, a specially designed headband, included an accelerometer, gyroscope, and magnetometer [22]. The device measured neck flexion, extension, and rotation every 200 milliseconds [22]. The device was capable of recording neck position for an extended period without failure. An adequate head position was recorded on average 17% of the time [22]. The medical wearables market is rapidly growing, with US market value of US$7.4 billion in 2018 and a compound annual growth rate of 18.3% [23]. As the medical wearables industry continues to expand, similar devices may be developed commercially. This will allow retinal surgeons to monitor patient positioning compliance and provide the opportunity to give encouragement and correction at follow-up visits.

New avenues in pneumatic retinopexy research focusing on postoperative anatomic changes have been explored. Muni and colleagues examined the anatomic basis behind the superior visual outcomes in pneumatic retinopexy compared with PPV in the PIVOT trial. Among the 176 patients enrolled in the trial, a total of 150 patients completed the 1-year follow-up visit. Postoperative retinal optical coherence tomography (OCT) scans of the PPV and pneumatic retinopexy groups were compared. About 24% of the foveal scans in the PPV group showed ellipsoid zone discontinuity versus 7% in the pneumatic retinopexy group [24]. About 20% of the PPV group versus 6% of the pneumatic retinopexy showed external limiting membrane discontinuity [24]. Improved photoreceptor preservation in pneumatic retinopexy compared with PPV, therefore, may explain the superior visual outcomes.

Kaderli and colleagues studied microvascular changes that occur in rhegmatogenous retinal detachments occurring after pneumatic retinopexy. OCT angiography was used to assess alterations in macular perfusion 1 and 3 months after pneumatic retinopexy in macula-on or macula-off rhegmatogenous retinal detachments, with fellow eyes serving as controls [25]. One month after pneumatic retinopexy, vessel density of the superficial and deep capillary plexuses was significantly lower in the macula-off group compared with the macula-on group. However, by the third month, vessel density increased significantly in the macula-off group, and no difference occurred in vessel density between the treated and fellow eyes in both the macula-on and macula-off groups

[25]. Similar results were seen when looking at the choriocapillaris flow area. The authors attributed the lack of difference between vessel density and choriocapillaris flow area between eyes treated with pneumatic retinopexy and fellow eyes at 3 months postoperatively to the relatively low invasiveness of the procedure, especially compared with PPV [25].

In addition to visual and anatomic success, the use of pneumatic retinopexy involves significant cost savings. Pneumatic retinopexy can readily be performed in an outpatient office and does not need the supplemental resources and staffing required in an operating room. The procedure is minimally invasive and, therefore, does not have the risks involved with sedation or general anesthesia. Furthermore, the easier accessibility equates to saved time and opportunity costs for patients and surgeons. In a study of 178 eyes treated with primary pneumatic retinopexy, the total average cost for the procedure in cases traditionally indicated for repair with the technique was US$1248.37 ± US$882.11 and the total average cost of the procedure for nontraditional indications (as described previously) was US$1471.91 ± US$942.84. This represented a cost savings of 62% when compared with scleral buckle and 61% when compared with PPV. In this study, all procedures were performed by the same surgeon, eliminating the effect of intersurgeon variability on the final total costs [26]. This, however, may not include the cost of the surgeon's time (repeated office visits/laser) and its remuneration.

Approximately 15% of all rhegmatogenous retinal detachments in the United States are currently repaired using pneumatic retinopexy [14]. In the period 2000–2014, the rates of scleral buckling and pneumatic retinopexy have both declined in the United States compared with PPV, which has increased significantly to 83% of all vitreoretinal surgeries [27]. However, cost analysis studies have shown pneumatic retinopexy is nearly 50% more favorable compared with PPV [28]. Increasing utilization to 20% to 35% has been hypothesized to save US$6 to 30 million worth of annual health costs [14].

Pneumatic retinopexy has established itself in vitreoretinal surgery during the past 4 decades. It allows for the repair of rhegmatogenous retinal detachments, particularly those with breaks that are small, located superiorly, and is otherwise uncomplicated, with the injection of intraocular gas and careful postoperative positioning. As it can be performed in the office, it obviates an operating room, operating staff, or anesthesia. Thus, it reduces the morbidity and financial costs associated with retinal detachment repair. It may also be effective as a rescue procedure for failed primary scleral buckles or pars plana vitrectomies. The indications for pneumatic retinopexy have expanded in the decades since its introduction, with numerous groups demonstrating success in cases that were previously thought to be contraindicated. In comparison to PPV and scleral buckling, final anatomic success rate has been found to be no different and visual outcomes may be superior. The tissue-level physiologic changes that occur after pneumatic retinopexy are an active area of investigation.

CLINICS CARE POINTS

- When considering pneumatic retinopexy for the repair of a retinal detachment, close attention should be paid to the characteristics of the detachment, including phakic status, location of breaks, presence of proliferative vitreoretinopathy, and patient compliance with instructions.
- A careful scleral depressed examination should be performed on all patients who are planned for pneumatic retinopexy.
- Close monitoring of intraocular pressure is critical during and after the procedure.
- Patients should be counseled that they make require numerous, potentially painful, laser treatments.
- Postoperative visits within 1 month are essential because most incidences of failure occur within 1 month of the procedure.
- A repeat pneumatic retinopexy should not be performed in the case of failure—consider PPV and/or scleral buckle as rescue instead.

DISCLOSURE

The authors have nothing to disclose.

References

[1] Hilton GF, Sanderson Grizzard W. Pneumatic retinopexy: a two-step outpatient operation without conjunctival incision. Ophthalmology 1986;93(5):626–41.

[2] Chan CK. Pneumatic retinopexy for the repair of retinal detachments: a comprehensive review (1986–2007). Surv Ophthalmol 2008;53(5):443–78.

[3] Hilton GF. Pneumatic retinopexy: principles and practice. Indian J Ophthalmol 1996;44(3): 131.

[4] Tornambe PE. Pneumatic retinopexy. Surv Ophthalmol 1988;32(4):270–81.

[5] Abecia E. Anatomic results and complications in a long-term follow-up of pneumatic retinopexy cases. Retina 2000;20(2):156–61, Philadelphia, Pa.

[6] Eter N, Böker T, Spitznas M. Long-term results of pneumatic retinopexy. Graefes Arch Clin Exp Ophthalmol 2000;238(8):677–81.

[7] Grizzard WS. Pneumatic retinopexy failures: cause, prevention, timing, and management. Ophthalmology 1995;102(6):929–36.

[8] Sharma T. A multivariate analysis of anatomic success of recurrent retinal detachment treated with pneumatic retinopexy. Ophthalmology 1997;104(12):2014–7.

[9] Chronopoulos A, Hattenbach L-O, Schutz JS. Pneumatic retinopexy: a critical reappraisal. Surv Ophthalmol 2021;66(4):585–93.

[10] Yoon YH, Marmor MF. Rapid enhancement of retinal adhesion by laser photocoagulation. Ophthalmology 1988;95(10):1385–8.

[11] Hillier RJ. The pneumatic retinopexy versus vitrectomy for the management of primary rhegmatogenous retinal detachment outcomes randomized trial (PIVOT). Ophthalmology 2019;126(4):531–9.

[12] Huang C-Y, Mikowski M, Wu L. Pneumatic retinopexy: an update. Graefes Arch Clin Exp Ophthalmol 2022;260(3):711–22.

[13] Holz ER, Mieler WF. View 3: the case for pneumatic retinopexy. Br J Ophthalmol 2003;87(6):787–9.

[14] Goldman DR, Shah CP, Heier JS. Expanded criteria for pneumatic retinopexy and potential cost savings. Ophthalmology 2014;121(1):318–26.
[15] Hwang J-F, Chen S-Ni, Lin C-J. Treatment of inferior rhegmatogenous retinal detachment by pneumatic retinopexy technique. Retina 2011;31(2):257–61.
[16] Petrushkin HJD, Elgohary MA, Sullivan PM. Rescue pneumatic retinopexy in patients with failed primary retinal detachment surgery. Retina 2015;35(9):1851–9.
[17] Tornambe PE. Pneumatic retinopexy: a multicenter randomized controlled clinical trial comparing pneumatic retinopexy with scleral buckling. Ophthalmology 1989;96(6): 772–84.
[18] Tornambe PE. Pneumatic retinopexy: two-year follow-up study of the multicenter clinical trial comparing pneumatic retinopexy with scleral buckling. Ophthalmology 1991;98(7): 1115–23.
[19] Gorovoy IR. Characterization of pneumatic retinopexy failures and the pneumatic pump: a new complication of pneumatic retinopexy. Retina 2014;34(4):700–4.
[20] Demircan A. Comparison of pars plana vitrectomy for retinal detachment after failed pneumatic retinopexy and primary pars plana vitrectomy. J Fr Ophtalmol 2019;42(2):146–52.
[21] Vidne-Hay O. Outcomes of rhegmatogenous retinal detachment repair after failed pneumatic retinopexy. Retina 2020;40(5):805–10.
[22] Velez-Montoya R, León AG-H, Hernández-Quintela E. Assessment of postural compliance after pneumatic retinopexy. Translational Vision Science & Technology 2019;8(3):4.
[23] Mück JE. Market and patent analyses of wearables in medicine. Trends Biotechnol 2019;37(6):563–6.
[24] Muni RH. Postoperative photoreceptor integrity following pneumatic retinopexy vs pars plana vitrectomy for retinal detachment repair: a post hoc optical coherence tomography analysis from the pneumatic retinopexy versus vitrectomy for the management of primary rhegmatogenous retinal detachment outcomes randomized trial. JAMA Ophthalmology 2021;139(6):620–7.
[25] Kaderli ST, Karalezli A, Sul S. Microvascular retinal alterations in rhegmatogenous retinal detachment after pneumatic retinopexy. Acta Ophthalmol 2021;99(4):383–9.
[26] Jung JJ. Anatomic, visual, and financial outcomes for traditional and nontraditional primary pneumatic retinopexy for retinal detachment. Am J Ophthalmol 2019;200:187–200.
[27] McLaughlin MD, Hwang JC. Trends in vitreoretinal procedures for medicare beneficiaries, 2000 to 2014. Ophthalmology 2017;124(5):667–73.
[28] Elhusseiney AM, Yannuzzi NA, Smiddy WE. Cost analysis of pneumatic retinopexy versus pars plana vitrectomy for rhegmatogenous retinal detachment. Ophthalmology Retina 2019;3(11):956–61.

Advances in Ophthalmology and Optometry 8 (2023) 191–211

ADVANCES IN OPHTHALMOLOGY AND OPTOMETRY

Ocular Toxicity of Immunotherapy and Targeted Antineoplastic Agents

Nancy Worley, MD[a], Kyle Hirabayashi, MD[b],
Robin Ginsburg, MD[a,b,*]

[a]Department of Ophthalmology, Icahn School of Medicine at Mount Sinai, 1 Gustave L. Levy Place, New York, NY 10029, USA; [b]Department of Ophthalmology, New York Eye and Ear Infirmary at Mount Sinai, 310 East 14th Street, New York, NY 10003, USA

Keywords
- Immunotherapy • Antineoplastic therapy • Ocular toxicity

Key points
- Targeted immunotherapy has been associated with a variety of ocular toxicities, including dry eye syndrome, uveitis, corneal abnormalities, retinopathy, and retinal vein occlusions.
- Ocular toxicity associated with targeted immunotherapy may require cessation or adjustments to therapy.
- It is important for oncologists and ophthalmologists to know and recognize ocular toxicities associated with antineoplastic therapy and to communicate with each other regarding treatment.

INTRODUCTION
In this article, the authors aim to review known and suspected ocular toxicities of rapidly expanding and increasingly used oncologic immunotherapies as well as targeted therapies.

Traditionally, the mainstays of cancer treatment have been cytotoxic chemotherapy, radiation, and surgical excision. It is well established that life-saving chemotherapeutic medications and radiation used to treat malignancy can have ocular side effects. In recent decades, however, molecular targeted agents

*Corresponding author. Department of Ophthalmology, Icahn School of Medicine at Mount Sinai, 1 Gustave L. Levy Place, New York, NY 10029, USA.Department of Ophthalmologylcahn School of Medicine at Mount Sinai1 Gustave L. Levy PlaceNew YorkNY10029USA

https://doi.org/10.1016/j.yaoo.2023.02.012

and immune-based therapies have significantly improved outcomes of patients with cancer and revolutionized the way oncologists treat malignancies [1]. Importantly, although targeted therapies and immunotherapies generally are more tolerable than classical chemotherapy, ocular toxicities have been observed with several of these novel agents. With the advent of targeted and immune therapies, it is essential that oncologists and ophthalmologists be aware of associated ocular adverse events.

The earliest form of immunotherapy was allogeneic bone marrow transplantation first used in the 1950s, through which donor T cells could ferret out and destroy residual leukemic blasts leading to durable remissions [2]. Donor immunity also could activate the recipients' healthy tissue (so-called graft-versus-host disease [GVHD]), with ocular GVHD being a common chronic manifestation [3]. As the molecular composition and biology of malignancies became better understood, therapies targeted to specific tumor antigens or signaling pathways emerged. Monoclonal antibodies, like *trastuzumab* for HER2-positive breast cancer and *rituximab* for non-Hodgkin lymphoma, became central components of cancer therapy. In recent years, oncologic immunotherapy has been revolutionized by the development of chimeric antigen receptor (CAR) T-cell therapy and immune checkpoint inhibitors, first offered to patients with cancer in the 2010s. Unfortunately, improved outcomes also come with unique and potentially serious side effects. In this article, the authors review a wide breadth of immunotherapies as well as targeted cancer treatments, specifically focusing on their ocular side effects (Table 1). It is imperative that ophthalmologists continue to become more knowledgeable in identifying and managing the complications of these immunotherapies, as their use continues to expand in the types of malignancies treated and utilization becomes more widespread.

SIGNIFICANCE
Biologic drug nomenclature
Traditionally, biologic therapy referred to medications that came from an organic source. More recently, the term "biologics" refers to medications produced by biotechnology methods. Many biologic drugs are named based on their molecular structure and mechanism of action.

The following is an example of a drug described later in this article:
Neci-tum-u-mab
The first segment of the name is determined by the drug developer [4].

The second segment describes the target or disease class with, at times, the addition of a vowel to aid in pronunciation [4]. "B" indicates bacterial, "c" is for cardiovascular, "f" is for antifungal, "k" is for interleukin, "l" is for immunomodulator, "n" is for neuron, "s" is for bone, "t" is for tumor, and "v" for virus [4]. The naming system has changed over time, and older drugs do not follow this current system exactly. In the example above, "tum" indicates that the target is a tumor, and, since that time, "tum" has been replaced by "t" [4].

Table 1
Ocular toxicities by medication class

Medication class	Agents	Ocular toxicities
Immune checkpoint inhibitors	CTLA-4 inhibitors: • Ipilimumab • Tremelimumab PD-1 inhibitors: • Pembrolizumab • Nivolumab • Cemiplimab PD-L1 inhibitors: • Atezolizumab • Avelumab • Durvalumab	• Dry eye [5] • Blepharitis [5] • Conjunctivitis [5] • Episcleritis [5] • Scleritis [5] • Ulcerative keratitis [5] • Corneal graft rejection [5] • Corneal perforation [5] • Uveitis [7] • Vogt-Koyanagi-Harada-like syndrome [7] • Acute macular neuroretinopathy, paracentral acute middle maculopathy with retinal vasculitis or venulitis [7]
MEK inhibitors	• Binimetinib • Cobimetinib • Selumetinib • Trametinib	• MEKAR [8] • Retinal vein occlusion [5] • Uveitis [5]
BRAF inhibitors	• Dabrafenib • Encorafenib • Vemurafenib	• Uveitis [10] • Conjunctivitis [10] • Dry eyes [10] • Retinal vein occlusion [5]
BCR-ABL inhibitors	• Imatinib • Nilotinib • Dasatinib • Bosutinib • Ponatinib • Asciminib	• Periorbital edema [5] • Epiphora [11] • Macular edema [5] • Optic neuritis [5]
SERMs	• Tamoxifen • Raloxifene • Toremifene	• Keratopathy [5,12] • Crystalline retinopathy ± macular edema [5] • Posterior subcapsular cataracts [5] • Retinal vein occlusion [5]
Aromatase inhibitors	• Anastrozole • Letrozole • Exemestane	• Blepharitis [13,14] • Meibomian gland dysfunction [13,14] • Dry eyes [13,14]
JAK2 inhibitors	• Ruxolitinib • Tofacitinib • Baricitinib • Fedratinib • Upadacitinib	• Eyelash growth [5] • Herpes zoster [5] • Toxoplasmosis retinitis [5] • Cytomegalovirus retinitis [5] • Aspergillosis-associated retinal necrosis [5]

(continued on next page)

Table 1
(continued)

Medication class	Agents	Ocular toxicities
FLT3 inhibitors	• Sorafenib • Sunitinib • Midostaurin • Gilteritinib • Regorafenib	• Periocular edema [15] • Dry eye [5] • Eyelash discoloration [15] • Retinal tears [15] • Retinal detachments [15] • Retinal vein occlusion [15] • Retinal artery occlusion [15] • Optic neuropathy [5] • Cataracts [16] • Retinal hemorrhages [15] • Uveitis [15] • Macular edema [15]
BTK inhibitors	• Ibrutinib • Acalabrutinib • Zanubrutinib	• Dry eye [17] • Red eye [17] • Branch retinal artery occlusion [17]
EGFR inhibitors	• Gefitinib • Erlotinib • Afatanib • Brigatinib • Cetuximab • Osimertinib • Dacomitinib • Panitumumab • Necitumumab	• Blepharitis [5] • Periorbital rash [5] • Periorbital edema [5] • Ectropion [5] • Conjunctivitis [5] • Dry eye [5] • Keratopathy (vortex) [5] • Persistent corneal epithelial defect [5] • Trichomegaly [5] • Corneal ulcer [5] • Corneal perforation [5] • Uveitis [5] • Macular edema [5]
FGFR inhibitors	• Ponatinib • Erdafitinib	• Central serous retinopathy [18] • Corneal thinning [19]
KIT inhibitors	• Avapritinib • Ripretinib	• Periorbital edema [20] • Increased lacrimation [20]
HER2 inhibitors	• Trastuzumab • Pertuzumab • Lapatanib • Neratinib • Tucatinib	• Infectious crystalline keratopathy [21] • Corneal ulceration [22] • Increased lacrimation [5]
VEGFR inhibitors	• Sorafenib • Sunitinib • Vandetanib • Lenvatinib • Axitinib • Bevacizumab • Ramucirumab • Cabozantinib • Pazopanib	• Retinal tears [15] • Retinal detachment [15] • Subconjunctival hemorrhage [5] • Retinal artery occlusion [5] • Retinal vein occlusion [5] • Ocular motility disorders [5] • Corneal abnormalities (vortex keratopathy) [5] • Increased lacrimation [5] • Optic neuropathy [5]

(continued on next page)

Table 1
(*continued*)

Medication class	Agents	Ocular toxicities
mTOR inhibitors	• Everolimus • Temsirolimus	• Eyelid edema [5]
CDK inhibitors	• Palbociclib • Ribociclib • Abemaciclib	• Dry eye [5] • Increased lacrimation [5]
Proteasome inhibitors	• Bortezomib • Carfilzomib • Ixazomib	• Chalazia [5,24–26] • Conjunctivitis [5]
Antibody-drug conjugates	• Trastuzumab deruxtecan • Belantamab mafodotin • Trastuzumab emtansine • Enfortumab vedotin • Gemtuzumab ozogamicin • Sacituzumab govitecan • Inotuzumab ozogamicin	• Lacrimal drainage stenosis [5] • Dry eye [5] • Microcyst-like corneal epithelial abnormalities [5]
CAR T therapy	• Axicabtagene ciloleucel	• oGVHD [27] • Acute retinal necrosis [27]

The third segment describes the source, with "o" indicating mouse, "u" indicating fully human, "xi" means chimeric (approximately two-thirds human and one-third mouse), and "z" means humanized (approximately 95% human) [4].

The final segment determines the structure. *Necitumumab* ends in "-mab," indicating that it is a monoclonal antibody, a large molecule drug produced with DNA technology from microorganisms, plant, or animal cells [4].

In contrast, drugs composed of small molecules are chemically synthesized and act intracellularly, and these drug names end in "-mib" or "-nib" [4]. Drugs with names that end in "-mib" slow proliferation intracellularly and increase apoptosis [4]. Specifically, the suffix "-zomib" is used to describe protease or proteasome inhibitors [4]. "-nib" is used to describe kinase enzyme inhibitors [4]. "-tinib" is designated for tyrosine kinase inhibitors; "-anib" is for angiogenesis inhibitors, and "-rafenib" is for rapidly accelerated fibrosarcoma (RAF) kinase inhibitors [4].

Immune checkpoint inhibitors

Immune checkpoint inhibitors are monoclonal antibodies that block proteins produced by T cells that downregulate the immune response, leading to up-regulation of T-cell antitumor activity [5]. This class of medications is categorized based on the ligand that is targeted, consisting of cytotoxic T-lymphocyte–associated antigen 4 (CTLA-4) inhibitors *ipilimumab* and *tremelimumab*, programmed cell death 1 (PD-1) inhibitors *pembrolizumab, nivolumab,* and *cemiplimab*, and programmed cell death ligand 1 (PD-L1) inhibitors *atezolizumab, avelumab,* and *durvalumab* [6]. These medications are used to treat metastatic melanoma, renal cell carcinoma, colon cancer, lung cancer, head and neck cancer, urothelial carcinoma, Merkel cell carcinoma, breast cancer, cervical cancer, and endometrial cancer [6].

Immune checkpoint inhibitors have been found to adversely affect the eyes in multiple ways. **Dry eye** is one of the most frequent ocular side effects of checkpoint inhibitors, with incidence ranging from 1% to 24% [5]. **Blepharitis, conjunctivitis, episcleritis, scleritis, ulcerative keratitis, corneal graft rejection**, and **corneal perforation** also have been associated with these medications [5].

Uveitis occurs in 1% of patients, with one literature review identifying 126 patients and 241 eyes with uveitis, including anterior (37.7%), intermediate (0.01%), posterior (25.7%), and panuveitis (34%), with 28 eyes from 15 patients found to have **Vogt-Koyanagi-Harada–like syndrome** [7]. Uveitis developed at a median of 9 weeks after initiation of checkpoint inhibitor therapy, and 83.6% of patients developed it within 6 months [7]. Of cases of uveitis, 93.5% were bilateral [7]. Systemic therapy was held in 11.4% of cases and discontinued in 51.4% of cases, with uveitis being the reason for holding or discontinuing therapy in 83% of these cases [7]. Of the few patients who restarted therapy, 58.3% had another episode of uveitis [7]. *Atezolizumab* was associated with a higher incidence of posterior uveitis (80%) compared with other immune checkpoint inhibitors (23.7%), with 10 of 15 eyes developing findings similar to **acute macular neuroretinopathy** or **paracentral acute middle maculopathy** with **retinal vasculitis or venulitis** [7].

Mitogen-activated extracellular kinase inhibitors

Mitogen-activated extracellular kinase (MEK) is a protein kinase that is part of the mitogen-activated protein kinase (MAPK) signal transduction cascade involved in cellular proliferation. MEK inhibitors include *binimetinib, cobimetinib, selumetinib,* and *trametinib* and are indicated for symptomatic, inoperable plexiform neurofibromas, anaplastic thyroid cancer, and ovarian carcinoma as well as BRAF mutation unresectable or metastatic melanoma, solid tumors, and non–small cell lung cancer [8,9].

Mitogen-activated extracellular kinase–associated retinopathy (MEKAR) is a characteristic ocular toxicity associated with MEK inhibitors [8]. MEKAR describes the presence of subretinal fluid that resembles central serous chorioretinopathy but is typically bilateral, multifocal, foveal-involving, and fairly symmetric (Fig. 1) [8]. Incidence has been reported as low as less than 1% to 2% and as high as 9% to 62% [5]. Subretinal fluid is seen on optical coherence tomography between the retinal pigmental epithelium and the interdigitation zone, although without gravitational dependent tracking, pigment

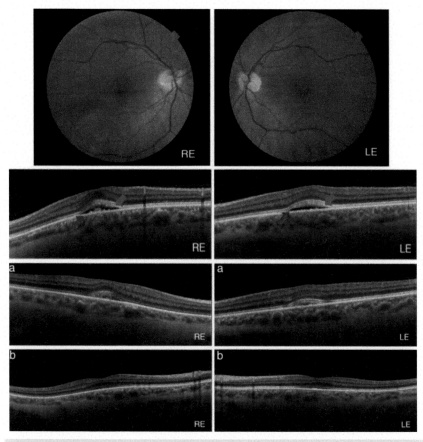

Fig. 1. MEKAR. Fundus photographs of the RE (right eye) and LE (left eye): subfoveal macular thickening in both eyes. Macular optical coherence tomography of the RE (right eye) and LE (left eye) at diagnosis: in both eyes there is thickening of the interdigitation zone (IZ) (*blue arrow*) with preservation of its hyper-refringence. Elongations of the IZ are also seen. The retinal pigments epithelium (*red arrow*) and the rest of the layers, including the choroid, remain unchanged. Macular optical coherence tomography of the RE (right eye) and LE (left eye) after treatment discontinuation: (**A**) at 10 days, with resolution of the neurosensory detachment and (**B**) at one month, with complete restructuring of the layers. (*From* Buenasmañanas-Maeso M, Gutiérrez-Montero Ó, Reche-Sainz JA, Badillo Arcones E, Monja-Alarcón N, Toledano-Fernández N. Mitogen-activated protein kinase inhibitor-associated retinopathy (MEKAR). A clinical case. *Arch Soc Esp Oftalmol (Engl Ed)*. May 2022;97(5):286 to 289.)

epithelial detachment, hyperreflective dots, or increase in choroidal thickness [8]. Most commonly, patients lose two lines on the Snellen visual acuity chart compared with their baseline with improvement after resolution of fluid [8].

Retinal vein occlusion has been reported with an incidence of 0.2% to 1% [5]. **Anterior, intermediate, posterior**, and **panuveitis** have all been reported as well [5].

BRAF inhibitors

BRAF inhibitors work through inhibition of protein kinase B-raf (BRAF) in the MAPK signal cascade to inhibit tumor cell growth. BRAF inhibitors include *dabrafenib, encorafenib,* and *vemurafenib* [5]. They often are used in combination with MEK inhibitors [5]. Indications include adjuvant therapy of melanoma with BRAF mutation, non–small cell lung cancer, metastatic anaplastic thyroid cancer, and metastatic colorectal cancer [5].

A retrospective review of patients treated with *vemurafenib* identified the most common ocular adverse events as **uveitis**, seen in 4% of patients, **conjunctivitis**, seen in 2.8%, and **dry eyes**, seen in 2% [10]. **Retinal vein occlusion** has also been reported [5].

Breakpoint cluster region–Abelson inhibitors

Breakpoint cluster region–Abelson (BCR-ABL) is a tyrosine kinase upregulated in some cancers, and BCR-ABL inhibitors include *imatinib, nilotinib, dasatinib, bosutinib, ponatinib,* and *asciminib* [5]. These medications are used to treat chronic myeloid leukemia and gastrointestinal stromal tumors [11].

Periorbital edema, ranging from mild to visually significant, has been reported, with incidence varied from 24% to 80% in patients taking *imatinib* [5]. **Epiphora** has been reported in 18% of patients, presumably secondary to periorbital edema and conjunctival chemosis [11].

Several cases of **macular edema** as well as **optic neuritis** have occurred [5].

Selective estrogen receptor modulators

Selective estrogen receptor modulators (SERMs) modulate estrogen receptors through either agonist or antagonist activity [5]. *Tamoxifen, raloxifene,* and *toremifene* are SERMs that are used to treat breast cancer and osteoporosis [5].

Keratopathy has a reported incidence as high as 72%, presenting as bilateral, whorl-like corneal opacities, which may be associated with brown horizontal subepithelial changes centrally [5,12]. **Crystalline retinopathy** presents as bilateral, small opacities in the inner retina sometimes associated with **macular edema**, with a prevalence of 0.9% to 12% (Figs. 2 and 3) [5]. Crystalline retinopathy is considered irreversible, although it often is asymptomatic. An association has been seen with *tamoxifen* and **posterior subcapsular cataracts**, with a prevalence of 9.2% to 23.8% [5]. **Retinal vein occlusion** also has been reported [5].

Aromatase inhibitors

Aromatase inhibitors decrease estrogen to treat hormone receptor–positive breast cancer [5]. Agents include *anastrazole, letrozole,* and *exemestane.* Aromatase inhibitors have been frequently associated with **blepharitis**, with a reported incidence of 73% to 75%, **meibomian gland dysfunction** in 42.5%, and **dry eyes** [13,14].

JAK2 inhibitors

JAK2 inhibitors inhibit and modulate mutated JAK2 tyrosine kinase activity in the JAK-STAT signaling pathway. Medications include *ruxolitinib, tofacitinib,*

Tamoxifen retinopathy

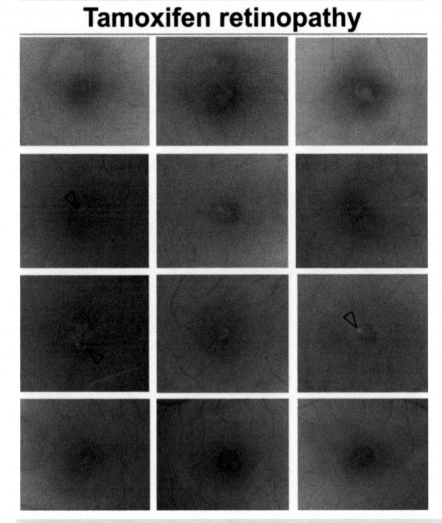

Fig. 2. Color fundus photographs of tamoxifen retinopathy with foveal lesions (pseudolamellar holes), central hypopigmentation (*arrowheads*), and crystalline deposits. (*From* Hess K, Park YJ, Kim HA, et al. Tamoxifen Retinopathy and Macular Telangiectasia Type 2: Similarities and Differences on Multimodal Retinal Imaging. Ophthalmol Retina. 2023;7(2):101-110.)

baricitinib, fedratinib, and *upadacitinib* to treat ulcerative colitis, myelofibrosis, polycythemia vera, GVHD, rheumatoid arthritis, and psoriatic arthritis [5].

JAK2 inhibitors have been associated with **eyelash growth** (Fig. 4) as well as with several infectious disease-related ocular adverse events, including **herpes zoster** with skin and ocular involvement, **toxoplasmosis retinitis**, **cytomegalovirus retinitis**, and **aspergillosis-associated retinal necrosis** [5].

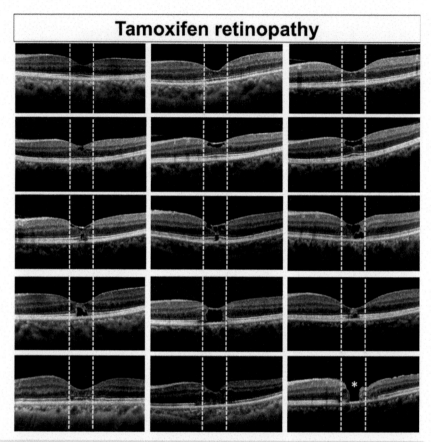

Tamoxifen retinopathy

Fig. 3. OCT of tamoxifen retinopathy with inner foveal crystalline deposits, hyporeflective cavities, foveal ellipsoid zone disruptions, pseudolamellar holes, and a full-thickness macular hole (*asterisk*). OCT, optical coherence tomography. (*From* Hess K, Park YJ, Kim HA, et al. Tamoxifen Retinopathy and Macular Telangiectasia Type 2: Similarities and Differences on Multimodal Retinal Imaging. Ophthalmol Retina. 2023;7(2):101-110.)

FMS-like tyrosine kinase 3 inhibitors

FMS-like tyrosine kinase 3 (FLT3) inhibitors inhibit mutated tyrosine kinase FLT3 in patients with acute myeloid leukemia, hepatocellular carcinoma, renal cell carcinoma, and metastatic thyroid carcinoma. Medications include *sorafenib, sunitinib, midostaurin, gilteritinib,* and *regorafenib* [5].

Sorafenib and *sunitinib* have multiple mechanisms of action. *Sorafenib* inhibits FLT3 as well as VEGF, c-KIT, PDGFR, ERK, and RAF-1, and *sunitinib* is also a multikinase inhibitor of vascular endothelial growth factor receptor (VEGFR) [15]. Fraunfelder and Fraunfelder [15] reviewed ocular side effects of *sorafenib, sunitinib,* as well as *pazopanib,* a VEGFR inhibitor. Notable associated ocular adverse events include **periocular edema and eyelash discoloration**

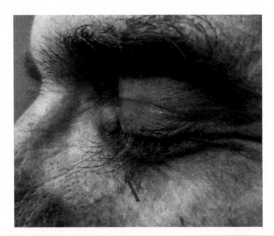

Fig. 4. Trichomegaly (*red arrow*) in a patient on EGFR inhibitor therapy. (*From* Goyal S, Uwaydat SH. Epidermal Growth Factor Receptor Inhibitor Induced Trichomegaly and Poliosis. Ophthalmology. 2018;125(2):294.)

[15]. Nine cases of **retinal tears** and **retinal detachments** were associated with *sorafenib*, and 24 cases were associated with *sunitinib* [15]. **Retinal vein occlusion** and **retinal artery occlusion** can occur [15]. *Gilteritinib* is associated with **dry eye**, with a rate of 6.3% to 9.76% [5]. **Optic neuropathy** has been reported [5], as have **cataracts** [5,16]. **Retinal hemorrhages** were identified in 7.72% of patients in one study as well as **uveitis** and **macular edema** [15].

Bruton tyrosine kinase inhibitors

Bruton tyrosine kinase (BTK) inhibitors provide inhibition of the BTK enzyme activity, and, thus, B-cell receptor and cytokine receptor pathways. Agents include *ibrutinib, acalabrutinib,* and *zanubrutinib,* which are used to treat mantle cell lymphoma, chronic lymphocytic leukemia, Waldenstrom macroglobulinemia, marginal zone lymphoma, and chronic GVHD [5,17]. Associated ocular toxicities include **dry eye, red eye,** and **branch retinal artery occlusion**. [17].

Epidermal growth factor receptor inhibitors

Epidermal growth factor receptor (EGFR) inhibitors inhibit EGFR tyrosine kinase, thus impacting multiple signaling pathways involved in carcinogenesis and also are the most associated with ocular side effects. Medications include *gefitinib, erlotinib, afatinib, brigatinib, cetuximab, osimertinib, dacomitinib, panitumumab,* and *necitumumab* [5]. Indications include colorectal cancer as well as cancers involving the head and neck, breast, lung, prostate, kidneys, pancreas, ovaries, and brain [5].

These medications have been associated with **blepharitis, periorbital rash, periorbital edema, ectropion,** and **conjunctivitis** in 1.4% to 14.5% of patients, and **dry eye** in 4% to 8.1% of patients [5]. **Keratopathy**, including a **vortex keratopathy** with bilateral whorl pattern of corneal deposits at the basal epithelium associated with *osimertinib*, persistent **corneal epithelial defect**, and **trichomegaly** have been noted [5]. **Corneal ulcers** have been observed with **corneal perforation** requiring penetrating keratoplasty as well as discontinuation of EGFR inhibitor therapy [5]. **Uveitis** and **macular edema** also were reported [5].

FGFR inhibitors

Fibroblast growth factor receptor (FGFR) inhibitors provide inhibition of FGFR tyrosine kinase enzyme activity. Medications include *ponatinib* and *erdafitinib*, which are used to treat urothelial carcinoma, hepatocellular carcinoma, ovarian cancer, and lung adenocarcinoma [5].

In one study [5], 21% of patients receiving FGFR inhibitor therapy were found to have **central serous retinopathy** [18]. **Corneal thinning** can be seen with an incidence of 7.3% [19].

Receptor tyrosine kinse (KIT) inhibitors

Receptor tyrosine kinase (KIT) inhibitors include avapritinib and ripretinib, which are used to treat gastrointestinal stromal tumors. [5]. Ocular toxicities include **periorbital edema** in 43.5% of patients taking *avapritinib* and **increased lacrimation** seen in 25.8% of patients [5,20].

Human epidermal growth factor 2 inhibitors

Human epidermal growth factor 2 (HER2) is an antigen associated with cancer, and HER2 inhibitors include *trastuzumab, pertuzumab, lapatinib, neratinib,* and *tucatinib* for the treatment of breast cancer and gastric adenocarcinoma [5]. **Infectious crystalline keratopathy, corneal ulceration,** and **increased lacrimation** with rates of 8% to 14% have been reported [5,21,22]. *Trastuzumab* has been associated with serous retinal detachment [23].

Vascular endothelial growth factor receptor inhibitors

VEGFR inhibitors provide inhibition of VEGFR and angiogenesis. Agents include s*orafenib, sunitinib, vandetanib, lenvatinib, axitinib, bevacizumab, ramucirumab, cabozantinib,* and *pazopanib* [5]. Indications include renal cell carcinoma, soft tissue carcinoma, medullary thyroid cancer, hepatocellular carcinoma, metastatic colorectal cancer, cervical cancer, glioblastoma, nonsquamous non–small cell lung cancer, and gastric adenocarcinoma [5].

One study reported 44 cases of **retinal detachment** or retinal **tears** associated with *pazopanib* [15]. **Subconjunctival hemorrhage, retinal artery** or **vein occlusion,** and **ocular motility disorders** can be observed [5]. Corneal abnormalities, most notably **vortex keratopathy, increased lacrimation,** and **optic neuropathy** may occur [5].

Mammalian target of rapamycin inhibitors

Agents that inhibit the mammalian target of rapamycin (mTOR) signaling pathway include *everolimus* and *temsirolimus,* which are used for the treatment of breast cancer, renal cell carcinoma, neuroendocrine tumors, renal angiomyolipoma, subependymal giant cell astrocytoma, and tuberous sclerosis [5]. **Eyelid edema** is a noted association [5].

Cyclin-dependent kinase inhibitors

Inhibition of cyclin-dependent kinase (CDK) decreases tumor burden. Agents include *palbociclib, ribociclib,* and *abemaciclib* for the treatment of metastatic breast cancer [5]. Associated ocular toxicities include **dry eye** and **increased lacrimation** [5].

Proteasome inhibitors

Bortezomib, carfilzomib, and *ixazomib* inhibit the ubiquitin proteasome pathway to treat multiple myeloma and mantle cell lymphoma [5]. **Chalazia** have been reported with an estimated incidence of 6.8% as well as **conjunctivitis** [5,24–26].

Antibody-drug conjugates

Antibody-drug conjugates are a combination of a monoclonal antibody with a cytotoxic drug that targets tumor cells and avoids healthy cells. Agents include *trastuzumab deruxtecan, belantamab mafodotin, trastuzumab emtansine, enfortumab vedotin, gemtuzumab ozogamicin, sacituzumab govitecan,* and *inotuzumab ozogamicin* [5]. Indications include breast cancer, multiple myeloma, metastatic breast cancer, metastatic urothelial cancer, acute myeloid leukemia, and B-cell acute lymphoblastic leukemia [5]. These medications are associated with **lacrimal drainage stenosis** and **dry eye** [5]. Unique to this drug class, microcyst-like **corneal epithelial abnormalities** have been reported [5].

Chimeric antigen receptor T-cell therapy

CAR T cells are T cells that have been genetically engineered to express anti-CD19 CARs that target CD19-positive tumor cells [27]. **Ocular graft-versus-host disease (oGVHD)** can occur [27]. **Acute retinal necrosis** also can be observed [27].

PRESENT RELEVANCE AND FUTURE AVENUES

Periorbital edema

BCR-ABL inhibitors, FTL3 inhibitors, KIT inhibitors, and *mTOR inhibitors* have been associated with periorbital edema [5]. Diuretics as well as surgical intervention can be employed [5,11]. Continued antineoplastic therapy, possibly with dose reduction, should be considered [5].

Ectropion

EGFR inhibitors have been associated with ectropion [5]. In the case of cicatricial ectropion, treatment recommendations include oral doxycycline, topical corticosteroids, and antibiotic ointment [5]. Antineoplastic therapy may need to be discontinued [5].

Lacrimal drainage stenosis

Antibody-drug conjugates have been associated with lacrimal drainage stenosis, which can be treated with topical tobramycin and dexamethasone and prophylactic silicone intubation [5].

Chalazia

Proteasome inhibitors have been linked to chalazia, which often are recalcitrant, multifocal, and bilateral and can be treated with hot compresses, topical antibiotics, and corticosteroids [5,24–26]. In more severe cases, oral antibiotics and discontinuation of targeted antineoplastic therapy may be necessary [5,24–26].

Conjunctivitis

Immune checkpoint inhibitors, BRAF inhibitors, EGFR inhibitors, and *proteasome inhibitors* have been associated with conjunctivitis, which most often can be managed with observation and symptomatic treatment [5].

Dry eye syndrome

Dry eye syndrome is one of the more common ocular adverse effects experienced by patients undergoing targeted antineoplastic therapy. *Immune checkpoint inhibitors, BRAF inhibitors, aromatase inhibitors, BTK inhibitors, EGFR inhibitors, CDK inhibitors, HER2 inhibitors,* and *antibody-drug conjugates* are all associated with dry eye syndrome [5]. Management may involve lubrication with artificial tears, punctal plugs, warm compresses, topical steroids, and cyclosporine [5]. Prophylaxis with preservative-free artificial tears has been suggested for patients taking the antibody-drug conjugate *belantamab mafodotin* [5]. Dose reduction and interruption can mitigate the keratitis in some cases, prolonging drug tolerance, although treatment cessation should be considered with more severe cases [5].

Ocular graft-versus-host disease

CAR T therapy has been associated with oGVHD, which can be treated with topical lubricants, autologous serum, steroids, and cyclosporine [27]. More aggressive cases may ultimately need to be managed with Prokera or systemic immunosuppression [27].

Corneal pathologic condition

Tamoxifen, a SERM, has been associated with reversible keratopathy that can be observed but may require discontinuation of SERM therapy [5,12].

EGFR inhibitors have been associated with significant anterior segment complications, including corneal erosions, which can be treated with eyelash epilation and holding or discontinuing the EGFR inhibitor [5]. Trichomegaly also can be seen and can be managed with eyelash trimming or observation [5]. Keratopathy may need to be treated with EGFR inhibitor discontinuation, antibiotics, steroids, and lubrication. Two cases of keratitis, including filamentary keratitis, were successfully managed with topical EGF drops, which could be considered [5]. *Osimertinib* is associated with a vortex keratopathy, which is asymptomatic and can be managed with lubrication [5].

Corneal ulcers can be seen with the use of *EGFR inhibitors,* which require antibiotics, and discontinuation of the EGFR inhibitor [5]. Ulcerative keratitis and corneal graft rejection can be seen with *immune checkpoint inhibitors* and treated with topical or systemic steroids [5]. Corneal perforation can occur with the use of both classes of medications and may require the use of glue, a bandage contact lens, or penetrating keratoplasty [5]. Antineoplastic therapy may need to be discontinued in these cases [5].

FGFR inhibitor therapy can be associated with corneal thinning, which resolves with discontinuation of therapy [19].

HER2 inhibitors can cause infectious crystalline keratopathy, which can be treated with topical antibiotics, and corneal ulceration, which can be treated with autologous serum and interrupting HER2 inhibitor therapy [21,22].

Corneal abnormalities, most notably vortex keratopathy, have been noted in patients undergoing *VEGFR inhibitor* therapy, which improves with dosage reduction and lubrication and resolves with discontinuation of therapy [5].

Antibody-drug conjugates have been associated with microcyst-like corneal epithelial abnormalities that need to be monitored for worsening of keratopathy and vision [19]. Baseline eye examination is recommended before initiation of *belantamab mafodotin* and before each dose [19]. Management of corneal abnormalities includes use of autologous serum, hyaluronic acid, and observation [19]. Dose reduction and interruption also can mitigate the keratitis in some cases, prolonging drug tolerance, although treatment cessation should be considered with more severe cases.

Cataracts

SERMs and *FLT3 inhibitors* have been associated with cataracts [5]. Cataracts can be removed with surgery once symptomatic without the need for discontinuation of therapy [5].

Uveitis

Cases of uveitis have been reported with use of *immune checkpoint inhibitors, MEK inhibitors, EGFR inhibitors, FLT3 inhibitors, and BRAF inhibitors* [5]. Management of uveitis includes the use of topical and/or periocular steroids, nonsteroidal anti-inflammatory drugs (NSAIDs), cycloplegics, and intraocular pressure–lowering agents when needed [5]. In some patients, systemic or intraocular steroids need to be used [5]. Targeted therapy can be continued in some cases, but dose reduction and medication cessation may be necessary [7]. More aggressive therapies include methotrexate, pars plana vitrectomy, and intravenous immune globulin [5]. Of note, the US Prescribing Information for the BRAF inhibitor, *encorafenib*, specifically recommends regularly scheduled ophthalmologic evaluations for new or worsening symptoms.

The Common Terminology Criteria for Adverse Events (CTCAE) provides a grading scale for severity of adverse events with guidelines for management based on severity (Table 2) [7]. Management varies and may include local steroids, systemic steroids, immunosuppression, and holding or discontinuing systemic immunotherapy [7]. Of note, the CTCAE scale does not consider baseline visual acuity and other baseline ocular pathologic conditions, which may need to be adjusted in the future [7].

In the case of uveitis associated with *immune checkpoint inhibitors*, most patients recover to within one line of baseline vision after management. The severity of patients' symptoms may not correlate with the severity of the uveitis, so it is important for clinicians to keep a high index of suspicion for ocular toxicity [7].

PD-L1 inhibitor associated uveitis was noted to have deep capillary ischemia, which could be studied in the future and carefully evaluated [7]. It also is important to remember that ocular metastases can masquerade as uveitis and must be taken into consideration. Heterogeneity of reported data can make classification difficult, highlighting the need for more specific classification of ocular pathologic conditions in future research studies.

Retinal tears and detachments

FLT3 inhibitor therapy and *VEGFR inhibitor* therapy have been associated with retinal tears and both serous and rhegmatogenous retinal detachments. It is possible that the cause of serous retinal detachments in these cases is changes in choroidal vascular permeability, microvascular events, or microemboli [15]. The importance of patient awareness of symptoms and prompt ophthalmic referral as well as consideration of discontinuation of systemic therapy should be emphasized with the use of these agents [5].

Retinopathy

MEKAR is typically self-limited. It has been thought that a thin choroid may be a predisposing risk factor for development of MEKAR, with a role for further studies [28]. With regard to *MEKAR*, emphasis has been placed on close monitoring to aid in early recognition, especially during the first 3 months of

Table 2
Common terminology criteria for adverse events grading scale and management of uveitis

	Presentation	Management
Grade 1	• Anterior uveitis with trace cells	• No intervention
Grade 2	• Anterior uveitis with 1 to 2+ cells	• Local or systemic steroids[a] • Hold systemic immunotherapy until uveitis has improved to grade 1 or less
Grade 3	• Anterior uveitis with 3+ or more cells or • Intermediate uveitis or • Posterior uveitis or • Panuveitis	• Local and high-dose systemic steroids[a] • Hold systemic immunotherapy for up to 6 weeks or discontinue immunotherapy • If no improvement, initiate immunosuppression • If uveitis improves to grade 1 or less, systemic immunotherapy may be reinitiated
Grade 4	• BCVA 20/200 or worse	• High-dose systemic steroids[a] • Discontinuation of immunotherapy

[a]Systemic steroid use should occur in combination with gastrointestinal and, if on an extended duration, *Pneumocystis carinii* pneumonia prophylaxis.
    Data from Ref. [7].

initiation of *MEK inhibitor therapy*, with monthly documentation of visual acuity [8]. Patients are given Amsler grids and either continued close follow-up if ME-KAR is diagnosed or as-needed visits with return precautions afterward [8]. The CTCAE Grading for Eye Disorders provides guidelines for grading retinopathy and indications to decrease dosing (Table 3) [8].

SERMs have been associated with crystalline retinopathy, which often is asymptomatic and can be observed [5]. Symptomatic retinopathy should prompt communication between oncology and ophthalmology regarding the possibility of decreasing the dose or discontinuing SERM therapy.

Patients undergoing *FGFR inhibitor* therapy have been found to have central serous retinopathy and may require dose reduction, interruption, or, less commonly, discontinuation of therapy. Serous detachments also have been reported with the HER2 inhibitor, *trastuzumab* [18,23]. Discontinuation of therapy can result in resolution with return of vision.

CAR T therapy has been associated with acute retinal necrosis, which should be managed with antiviral therapy [27].

Retinal artery and vein occlusion

BRAF inhibitors, SERMs, FLT3 inhibitors, and *MEK inhibitors* should be discontinued in cases of retinal vein occlusion [5]. Retinal artery occlusion has been associated with *FLT therapy, VEGFR inhibitor therapy,* and *BTK inhibitor therapy* and should prompt consideration for withdrawal of therapy [5].

Macular edema

Macular edema can be seen in association with *BCR-ABL inhibitors, FLT3 inhibitors,* and *EGFR inhibitors* and can be treated in several ways [5]. A course of topical NSAIDs and corticosteroids can be trialed as well as oral acetazolamide, oral prednisone, and/or intravitreal corticosteroids [5]. Cases have resolved with discontinuation of antineoplastic therapy [5].

Optic neuritis

Optic neuritis has been reported in patients using *BCR-ABL inhibitors,* which might require treatment with oral steroids and drug discontinuation [5]. Optic

Table 3		
Common terminology criteria for adverse events grading scale and management of mitogen-activated extracellular kinase-associated retinopathy		
	Presentation	Management
Grade 1	• Asymptomatic	• No intervention
Grade 2	• Symptomatic and	• No intervention
	• BCVA 20/40 or better	
Grade 3	• Symptomatic and disabling and	• Decrease dose of MEK inhibitor
	• BCVA worse than 20/40	
Grade 4	• BCVA 20/200 or worse	• Decrease dose of MEK inhibitor
Data from Ref. [8].		

neuropathy has been observed in patients using *FLT3 inhibitor* therapy and in *VEGFR inhibitor* therapy, in which therapy can be discontinued, and in some cases, oral prednisone or intravenous methylprednisolone should be initiated [5].

Infectious pathologic condition

Infectious disease–related ocular adverse events may occur with *JAK2 inhibitor* therapy, in which case, therapy cessation may need to be considered as well as prompt initiation of appropriate local or systemic therapies [5].

SUMMARY

With advances in life-prolonging immunotherapy and targeted antineoplastic agents, the potential exists for malignancies to become chronically managed. However, these medications not uncommonly are associated with a myriad of ocular side effects. Thus, it is paramount for oncologists and ophthalmologists to know and recognize early associated ocular toxicities, many of which can be treated conservatively. Communication between oncologists and ophthalmologists is crucial to provide the best care for these patients. Some ocular adverse events may lead to permanent vision loss and necessitate discontinuation of life-preserving measures, which should be discussed between physicians in an interdisciplinary manner.

The treatments for some of the ocular toxicities, such as corticosteroids, can be associated with other ocular adverse events as well as systemic toxicity. Identification of risk factors for ocular adverse events associated with systemic cancer therapy could pave the way for future studies as well as new screening tools for patients before initiation of targeted cancer therapy. Francis and colleagues [29] reported an association with hyperhomocysteinemia and gene variants of methylene tetrahydrofolate reductase, which could help identify patients at risk for central retinal vein occlusion, one of the more devastating ocular toxicities associated with *MEK inhibitors*. Pretherapy screening could identify patients at risk, preventing vision-threatening complications in the future. Similarly, it has been thought that a thin choroid may be a predisposing risk factor for development of MEKAR, with a role for further studies and opportunities for future pretherapy screening [28]. Given that administration of these life-sustaining antineoplastic therapies may otherwise continue if they are tolerated, screening may be useful before initiation of therapy in order to prevent frequent ophthalmology visits. There may be a role for future studies to evaluate remote screening tools for ocular toxicity, including the use of non-mydriatic cameras and optical coherence tomography at infusion or oncology offices with remote reading centers or artificial intelligence technology. These tools could have the potential to improve quality of life by limiting what may be frequent and time-consuming monitoring office visits.

With novel cancer treatments, such as CAR T therapy, it will be important for oncologists and ophthalmologists to continue to report adverse events as well as to contribute case reports and larger studies over time to add to the current knowledge base. Furthermore, it would be beneficial to improve standardization of the classification of ocular adverse events. The CTCAE provides a standardized grading system for eye disorders with recommendations for management; however, not all clinical trials use the CTCAE, possibly because of the lack of specificity of certain terms [8].

Knowledge of ocular toxicities associated with cancer therapy can help improve understanding of the physiology and pathophysiology underlying these ocular abnormalities. For example, given the frequency of uveitis episodes seen in patients undergoing MEK inhibitor therapy, there may be a role of the MEK/ERK pathway in the pathophysiology of ocular inflammation. There may be room for the development of novel therapies exploiting certain side effects. JAK2 inhibitors and EGFR inhibitors, for example, have been associated with eyelash growth. A study of patients with alopecia areata showed that many patients benefited from eyelash and eyebrow growth with the use of a JAK2 inhibitor [30].

As ophthalmologists diagnose and treat patients with cancer, it is important for them to identify patients undergoing antineoplastic therapy to determine any associations between ocular pathologic conditions and such treatment. Often, medical records are not easy to navigate, and therapeutic protocols are not obvious in the medication record. There is room to develop systems in which the medical record of patients undergoing antineoplastic therapy are appropriately updated in such a way that ophthalmologists can easily identify patients who are undergoing antineoplastic therapy with specific agents that may be associated with ocular adverse events. It also is beneficial for oncologists to educate patients on potential ocular toxicities known to be associated with their cancer therapy, so that they can be proactive in their own care, reporting early symptoms and seeking appropriate follow-up. The increasing use of these potentially lifesaving, but possibly toxic, treatments demands a coordinated effort between oncologists, ophthalmologists, and patients to maximize outcomes and mitigate any potential ocular toxicities, thereby ensuring the best quality of life for these patients.

CLINICS CARE POINTS

- Patients undergoing targeted immunotherapy should be educated regarding the associated ocular adverse events to aid in early recognition.
- Chemotherapeutic protocols and agents should be easily accessible in the medical record to aid in the ophthalmologist's evaluation of patients with the appropriate focus and auxiliary testing.
- In the event of potential ocular toxicity associated with targeted immunotherapy, close communication between the patient's oncologist and ophthalmologist is necessary, as management may require cessation or adjustments to therapy.
- Improved standardization of classification of adverse events with treatment strategies is critical to mitigate ocular toxicities, making reporting side effects to a centralized database another crucial role of the ophthalmologist.

- Development of improved screening strategies to determine patients at risk and minimize office visits is essential for improving quality of life for these patients undergoing long-term care.

DISCLOSURE

The authors have nothing to disclose.

References

[1] Dobosz P, Dzięciątkowski T. The Intriguing History of Cancer Immunotherapy. Front Immunol 2019;10:2965.

[2] Ueda N, Cahen M, Danger Y, et al. Immunotherapy perspectives in the new era of B-cell editing. Blood Adv 2021;5(6):1770–9.

[3] Hessen M, Akpek EK. Ocular graft-versus-host disease. Curr Opin Allergy Clin Immunol 2012;12(5):540–7.

[4] Scott GN. Sorting Through the Confusion of Biologic Drug Names. Commentary. Medscape 2016;19:1–3.

[5] Fortes BH, Tailor PD, Dalvin LA. Ocular Toxicity of Targeted Anticancer Agents. Drugs 2021;81(7):771–823.

[6] Ai L, Chen J, Yan H, et al. Research Status and Outlook of PD-1/PD-L1 Inhibitors for Cancer Therapy. Drug Des Devel Ther 2020;14:3625–49.

[7] Dow ER, Yung M, Tsui E. Immune Checkpoint Inhibitor-associated Uveitis: Review of Treatments and Outcomes. Ocul Immunol Inflamm 2021;29(1):203–11.

[8] Méndez-Martínez S, Calvo P, Ruiz-Moreno O, et al. Ocular adverse events associated with MEK inhibitors. Retina 2019;39(8):1435–50.

[9] Cheng Y, Tian H. Current Development Status of MEK Inhibitors. Molecules 2017;22(10); https://doi.org/10.3390/molecules22101551.

[10] Choe CH, McArthur GA, Caro I, et al. Ocular toxicity in BRAF mutant cutaneous melanoma patients treated with vemurafenib. Am J Ophthalmol 2014;158(4):831–7.e2.

[11] Breccia M, Gentilini F, Cannella L, et al. Ocular side effects in chronic myeloid leukemia patients treated with imatinib. Leuk Res 2008;32(7):1022–5.

[12] Muftuoglu O, Uçakhan OO, Kanpolat A. Clinical and in vivo confocal microscopy findings in patients receiving tamoxifen citrate. Eye Contact Lens 2006;32(5):228–32.

[13] Chatziralli I, Sergentanis T, Zagouri F, et al. Ocular Surface Disease in Breast Cancer Patients Using Aromatase Inhibitors. Breast J 2016;22(5):561–3.

[14] Turaka K, Nottage JM, Hammersmith KM, et al. Dry eye syndrome in aromatase inhibitor users. Clin Exp Ophthalmol 2013;41(3):239–43.

[15] Fraunfelder FT, Fraunfelder FW. Oral Anti-Vascular Endothelial Growth Factor Drugs and Ocular Adverse Events. J Ocul Pharmacol Ther 2018;34(6):432–5.

[16] Bhatia S, Moon J, Margolin KA, et al. Phase II trial of sorafenib in combination with carboplatin and paclitaxel in patients with metastatic uveal melanoma: SWOG S0512. PLoS One 2012;7(11):e48787.

[17] Kunkler AL, Binkley EM, Mantopoulos D, et al. Known and novel ocular toxicities of biologics, targeted agents, and traditional chemotherapeutics. Graefes Arch Clin Exp Ophthalmol 2019;257(8):1771–81.

[18] Loriot Y, Necchi A, Park SH, et al. Erdafitinib in Locally Advanced or Metastatic Urothelial Carcinoma. N Engl J Med 2019;381(4):338–48.

[19] Bauters G, Paques M, Borderie V, et al. Reversible corneal stromal thinning, acute-onset white cataract and angle-closure glaucoma due to erdafitinib, a fibroblast growth factor receptor inhibitor: Report of three cases. J Fr Ophtalmol 2021;44(1):67–75.

[20] Heinrich MC, Jones RL, von Mehren M, et al. Avapritinib in advanced PDGFRA D842V-mutant gastrointestinal stromal tumour (NAVIGATOR): a multicentre, open-label, phase 1 trial. Lancet Oncol 2020;21(7):935–46.

[21] Sridhar MS, Laibson PR, Rapuano CJ, et al. Infectious crystalline keratopathy in an immuno-suppressed patient. Clao J 2001;27(2):108–10.

[22] Orlandi A, Fasciani R, Cassano A, et al. Trastuzumab-induced corneal ulceration: successful no-drug treatment of a "blind" side effect in a case report. BMC Cancer 2015;15:973.

[23] Saleh M, Bourcier T, Noel G, et al. Bilateral macular ischemia and severe visual loss following trastuzumab therapy. Acta Oncol 2011;50(3):477–8.

[24] Fraunfelder FW, Yang HK. Association Between Bortezomib Therapy and Eyelid Chalazia. JAMA Ophthalmol 2016;134(1):88–90.

[25] Sklar BA, Gervasio KA, Leng S, et al. Management and outcomes of proteasome inhibitor associated chalazia and blepharitis: a case series. BMC Ophthalmol 2019;19(1):110.

[26] Dennis M, Maoz A, Hughes D, et al. Bortezomib ocular toxicities: Outcomes with ketotifen. Am J Hematol 2019;94(3):E80–2.

[27] Mumtaz AA, Fischer A, Lutfi F, et al. Ocular adverse events associated with chimeric antigen receptor T-cell therapy: a case series and review. Br J Ophthalmol 2022; https://doi.org/10.1136/bjophthalmol-2021-320814.

[28] Stjepanovic N, Velazquez-Martin JP, Bedard PL. Ocular toxicities of MEK inhibitors and other targeted therapies. Ann Oncol 2016;27(6):998–1005.

[29] Francis JH, Diamond EL, Chi P, et al. MEK Inhibitor-Associated Central Retinal Vein Occlusion Associated with Hyperhomocysteinemia and MTHFR Variants. Ocul Oncol Pathol 2020;6(3):159–63.

[30] Liu LY, King BA. Response to tofacitinib therapy of eyebrows and eyelashes in alopecia areata. J Am Acad Dermatol 2019;80(6):1778–9.

Glaucoma

Advances in Ophthalmology and Optometry 8 (2023) 213–237

ADVANCES IN OPHTHALMOLOGY AND OPTOMETRY

Virtual Perimetry

Wesam Shamseldin Shalaby, MD[a,b],
Sapna Sinha, MD[a], Jonathan S. Myers, MD[c],
Reza Razeghinejad, MD[c],*

[a]Glaucoma Research Center, Wills Eye Hospital, 11th Floor, 840 Walnut Street, Philadelphia, PA 19107, USA; [b]Tanta Medical School, Tanta University, Tanta University Ophthalmology Hospital, 3rd Floor, Al-Geish Street, Tanta, Gharbia 31527, Egypt; [c]Glaucoma Service, Wills Eye Hospital, 11th Floor, 840 Walnut Street, Philadelphia, PA 19107, USA

Keywords
- Glaucoma • Perimetry • Telemedicine • Visual field • Virtual reality
- Virtual perimetry

Key points
- Virtual perimetry is a promising technology that could make a significant change in glaucoma screening and teleglaucoma management.
- Wheelchair-bound patients, patients admitted in the hospital with various neuro-ophthalmic or neurosurgical issues, and those with musculoskeletal issues, who cannot do the standard perimetry, are all able to do virtual perimetry.
- Studies on virtual perimeters have shown promising reliability and reproducibility compared with standard perimetry.
- Virtual perimeters still have their own limitations, needing further refining, expanding the database, and adding progression analysis modules.

INTRODUCTION

The first record of a visual field defect dates back to the late fifth century BCE, wherein Hippocrates described hemianopia. Ptolemy (150 BCE) first attempted to quantify the visual field and noted its circular form [1]. Leonardo da Vinci recognized the temporal extent of visual field to exceed beyond 90° of fixation [2]. Later, in 1825, Thomas Young described the lateral limits to be 100°, the nasal 60°, upper 60°, and lower 80° [3]. Scotomas were first described by Boerhaave in

*Corresponding author. Glaucoma Research Center, Wills Eye Hospital, 11th Floor, 840 Walnut Street, Philadelphia, PA 19107, USA. E-mail address: reza@willseye.org

https://doi.org/10.1016/j.yaoo.2023.03.008
2452-1760/23/

1708 [4]. Their shape and location of scotomas were later characterized by Beer in 1817 [5].

Purkinje was the first to apply a curved surface for measuring visual fields [1]. Albrecht von Graefe is credited with introducing perimetry into clinical ophthalmology. He published examples of visual field losses associated with many ocular and neurologic diseases [6]. Jannik Bjerrum popularized campimetry and used a tangent screen to map the central 30°of the visual field [3].

In 1945, Hans Goldmann developed a hemispherical bowl perimeter that provided a uniform background illumination [3]. In the late 1950s and early 1960s, Elfriede Aulhorn and Heinrich Harms designed the Tubinger perimeter to perform static perimetry, although kinetic testing could also be performed [7,8]. The Octopus, an automated perimetry was introduced by Franz Fankhauser in 1975 [9]. The Humphrey field analyzer (HFA), an automated perimeter was introduced by Anders Heijl and his colleagues in 1982 [10]. The HFA was shown to detect visual field loss earlier than Goldmann perimetry in glaucoma, and clinical monitoring of glaucoma has been primarily based on static perimetry for decades [11]. Although both Octopus perimeter and HFA are types of static perimeters, they have some differences. Octopus perimeter uses direct projection with Goldmann stimulus size III or V, stimulus duration of 100 milliseconds, and luminance of 4800 asb. Test strategies include normal, dynamic, and tendency oriented perimetry. However, HFA uses aspherical bowl with Goldmann stimulus size I to V, stimulus duration of 200 milliseconds, and luminance of 10,000 asb. Test strategies include full threshold, Swedish interactive thresholding algorithm (SITA) standard, SITA fast, and SITA faster. Both devices use background luminance of 31.5 asb, and have measuring range of 0 to 40 dB [12].

Virtual reality (VR) perimetry is a developing technology that has improved affordability, and compliance, with wide applications in telemedicine and home perimetry. These devices require less room than tabletop instruments, and in some cases are more comfortable for elderly patients with ergonomic challenges. Tablet-based strategies and VR headsets show promise for remote monitoring of patients with glaucoma and glaucoma screening [13]. Tablet perimeters such as the Visual Fields Easy (VFE) [14], Melbourne Rapid Fields (MRFs) [15], or Eyecatcher [16] use either gaze-based or touch-based feedback systems with fairly comparable test–retest variability compared with the automated perimeters. Head-mounted devices (HMDs) include 2 feedback options, namely manual (ie, mouse click) and visual grasp (ie, directing the gaze to the target). Vivid vision perimetry (VVP; Vivid Vision, Inc., San Francisco, CA) uses a VR platform and oculokinetic perimetry [17]. The VisuALL (Olleyes Inc., Summit, NJ) HMD showed excellent correlation with standard automated perimetry (SAP) in normal individuals and in patients with glaucoma [18].

Virtual perimetry has been shown to be a reliable aid in glaucoma screening, diagnosis, and monitoring [19]. Given the good correlation with HFA in classic neurologic fields such as hemianopias, this can be used as an alternative in the elderly, bedbound, disabled, individuals with stroke or neurologic disorders [20,21].

VIRTUAL PERIMETRY APPLICATIONS

The current SAP devices have their own limitations. SAP may be a difficult test to administer, time-consuming, and more demanding burden on the patient's attention and performance. It requires that patients travel to a specialized eye center, necessitates a skilled technician and dedicated examination room and lighting, and can create an uncomfortable and fatiguing experience for patients [22,23]. Furthermore, SAP has a high-inherent variability in its output data that obligate patients to return for repeated testing to generate clinically reliable results [24]. Despite being the only standard test to assess the visual field, it has not evolved much with the rapid advancements in technology. VR technology has created an opportunity for advances in perimetric testing concerning the data obtained and the patient experience.

Glaucoma screening

No single test has ever been found to be completely satisfactory for glaucoma screening, a combination of structural and functional evaluations is necessary. Visual field testing should always be part of the initial evaluation of glaucoma. The current approach for evaluating the visual field in glaucoma screening is taking the perimeter to the screening locations or having the patients in the ophthalmic centers equipped with computerized perimeters [25]. Although this approach may work well in cities, it is not a practical solution in developing countries. Glaucoma screenings in developing nations would be best served by a field machine that is ultraportable, does not require electricity, and can be performed rapidly [26]. Current SAP devices have great limitations with regards to screening efforts for glaucoma. They are cumbersome and require plug in electricity. SAP in novice test takers is neither sensitive nor specific for the detection of glaucoma. These and other issues have limited their use and utility in screening efforts and have precluded their use in many rural areas and developing countries for screening efforts.

Perimetry in special situations

Assessment of visual fields using SAP is routinely performed in neurologic diseases affecting the visual pathway. Such assessment is necessary in planning the medical and surgical interventions in some patients. SAP cannot be performed in patients who are bed-bound or unable to sit for the test. As the virtual perimetry is portable, the visual field can be completed everywhere (clinic, hospital, nursing homes, and patient homes) and in any position [27].

Test positioning is more flexible in virtual perimetry, which makes this perimetry method very useful for patients with restrictive neck conditions that preclude satisfactory positioning at the automated perimeter, and for children and short adults. The current SAPs are designed for adults and positioning a child behind the machine is challenging. Many children are familiar with virtual headsets and adding children's specific testing strategies should improve our ability in following the children with glaucoma and various optic neuropathies or neurologic diseases. The Olleyes VisuALL has a pediatric-specific testing algorithm. It uses a game-based format that engages the attention of children [28].

The improved ergonomics also translate to patients that are unable to fully sit up, such as patients who are either bed or wheelchair-bound patients. The ability to acquire for mal visual fields in a myriad of environments provides tremendous utility [27]. Nesaratnam and colleagues reported that a portable tablet device (MRF) was used at the bedside to assess a patient with a suspected pituitary tumor [29]. The test confirmed a dense superior bitemporal field loss with an early involvement of the inferior bitemporal fields in addition to foveal field loss. Accordingly, the patient underwent an endonasal endoscopic resection of the pituitary mass [29].

Teleglaucoma

Many factors seem to be driving the momentum of the development and adoption of virtual perimetry. The COVID-19 pandemic has broadly affected society, including illuminating the vulnerability of clinic-based medical care. With emerging technologies, diseases can be monitored in the safety of one's home [27]. Telemedicine has expanded in other subspecialties but still has been limited in ophthalmology practice due to the dependence on device-based data gathering (intraocular pressure, optical coherence tomography [OCT], visual fields, fundus photography). Advancements in virtual visual field testing and similar technologies addressing other aspects of clinical testing such as cell phone-based imaging and acuity testing, telemedicine protocols in ophthalmology will gain more popularity [27]. The American Academy of Ophthalmology has recognized the value of telemedicine and has sponsored a task force on tele-ophthalmology. For example, teleophthalmology has proven to successfully improve and extend ophthalmic care in diabetic retinopathy and retinopathy of prematurity [30]. With advances in intraocular pressure monitoring and optic nerve evaluation, the Academy's goal is to expand this successful initiative to the realm of teleglaucoma to improve the detection and treatment of glaucoma and have a positive impact on quality of life and patient outcomes [30].

Even in normal circumstances before and after the pandemic, there are many barriers that prevent patients from seeking appropriate eye care including but not limited to, geographic, educational, socioeconomic, and cultural considerations [31,32]. Teleglaucoma may help overcome these barriers through remote consultation allowing patients with glaucoma to be followed and monitored remotely. Virtual perimetry is a cornerstone of teleglaucoma and can be used for home-based visual field testing for those who cannot travel to eye centers with full-scale visual field. The lower cost and greater portability of the headsets may also create opportunities for screening and testing in general medicine clinics in areas and populations without routine access to ophthalmic care, rural or urban.

VIRTUAL PERIMETERS
Tablet-based virtual perimetry

Tablet-based virtual perimetry has the advantage that unlike traditional SAP, both the visual stimuli and the patient's response can be administered by a touch screen tablet [33]. Tablet-based perimetry may improve device cost and portability but challenges include nonstandardized ambient lighting and test distance. Different types of tablets based virtual perimeters and their characteristics are displayed in Table 1.

Melbourne rapid fields

MRF (GLANCE Optical Pty Ltd., Melbourne, Australia; Fig. 1) is a tangent perimeter on an iPad platform (Apple, Inc.), which maps the central and peripheral visual fields using fast threshold strategies. The MRF test pattern has either a modified 24-2 grid or a radial orientation assessing 66 locations [34].

The testing is performed in a dimly lit room, with the screen brightness set to maximum (100%) by the software and iPad. Each eye is tested separately with the patient wearing near spectacle correction if required. Fixation is maintained with a central fixation target, which can move to the peripheries of the tablet to further test the extremities. A computed voice prompt guides the patient throughout the test [35]. In a preliminary study, the iPad perimeter could detect early and mild simulated scotoma with mean deviation (MD) of -3 to -6 dB. Moreover, the MRF could return thresholds that were robust to variation in pupil size, blur, viewing distance, and ambient illumination [34]. Compared with HFA in patients with glaucoma, the MRF test duration was shorter and had a high level of concordance and test–retest reliability [32]. Comparable test–retest variability suggests minimal learning effect between test and retest. However, the lack of learning effect may indicate that patients in this study who were experienced in HFA perimetry may carry their experience over to the MRF [35]. Strong agreement between MRF and HFA was reported for MD and pattern deviation, although the MRF tended to give a less-negative MD. This level of agreement was similar to the degree of agreement between other SAPs and HFA [36,37].

Eyecatcher: tablet perimetry with gaze-tracking

Eyecatcher is a tablet perimeter with the stimuli displayed on a Microsoft Surface Pro 3 (Microsoft, Redmond, WA), at a viewing distance of 50 cm. Eye movements are recorded monocularly at 50 Hz using a Tobii EyeX eye-tracker (Tobii Technology, Stockholm, Sweden). The measurement grid consisted primarily of the points on standard 24-2 pattern [16,38]. Eyecatcher was able to clearly separate patients from controls, and the results were consistent with SAP. In particular, mean Eyecatcher scores were strongly correlated with MD scores, and there was a good concordance between corresponding visual field defects [38]. The Eyecatcher was further evaluated to examine its feasibility in a busy glaucoma clinic to determine whether it can be used as a rapid test to identify high-risk individuals (MD < -6 dB) and "false-positive" referrals. The authors used "false positive" to denote patients referred for glaucoma evaluation who proved not to have glaucoma [16]. The sample included established patients with glaucoma and false-positive new referrals (no visual field or optic nerve abnormalities). The results showed that Eyecatcher was fast (median: 2.5 min), produced results in good agreement with SAP, and

Table 1
Tablet-based virtual perimeters

	Dimensions	Stimulus duration	Stimulus color	Stimulus size	Testing features	Test strategies	Test patterns	Test duration	Laterality	Other functions
MRFs	9.7°	300 ms	White on white	Variable with eccentricity (Goldman III-V)	Tangent perimeter	Full threshold Fast threshold	10-2 24-2 30-2	4–5 min (full) 100 s (fast)	Monocular (Near spectacle correction)	–
Eyecatcher	28.5° × 19.2°	1500 ms	White on white	Goldman III	Open-source eye-movement perimeter	Full threshold	24-2	5 min	Monocular (Patient's glasses)	• Near-IR, remote eye-tracker • Integrated head-tracking
Visual Fields Easy App (VFE)	Free iPad app	1000 ms	White on white	Goldman V	iPad perimeter	Suprathreshold	30-2	3–4 min	Monocular (Near spectacle correction)	–

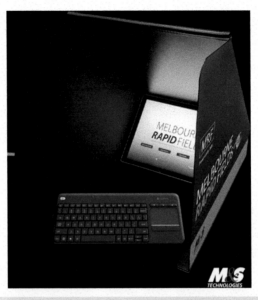

Fig. 1. Melbourne rapid fields (MRF). (*Courtesy of* GLANCE optical Pty Ltd., Melbourne, Australia.)

was rated as more enjoyable and less tiring. It exhibited good separation ability between eyes with advanced field loss (MD < −6 dB) and normal visual field (MD > −2 dB). It was able to flag two-thirds of false-positive referrals as functionally normal. However, 7 people (9%) failed to complete the test due to the hardware being unable to track their eyes reliably, the authors thought that the recent cataract surgery was the cause in 5 cases [16].

Visual fields easy app
VFE is a free of cost application that uses the iPad screen to perform a fast-screening test of the visual fields (Fig. 2). This app uses the suprathreshold strategy to detect gross abnormalities in the visual field [39]. The VFE program tests 96 points within the central 30°, using a background luminance of 31.5 apostilbs, a size V target (when placed at a 33-cm test distance) and a 16 dB suprathreshold static perimetry target for screening purposes. An analytical study enrolled subjects requiring visual field examination as part of the comprehensive ophthalmologic evaluation. Each subject was tested using the HFA and the VFE application loaded in an iPad 2 version 8.3. Although the application was not intended to replace SAP machines, the authors suggested that it may have a role in detecting, documenting, and monitoring visual field defects in low resource settings where visual field tests are not available [40].

Ichhpujani and colleagues [39] compared the perimetric outcomes of VFE and HFA in normal as well as eyes with glaucomatous damage of varying severity. The Spearman correlation coefficient showed a significant inverse

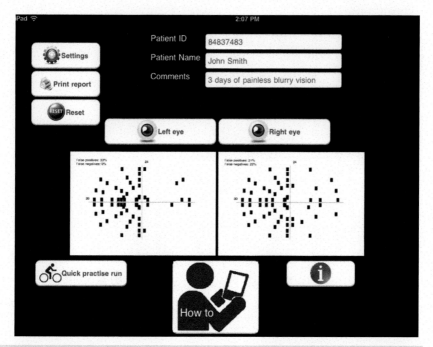

Fig. 2. VFE iPad-based app user interface. (*Courtesy of* GLANCE Optical Pty Ltd., Melbourne, Australia.)

relationship between missed points on the VFE with MD and a parabolic relationship with pattern standard deviation values obtained with the HFA. For mild glaucoma, missed points were 37.5 (sensitivity 77.8% and specificity 52.6%); for moderate glaucoma, missed points were 33.5 (sensitivity 90% and specificity 48%); whereas for severe glaucoma, missed points were 23 (sensitivity 97% and specificity 70%). Accordingly, the authors concluded that VFE is not suitable screening tool for mass screening of glaucoma. Additionally, it cannot be used as a substitute for HFA in clinic.

Head-mounted virtual perimetry
Different types of head-mounted virtual perimeters and their characteristics are displayed in Table 2. These devices also use portable and often more affordable technology but avoid challenges with regard to background illumination and standardization of test distance. The VR technology approach may present issues on rare occasions for patients with tendencies to motion sickness or claustrophobia.

Vivid vision perimetry
The VVP (Vivid Vision, Inc., San Francisco, CA) Swift test (Fig. 3) is a VR-based visual field assessment that uses Oculus Go mobile VR headset

Table 2
Head-mounted virtual perimeters

	Weight	Stimulus duration	Stimulus color	Stimulus size	Testing features	Test strategies	Test patterns	Test duration	Cloud-based server	Eye tracking	Laterality	Other functions
C3 field analyzer (CFA)	600 gm	200 ms	White on white	Goldman III	–	Supra threshold Fast threshold	10-2 24-2	20 min	Yes	–	Monocular	–
VVP	–	300 ms	Black on white	Diameter of 0.43°	Oculokinetic perimetry methods	Full threshold	24-2	8.5 min	–	–	Binocular	• Stereopsis • Oculomotor control • Amblyopia screening
Olleyes VisuALL	333 gm	150 ms	White on black	Goldman III and V	Multi-testing Virtual Reality Platform	Threshold Screening	10-2 24-2 30-2 24-2c	3 min for Threshold 45 s for Screening	Yes	- IMUs - IR-based position tracking	Binocular	• Visual acuity • Color vision • Contrast sensitivity • Low-contrast visual acuity • Pupillometry • Extraocular motility
AVA	500 gm	200 ms	White on white	Goldman III	Customized Elisar Standard Algorithm	Screening Full Threshold Elisar Standard Elisar Fast	10-2 24-2 30-2	6–8 min	Yes	Yes	Monocular Binocular	–
GlauCUTU	350 gm	Adjustable	White on white or black	Goldman I, II, and III	Time until perceived perimeter	Time until response strategy	24-2	7–9 min	–	–	Binocular	• Amblyopia screening • Contrast sensitivity
Oculus Quest VR headset	503 gm	100–200 ms	White on white	Goldman III	Octopus 900 test principles	G testing pattern	30-2	6–7 min	Secure web-based electronic data	No	Monocular	–

(continued on next page)

Table 2
(continued)

	Weight	Stimulus duration	Stimulus color	Stimulus size	Testing features	Test strategies	Test patterns	Test duration	Cloud-based server	Eye tracking	Laterality	Other functions
HTC Vive Pro Eye	550 gm	200 ms	White on white	Goldman III	LUXIE test grids	Bisection strategy	30-2	10 min	–	Tobii eye tracker	Monocular	• Pupillometry • Not able to detect retinal sensitivity less than 14 dB
Palm Scan VF2000		200 ms	White on white	Goldman III		Threshold	24-2	0.5 min	–	Active eye tracking in VF2000 Neo	Monocular	• Stereopsis • Visual acuity • Contrast sensitivity • Pupillometry • Color testing
Virtual Field VF3 – VF3 Pro	490 gm (VF3) 620 gm (VF3 pro)		White on white	Goldman III		Full Threshold Screening BOLT Strategy	10-2 24-2 30-2	3–6 min for full threshold BOLT Strategy is 2–4 min shorter	Data export (PDF, JPEC, DICOM)	Active eye tracking in VF3 Pro	Monocular Binocular	• Progression analysis • Pupillometry • Color testing • Ptosis screening • Magnetic trial lens adapters or patients can wear their glasses

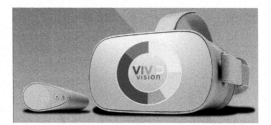

Fig. 3. Vivid vision perimetry (VVP). (*Courtesy of* Vivid Vision, Inc., San Francisco, CA.)

(Facebook, Inc) with oculokinetic perimetry methods. VVP assesses patient's visual fields across 54 points in a 24-2 pattern. Both eyes are tested during a single session using randomly alternating left-eye and right-eye stimuli. Stimuli are decremental with small black spots of luminance 0.2 cd/m^2 on a white background of luminance 25 cd/m^2 [17]. A cross-sectional study by Greenfield and colleagues [17] examined the reproducibility of VVP and compared its results with conventional SAP and OCT in glaucomatous eyes. The mean test duration of VVP was significantly shorter than SAP. The average absolute difference of the mean sensitivity between the 2 VVP sessions was found to be 0.73 dB. Relative to the HFA, the VVP test showed a test–retest variability that was comparable with reported values for moderately reliable test-takers with glaucoma [41]. A statistically significant association was found between average mean sensitivity of VVP, and HVF-MD. Mean visual sensitivity measurements from the VVP test were significantly associated with average retinal nerve fiber layer thickness and ganglion cell complex. The correspondence identified in this study is comparable with the known structure–function relationship demonstrated by SAP and OCT [41].

C3 fields analyzer

The C3 fields analyzer (CFA) (Fig. 4) is a head-mounted VR perimeter, which uses 0.55 mm circular stimuli placed in 24-2 pattern. Background brightness is 10 cd/m^2, which is equivalent to 31.5 apostilbs and stimuli brightness is 60 cd/m^2 (suprathreshold), using an HTC Instrument LX-101A Light Meter Luxmeter (HTC, Taoyuan City, Taiwan), approximating an 18-dB contrast on the HFA scale. Patients are instructed to focus on a central yellow fixation point and respond to the stimuli using a handheld clicker [21]. The number of stimuli missed on the CFA correlated well with HFA MD and with pattern standard deviation. The area under the curve was 0.77 ± 0.06 for mild and 0.86 ± 0.04 for moderate-advanced glaucoma. Patients with an 18 dB or worse deficit at a point on the HFA failed to see the CFA stimulus at the same position 38% of the time. Further refinements to the device will be required to improve point-by-point testing performance and screening performance. The CFA results were compared with the HFA in neuro-ophthalmic patients, and the correlation of the pattern of the field defect was assessed by an independent masked physician

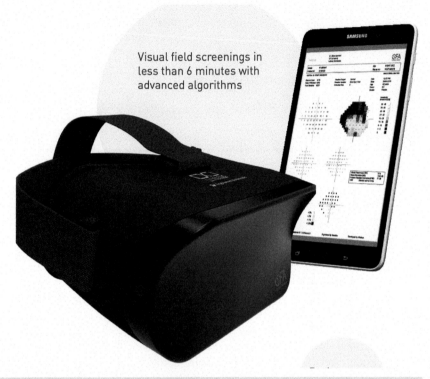

Visual field screenings in less than 6 minutes with advanced algorithms

Fig. 4. C3 fields analyzer (CFA). (*Courtesy of* Remidio Innovative Solutions Pvt Ltd., and Alfaleus Technologies Pvt Ltd, India.)

[20]. CFA was found to have greater proportion of reliable fields (81.4%) than HFA (59.3%). There were less false negatives but more false positives in CFA among neuro-ophthalmic patients compared with controls. Regarding the pattern of the field defects, there was almost 70% correlation of CFA with HFA, which increased up to 87.5% in classic neurologic fields such as hemianopia.

VisuALL

The VisuALL (Olleyes, Inc., Summit, NJ) (Fig. 5) is a US Food and Drug Administration-registered, VR-based perimeter. The hardware includes 3 main components: a VR headset, a web-capable device (laptop, phone, or tablet) and a Bluetooth connected handpiece. The HMD is powered by Pico (Pico Interactive, Inc., San Francisco, CA). The display is placed at a distance that subtends a field of view up to 100°. The HMD includes several tracking systems: inertial measurement units (IMUs) consisting of gyroscopes and accelerometers, and infrared (IR)-based position tracking with 2 arrays of 6 IR sensors. The VisuALL software includes the Olleyes cloud-based server, the VisuALL web application, and the Unity algorithms. All the VisuALL data

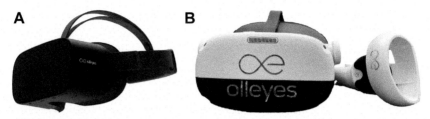

Fig. 5. VisuALL perimeter. (*Courtesy of* Olleyes, Inc., Summit, NJ.)

are stored in HIPAA-compliant cloud services hosted at Microsoft's Azure (Microsoft Corp., Redmond, WA) data centers [42].

The VisuALL uses Goldmann size III and V test stimuli in each virtual field (VF) protocol and has 2 displays (one for each eye) allowing it to test both eyes simultaneously but separately with similar test duration. The presentation of results for the Olleyes VisuALL with the stimulus sizes III and V are shown in Fig. 6. The device uses scotopic 1 cd/m^2 testing conditions in which a white stimulus is shown against a black background (1 cd/m^2). It uses a double crossover method to establish the threshold for 4 anchor points (one in each quadrant) after which it uses proprietary testing strategy to determine the threshold values for predetermined adjacent locations. The T-24 protocol tests 50 points of the central 24° (with test locations 6° apart) and the T-10 tests 68 points of the central 10° (with test locations 2° apart) [42]. In a study on normal individuals and glaucoma patients, all participants had visual field testing with VisuALL and the HFA. The global mean sensitivity of the VisuALL and the HFA correlated significantly in both normal and glaucoma groups. The

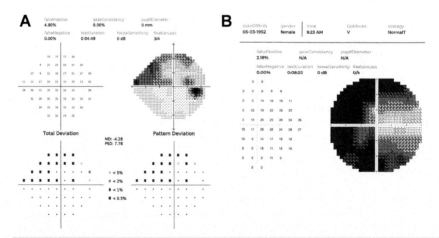

Fig. 6. VisuALL printouts showing superior arcuate defect with Goldmann size III stimulus **(A)** and advanced glaucomatous defect with Goldmann size V stimulus **(B)**. (*Courtesy of* Olleyes, Inc., Summit, NJ.)

mean sensitivity of all quadrants also correlated significantly in both groups. The VisuALL mean sensitivity had a greater (0.98) receiver operating characteristic curve than HFA (0.93) mean sensitivity in discriminating normal versus glaucoma [18]. The eye tracking system of VisuALL may improve the reliability of the visual field testing—it adjusts stimuli location for small changes in eye position and pauses testing with large eye-position deviations. The printout of the visual field of a patient with poorly reliable Octopus results who did a reliable test with VisuALL is shown in Fig. 7. In addition to checking the 24-2 and 10-2 visual field with stimulus size III and V, it evaluates Esterman, ptosis, pediatric field, visual acuity, low-contrast visual acuity, color vision, and contrast sensitivity.

Advanced vision analyzer
Advanced Vision Analyzer (AVA; Elisar Vision Technology) incorporates a customized Elisar Standard Algorithm that allows visual field evaluation under

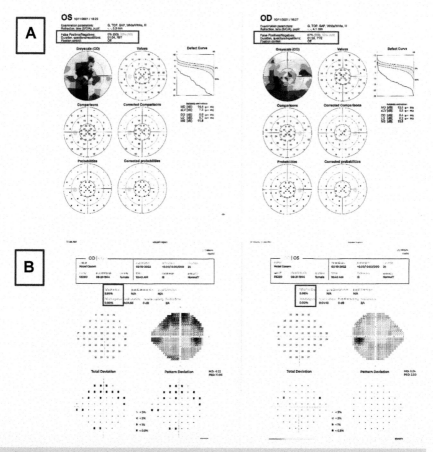

Fig. 7. Comparison between bad reliability indices of Octopus perimetry (**A**) versus very good reliability of VisuALL (**B**) in the same patient. (*Courtesy of* Olleyes, Inc., Summit, NJ.)

test conditions compatible with SAP with eye-tracking and a cloud-based storage system. It comprises of 4 main components: a 500-g HMD, a patient response button, a test controller device, and a backend cloud server. The HMD incorporates an optic and display subsystem that comprises a spectroscope with a liquid crystal display (LCD). The screen is coupled with a convex lens system that presents a magnified virtual image at 60 cm. The monocular field of view achieved for each eye is 60°, which allows conducting the standard 30-2, 24-2, and 10-2 tests. The algorithms incorporated in the AVA include Full Threshold, Elisar Standard, and Elisar Fast. The eye-tracking subsystem consists of 2 IR metal-oxide-semiconductor cameras placed for each eye and an array of IR LEDs is reflected in the pupil. Background illumination of the display is maintained at 9.6 cd/m^2, which can be controlled by changing the brightness and luminance of the screen. Goldman III size stimuli are presented for the range of 40 to 9 dB.

In a cross-sectional case series, AVA was evaluated and compared with HFA in normal and patients with glaucoma. The mean test duration with the AVA was slightly longer than HFA. The correlation coefficients for pointwise threshold values were moderately to strongly correlated with HFA, suggesting substantial equivalence between the AVA and HFA and implying that AVA may allow accurate assessment of visual field. Regarding test–retest variability, response variability decreased with an increase in sensitivity and increased with eccentricity. Blind spot location was accurate, and global indices of testing methods correlated well [43].

GlauCUTU virtual field test

GlauCUTU (Fig. 8) is a time until perceived perimeter using a portable VR headset with progressively increasing intensity of stimuli. The headset comprises of 2 separate LCD systems to provide a binocular view, which enables adequate positioning and increases the subject's field of view. The test reports real-time results including fixation loss and false-positive rate, as well as parameters such as stimulus presentation rate. GlauCUTU 24-2 tests 54 points that are 6° apart and 12 points are located in the central 10°. Responses are collected in terms of TUR, which is used to calculate time unit perceived and reported in terms of GlauCUTU sensitivity.

An automated transformation was developed to convert GlauCUTU sensitivity into HFA sensitivity using machine learning and deep learning algorithms. Results demonstrate no significant difference between HFA and GlauCUTU with machine learning transformation (GlauCUTU-ML) in all glaucoma stages [44]. Kunumpol and colleagues [44], investigated the accuracy of GlauCUTU test, and found that the system effectively differentiated glaucomatous from normal eyes. When compared with the HFA, the GlauCUTU test produced a significantly shorter average test duration by 354 seconds (254.41 seconds for GlauCUTU and 609 seconds for HFA).

Oculus quest virtual reality headset

Oculus Quest VR headset (Facebook Technologies, LLC, Bern, Switzerland;) is designed to simulate a standard visual field test by implementing the testing

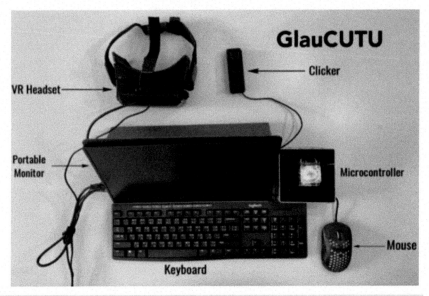

Fig. 8. Components of GlauCUTU showing a portable virtual reality headset, clicker, and a monitor with keyboard and mouse set. (*Courtesy of* GlauCUTU.)

principles used in Octopus 900. The light stimuli size III is presented, and subject feedback is provided with a remote clicker connected via Bluetooth. Noninferiority of Oculus Quest VR headset compared with SAP was investigated by Stapelfeldt and colleagues [45]. The participants underwent perimetry tests with Octopus 900 (Haag-Streit, Köniz, Switzerland) as the standard method. The standard dynamic strategy was used in conjunction with the G testing pattern. The results showed high mean MD correlations between the 2 systems. The VR system visual field defects in subjects with glaucoma were 1.4 dB less compared with the Octopus 900. No significant bias was found with respect to eccentricity or subject age. A similar number of stimuli presentations per visual field was necessary when measuring in patients with glaucoma and healthy subjects.

HTC vive pro eye with LUXIE software
HTC Vive Pro Eye (Fig. 9) comprises of 2 active-matrix organic light-emitting diode screens in Fresnel lenses and a field of view of 110° per eye with a Tobii eye tracker. The LUXIE test grids contain 76 points in the central 30° of visual field. The stimulus is 4 mm², corresponding to the Goldmann size III stimulus, and is displayed in a virtual bowl (radius 33 cm) using trigonometry adjustment. Each eye is tested separately without eye patching. LUXIE is not able to detect retinal sensitivity less than 14 dB.

Comparing the LUXIE with HFA, LUXIE demonstrated strong correlation with HFA in global mean sensitivity but the peripheral test locations had a

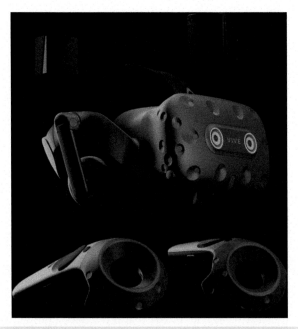

Fig. 9. HTC Vive Pro Eye head-mounted device with controller. (*Courtesy of* HTC Corporation. All rights reserved.)

weaker correlation with HFA. The test locations adjacent to the blind spot also showed weaker correlations in this study. The LUXIE has built-in eye-tracking, which adjusts the display of stimulus according to eye movement, and this may be part of the reason for these differences. The user survey showed that the participants were more satisfied with LUXIE in terms of operating difficulty, comfortability, time perception, concentration, and overall satisfaction [46].

Palm scan VF2000
The Palm Scan VF 2000 (Fig. 10) comprises of VR goggles; the controller device operated by the health-care staff who sets the testing strategy and the clicker. In a cross-sectional study, the sensitivity, specificity, positive predictive value, and negative predictive value for classification of individuals as glaucoma/nonglaucoma was 100%. The general agreement for the classification of glaucoma between Palm Scan and HFA was 0.63. The agreements for mild, moderate, and severe glaucoma were 0.76, 0.37, and 0.70, respectively. About 28% of moderate glaucoma cases were misclassified as mild and 17% as severe. Furthermore, 20% of severe cases were misclassified as moderate. Although the authors concluded that Palm Scan was 100% sensitive and specific in detecting glaucoma in this study, there is a relatively high proportion of misclassification in glaucoma severity [47].

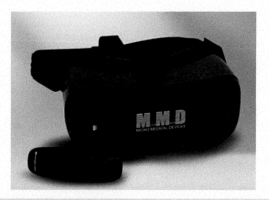

Fig. 10. Palm Scan VF2000 head-mounted device with controller. (*Courtesy of* Micro Medical Devices Inc., Calabasas, CA.)

Virtual field

Virtual Field (VF3 and VF3 Pro; Fig. 11) is a head-mounted VR perimeter that offers many features in addition to visual field-testing including color vision and pupillometry for relative afferent defect screening. It incorporates a special software for testing patients with ptosis. It also provides a progression analysis printout (Fig. 12). The test can be done monocular or binocular. Magnetic trial lens adapters are available for patients with refractive errors, or patients can wear their own glasses. Active eye tracking is available in the newer version VF3 Pro. Studies have shown that VF had good correlation with the HFA measurements [48,49].

nGoggle

The nGoggle (nGoggle, Inc., San Diego, CA; Fig. 13) integrates wearable wireless electroencephalogram (EEG) and electrooculogram (EOG) systems and a

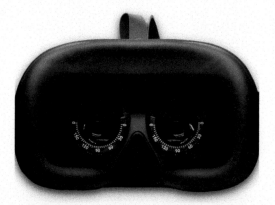

Fig. 11. Virtual Field VF3 head-mounted device. (*Courtesy of* Virtual Field, Inc., New York City, NY.)

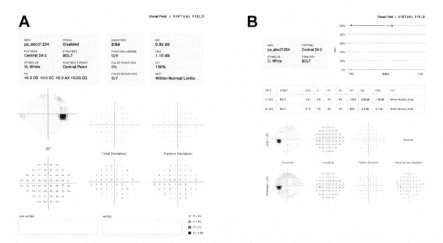

Fig. 12. Virtual field printouts showing superior arcuate defect with Goldmann size III stimulus (**A**) and progression analysis (**B**). (*Courtesy of* Virtual Field, Inc. New York City, NY.)

cellphone-based head-mounted display. The portable device is capable of objectively assessing visual function loss through detection of multifocal steady-state visual-evoked potentials associated with visual field stimulation. Earlier work with nonwearable EEG and EOG-based testing for glaucoma has not proven clinically useful for routine testing and patient care.

In a case control study including patients with glaucoma and healthy controls, the nGoggle demonstrated good agreement with SAP. The device was able to distinguish glaucomatous eyes from healthy eyes. No statistically significant differences were seen for the sectoral measurements between the nGoggle

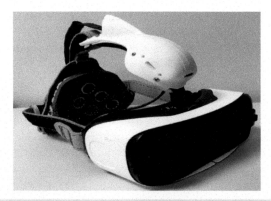

Fig. 13. nGoggle portable brain computer interface incorporating a dry EEG and EOG systems in the head-mounted device. (*Courtesy of* nGoggle, Inc., San Diego, CA.)

and SAP [50]. The study further investigated the ability of the nGoggle in detecting glaucomatous damage, by comparing its diagnostic accuracy to that of retinal nerve fiber layer thickness measurements obtained with spectral-domain OCT. The nGoggle global parameter had specificity and sensitivity, which were comparable to the retinal nerve fiber layer [50].

Toronto portable perimeter
The Toronto Portable Perimeter (TPP; VEM Medical Technologies, Toronto, Canada) is based on a cell phone, VR headset, handheld controller, and software app. Background illumination is 10 Cd/m^2, similar to the HFA. Goldmann size III stimuli are used to test high-threshold sensitivities, and Goldmann sizes IV and V stimuli are used for lower threshold stimuli. Sensitivity thresholds are measured at 54 points in the VF.

In a study of 91 patients and 150 eyes, the TPP showed similar results to the HFA SITA Standard 24-2 with similar test duration. A questionnaire revealed a preference by patients for the TPP over the HFA with patients finding the instructions easier to understand and the test easier to complete on the TPP [51].

BENEFITS AND LIMITATIONS

Although virtual perimetry is a new promising technology that has many advantages over the traditional SAP, including being portable, affordable, and a convenient device especially for bedridden, wheelchair-bound patients, and in teleglaucoma, it still has its own limitations.

One of the major drawbacks is the relatively lower sensitivity of some devices as compared with SAP especially in early glaucoma. Accordingly, the results are not robust enough to support using all types of virtual perimetry for screening general populations, although using this tool for high-risk groups, such as for people with limited or no access to eyecare and nonambulatory or debilitated elderly is useful, at least the patients with advanced glaucoma will not be missed.

Cost-effectiveness of glaucoma home monitoring has also yet to be demonstrated, and it would be helpful to perform an economic evaluation of its utility, similar to that reported recently for age-related macular degeneration home monitoring [52]. Combining home perimetry and tonometry with the technology advancement seems increasingly practicable [53].

Tablet-based perimeters
The major limitations of tablet perimeters include the testing environment. Most studies were conducted in a controlled environment in the clinic on patients with earlier SAP-testing experience with strict control of viewing distance and ambient light. These factors are less likely to be as controlled in the home environment. Moreover, the performance of patients who are not experienced in visual field testing needs to be evaluated in both supervised and unsupervised (home) environments, especially with the absence of effective eye tracking system in tablet perimeters, although HFA lacks adjustments for eye tracking. Furthermore, technical problems were sometimes experienced were

related to the device, software, or the patient. The instructions and training required for these patients to achieve reliable visual field results needs to be developed.

The future development of an effective tracking system for monitoring head and eye positions using the camera/eye tracker would allow fixation monitoring during field testing.

Head mounted perimeters

Notwithstanding the myriad benefits of the head-mounted perimeters, there are also specific limitations. Foremost is the lack of large database for both normal and glaucomatous visual fields. Normative database is still new and need to be expanded and updated. Not all of the mentioned studies had adequate sample

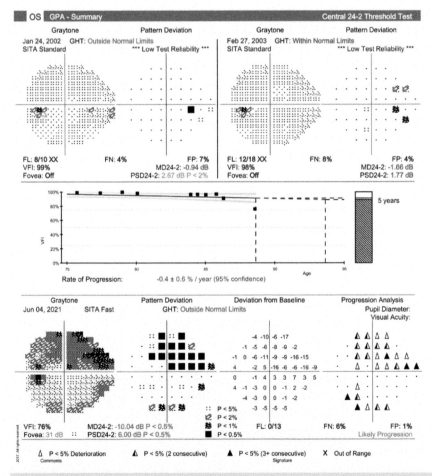

Fig. 14. Glaucoma progression analysis summary of Humphrey Field Analyzer 24-2 test.

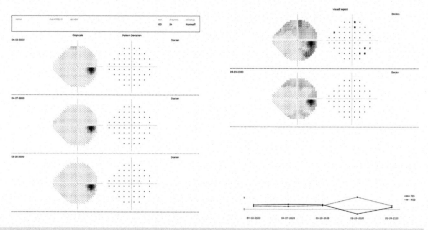

Fig. 15. VisuALL follow-up report with trend analysis for mean deviation and pattern standard deviation. (*Courtesy* of Olleyes, Inc., Summit, NJ.)

size and diversity to strongly validate the test results. Additionally, progression analysis is not yet available for many devices. The glaucoma progression analysis of HFA is shown in Fig. 14. The VisuALL follow-up printout showing the trend analysis for the MD and pattern standard deviation is shown in Fig. 15. Some of the virtual perimeters require refractive error correction by the trial lenses, which may result in lens-rim artifact (Fig. 16). Test duration may be longer than in SAP in some versions, and newer testing strategies are needed to reduce the duration of the test. The HMDs may not be tolerated by claustrophobic patients, and these patients may benefit from the updated tablet-based perimeters.

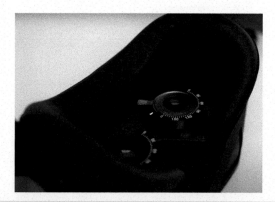

Fig. 16. Head-mounted device with corrective lens holders, which may result in lens-rim artifact. (*Courtesy of* Virtual Field, Inc. New York City, NY.)

SUMMARY

Virtual perimetry is a promising technology that could expand the visual field testing and monitoring of glaucoma and neurologic patients and decrease the burden of visual field testing for physicians and patients. Further refinements of the available devices, with better screening and monitoring strategies, software improvements, and development of normative databases should improve detection and monitoring of glaucoma and nonglaucomatous optic neuropathies, particularly in resource-limited settings.

FINANCIAL DISCLOSURE

J.S. Myers: Consultant: AbbVie, Aerie, Avisi, Embark Neuro, Glaukos, Haag Streit, MicroOptx, Olleyes. Research: AbbVie, Aerie, Equinox, Glaukos, Guardian, Haag Streit, Laboratories Thea, Nicox, Olleyes, Santen. R. Razeghinejad: Equinox, Olleyes, New World Medical.

References

[1] Koehler PJ. The historical roots of the visual examination. Semin Neurol 2002;22(4): 357–66.

[2] Thompson H, Wall M. History of Perimetry. Imaging and Perimetry Society (IPS). Available at: http://webeye.ophth.uiowa.edu/ips/PerimetryHistory/. Published 2008. Accessed January 2023.

[3] Johnson CA, Wall M, Thompson HS. A history of perimetry and visual field testing. Optom Vis Sci 2011;88(1):E8–15.

[4] LLOYD RI. Evolution of perimetry. Arch Ophthalmol 1936;15(4):713–32.

[5] Lascaratos J, Marketos S. A historical outline of Greek ophthalmology from the Hellenistic period up to the establishment of the first universities. Doc Ophthalmol 1988;68(1–2): 157–69.

[6] Graefe A v. Ueber die Untersuchung des Gesichtsfeldes bei amblyopischen Affectionen. Archiv für Ophthalmologie. 1856;2(2):258–98.

[7] Verriest G, Padmos P, Greve EL. Calibration of the Tübinger perimeter for colour perimetry. Mod Probl Ophthalmol 1974;13(0):109–12.

[8] Sloan LL. The Tubinger perimeter of Harms and Aulhorn. Recommended procedures and supplementary equipment. Arch Ophthalmol 1971;86(6):612–22.

[9] Gloor BP. Franz Fankhauser: the father of the automated perimeter. Surv Ophthalmol 2009;54(3):417–25.

[10] Ruia S., Tripathy K., Humphrey Visual Field. [Updated 2023 Feb 22]. In: StatPearls [Internet]. Treasure Island (FL): StatPearls Publishing; 2023. https://www.ncbi.nlm.nih.gov/books/NBK585112/.

[11] Katz J, Tielsch JM, Quigley HA, et al. Automated perimetry detects visual field loss before manual Goldmann perimetry. Ophthalmology 1995;102(1):21–6.

[12] Weijland A, Fankhauser F, Bebie H, et al. Automated perimetry : visual field digest, . S.l. 5th ed. Belgium: Haag Streit International; 2004.

[13] Prager AJ, Kang JM, Tanna AP. Advances in perimetry for glaucoma. Curr Opin Ophthalmol 2021;32(2):92–7.

[14] Johnson CA, Thapa S, George Kong YX, et al. Performance of an iPad Application to Detect Moderate and Advanced Visual Field Loss in Nepal. Am J Ophthalmol 2017;182:147–54.

[15] Kumar H, Thulasidas M. Comparison of Perimetric Outcomes from Melbourne Rapid Fields Tablet Perimeter Software and Humphrey Field Analyzer in Glaucoma Patients. J Ophthalmol 2020;2020:8384509.

[16] Jones PR, Lindfield D, Crabb DP. Using an open-source tablet perimeter (Eyecatcher) as a rapid triage measure for glaucoma clinic waiting areas. Br J Ophthalmol 2021;105(5):681–6.

[17] Greenfield JA, Deiner M, Nguyen A, et al. Virtual Reality Oculokinetic Perimetry Test Reproducibility and Relationship to Conventional Perimetry and OCT. Ophthalmol Sci 2022;2(1): 100105.

[18] Razeghinejad R, Gonzalez-Garcia A, Myers JS, et al. Preliminary Report on a Novel Virtual Reality Perimeter Compared With Standard Automated Perimetry. J Glaucoma 2021;30(1):17–23.

[19] Ma MKI, Saha C, Poon SHL, et al. Virtual reality and augmented reality- emerging screening and diagnostic techniques in ophthalmology: A systematic review. Surv Ophthalmol 2022;67(5):1516–30.

[20] Odayappan A, Sivakumar P, Kotawala S, et al. Comparison of a New Head Mount Virtual Reality Perimeter (C3 Field Analyzer) With Automated Field Analyzer in Neuro-Ophthalmic Disorders. J Neuro Ophthalmol 2022; https://doi.org/10.1097/WNO. 0000000000001714.

[21] Mees L, Upadhyaya S, Kumar P, et al. Validation of a Head-mounted Virtual Reality Visual Field Screening Device. J Glaucoma 2020;29(2):86–91.

[22] Hudson C, Wild JM, O'Neill EC. Fatigue effects during a single session of automated static threshold perimetry. Invest Ophthalmol Vis Sci 1994;35(1):268–80.

[23] Schimiti RB, Avelino RR, Kara-Jose N, et al. Full-threshold versus Swedish Interactive Threshold Algorithm (SITA) in normal individuals undergoing automated perimetry for the first time. Ophthalmology 2002;109(11):2084–92 [discussion: 2092].

[24] Wu Z, Saunders LJ, Daga FB, et al. Frequency of Testing to Detect Visual Field Progression Derived Using a Longitudinal Cohort of Glaucoma Patients. Ophthalmology 2017;124(6): 786–92.

[25] Hark L, Waisbourd M, Myers JS, et al. Improving Access to Eye Care among Persons at High-Risk of Glaucoma in Philadelphia–Design and Methodology: The Philadelphia Glaucoma Detection and Treatment Project. Ophthalmic Epidemiol 2016;23(2):122–30.

[26] Glaucoma Today; Henderer JD. Visual Fields as Screening Tools. Available at: https://glaucomatoday.com/articles/2016-may-june/visual-fields-as-screening-tools. Published 2016. Accessed 2022.

[27] Groth SL. New Strategies for Automated Perimetry: Historical Perspective and Future Innovations. J Curr Glaucoma Pract 2021;15(3):103–5.

[28] Groth SL, Linton E, Brown E, et al. Novel Virtual-Reality Perimetey in normal children compared to Humprey Field Analyzer. Investigative Ophthalmology & Visual Science. 2021;62(8):3391.

[29] Nesaratnam N, Thomas PBM, Kirollos R, et al. Tablets at the bedside - iPad-based visual field test used in the diagnosis of Intrasellar Haemangiopericytoma: a case report. BMC Ophthalmol 2017;17(1):53.

[30] Ophthalmology AAo. Telemedicine for Ophthalmology Information Statement - 2018. Available at: https://www.aao.org/clinical-statement/telemedicine-ophthalmology-information-statement. Published 2018. Accessed2022.

[31] Kassam F, Yogesan K, Sogbesan E, et al. Teleglaucoma: improving access and efficiency for glaucoma care. Middle East Afr J Ophthalmol 2013;20(2):142–9.

[32] Damji KF. Strengthening institutional capacity for glaucoma care in sub-Saharan Africa. Middle East Afr J Ophthalmol 2013;20(2):107–10.

[33] Skalicky SE, Kong GY. Novel Means of Clinical Visual Function Testing among Glaucoma Patients, Including Virtual Reality. J Curr Glaucoma Pract 2019;13(3):83–7.

[34] Vingrys AJ, Healey JK, Liew S, et al. Validation of a Tablet as a Tangent Perimeter. Transl Vis Sci Technol 2016;5(4):3.

[35] Kong YX, He M, Crowston JG, et al. A Comparison of Perimetric Results from a Tablet Perimeter and Humphrey Field Analyzer in Glaucoma Patients. Transl Vis Sci Technol 2016;5(6):2.

[36] Landers J, Sharma A, Goldberg I, et al. A comparison of perimetric results with the Medmont and Humphrey perimeters. Br J Ophthalmol 2003;87(6):690–4.

[37] Fredette MJ, Giguere A, Anderson DR, et al. Comparison of Matrix with Humphrey Field Analyzer II with SITA. Optom Vis Sci 2015;92(5):527–36.

[38] Jones PR, Smith ND, Bi W, et al. Portable Perimetry Using Eye-Tracking on a Tablet Computer-A Feasibility Assessment. Transl Vis Sci Technol 2019;8(1):17.

[39] Ichhpujani P, Thakur S, Sahi RK, et al. Validating tablet perimetry against standard Humphrey Visual Field Analyzer for glaucoma screening in Indian population. Indian J Ophthalmol 2021;69(1):87–91.

[40] Santos AS, Morabe ES. VisualFields Easy'': an iPad application as a simple tool for detecting visual field defects. Philipp J Ophthalmol 2016;41:22–6.

[41] Kitayama K, Young AG, Ochoa A 3rd, et al. The Agreement Between an iPad Visual Field App and Humphrey Frequency Doubling Technology in Visual Field Screening at Health Fairs. J Glaucoma 2021;30(9):846–50.

[42] Montelongo M, Gonzalez A, Morgenstern F, et al. A Virtual Reality-Based Automated Perimeter, Device, and Pilot Study. Transl Vis Sci Technol 2021;10(3):20.

[43] Narang P, Agarwal A, Srinivasan M. Advanced Vision Analyzer-Virtual Reality Perimeter: Device Validation, Functional Correlation and Comparison with Humphrey Field Analyzer. Ophthalmol Sci 2021;1(2):100035.

[44] Kunumpol P, Lerthirunvibul N, Phienphanich P, et al. GlauCUTU: Virtual Reality Visual Field Test. Annu Int Conf IEEE Eng Med Biol Soc 2021;2021:7416–21.

[45] Stapelfeldt J, Kucur SS, Huber N, et al. Virtual Reality-Based and Conventional Visual Field Examination Comparison in Healthy and Glaucoma Patients. Transl Vis Sci Technol 2021;10(12):10.

[46] Chen YT, Yeh PH, Cheng YC, et al. Application and Validation of LUXIE: A Newly Developed Virtual Reality Perimetry Software. J Pers Med 2022;12(10).

[47] Shetty V, Sankhe P, Haldipurkar SS, et al. Diagnostic Performance of the PalmScan VF2000 Virtual Reality Visual Field Analyzer for Identification and Classification of Glaucoma. J Ophthalmic Vis Res 2022;17(1):33–41.

[48] Phu J, Kalloniatis M. Static automated perimetry using a new head-mounted virtual reality platform, Virtual Field, compared with the Humphrey Field Analyzer in glaucoma and optic nerve disease. Investigative Ophthalmology & Visual Science 2021;62(8):3364.

[49] Nanti NB, Lenoci J. Comparison of Virtual Reality Visual Field Testing to Humphrey Visual Field Testing in an Academic Ophthalmology Practice. Investigative Ophthalmology & Visual Science. 2021;62(8):3486.

[50] Nakanishi M, Wang YT, Jung TP, et al. Detecting Glaucoma With a Portable Brain-Computer Interface for Objective Assessment of Visual Function Loss. JAMA Ophthalmol 2017;135(6):550–7.

[51] Ahmed Y, Pereira A, Bowden S, et al. Multicenter Comparison of the Toronto Portable Perimeter with the Humphrey Field Analyzer: A Pilot Study. Ophthalmol Glaucoma 2022;5(2):146–59.

[52] Wittenborn JS, Clemons T, Regillo C, et al. Economic Evaluation of a Home-Based Age-Related Macular Degeneration Monitoring System. JAMA Ophthalmol 2017;135(5):452–9.

[53] Mudie LI, LaBarre S, Varadaraj V, et al. The Icare HOME (TA022) Study: Performance of an Intraocular Pressure Measuring Device for Self-Tonometry by Glaucoma Patients. Ophthalmology 2016;123(8):1675–84.

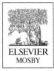

Advances in Ophthalmology and Optometry 8 (2023) 239–248

ADVANCES IN OPHTHALMOLOGY AND OPTOMETRY

Minimally Invasive Glaucoma Surgery: Past, Present, and Future

Lea Carter, BS, DO[a,1], Leon W. Herndon, MD[b,*]

[a]Campbell University School of Osteopathic Medicine, Leon Levine Hall of Medical Sciences, 4350 US Hwy 421 South, Lillington, NC 27546, USA; [b]Duke Eye Center, 2351 Erwin Road, Durham, NC 27705, USA

Keywords
- Minimally invasive glaucoma surgery • Trabeculectomy • Trabeculotomy
- Goniotomy • Future of MIGS

Key points
- Minimally invasive glaucoma surgery (MIGS) is the newest group of glaucoma surgical procedures that are known for their high safety profile.
- MIGS is commonly used in mild to moderate glaucoma, providing surgical options for patients before advanced stages.
- The future of MIGS surgery involves innovation to further improve intraocular pressure reduction while maintaining high safety and lack of post-operative complications.

Video content accompanies this article at http://www.advancesinophthalmology.com.

INTRODUCTION

Glaucoma remains one of the top causes of chronic vision loss throughout the world, affecting approximately 76 million people [1]. Even with the innovations of new medical, laser, and surgical techniques, glaucoma is still one of the leading causes of blindness, with an estimated 12 million people blind from glaucoma worldwide [1]. Glaucoma is defined as the degeneration and death of retinal ganglion cells, which results in progressive visual field loss [2]. Although age, race, family history, systemic disease, and corneal thickness are all risk

[1]Present address: 1300 South Harding Drive, Apartment 1103, Goldsboro, NC 27534.

*Corresponding author. Leon Levine Hall of Medical Sciences, 4350 US Hwy 421 South, Lillington, NC 27546. E-mail address: leon.herndon@duke.edu

https://doi.org/10.1016/j.yaoo.2023.03.005

factors for glaucoma, elevated intraocular pressure (IOP) is the only risk factor we can treat [2]. Glaucoma treatment is centered on maintaining a target IOP, which can be different for each patient. Although IOP between 10 to 21 mm Hg is statistically normal, target IOP is defined as the pressure at which there is no further progression of glaucomatous damage.

Minimally invasive glaucoma surgery, otherwise known as MIGS, is the newest branch of glaucoma surgical treatments offered today and allows surgical options for patients in all stages of glaucoma. Traditional glaucoma surgery (trabeculectomy and glaucoma drainage device surgery) is still the most effective option for large IOP reduction, but the risk of complications limits its use in milder stages of glaucoma. MIGS procedures are aimed at minimizing intraocular trauma, and, therefore, have a safer and quicker post-operative recovery period [2]. The advantage of MIGS comes from the safety profile, but also from the opportunity to intervene earlier in the course of glaucoma. Surgically intervening in the mild to moderate stages of glaucoma allows an intermediate and sometimes long-term solution for patients in pressure management and also can decrease the number of topical medications needed. Earlier surgical intervention ultimately is aimed at preventing progression of glaucoma to advanced stages.

SIGNIFICANCE

Traditional glaucoma surgical procedures create a new surgical pathway for aqueous humor to flow. Trabeculectomy has been the foundation for glaucoma surgery since its introduction almost 60 years ago [2,3]. Trabeculectomy has provided a consistent long-term pressure control for patients, but has a relatively higher risk profile, as serious complications have been known to occur. Glaucoma tube shunt surgery has made a comparable attempt in pressure control in relation to trabeculectomy, but is still an invasive technique requiring extensive tissue dissection. Compared to MIGS procedures, trabeculectomy and tube shunts provide a more reliable and effective IOP reduction, but also come with higher risk.

Trabeculectomy

Trabeculectomy is considered the gold standard for surgical glaucoma treatment but has gradually decreased in use over recent years since the introduction of MIGS [4]. Trabeculectomy creates a new pathway for aqueous humor to flow through a partial thickness scleral flap into a sub-conjunctival reservoir called a bleb. Trabeculectomy commonly is considered the primary surgical intervention in advanced glaucoma where a large reduction in IOP is necessary [2,3]. The routine use of antimetabolites and releasable sutures has improved management of post-operative scarring and flow rate, but the risk of serious complications, such as blebitis, bleb leakage, hypotony, hyphema, and endophthalmitis poses a hindrance to the universal use of trabeculectomy in the earlier stages of glaucoma [3]. Trabeculectomy is at higher risk for failure in patients with previous eye surgery, inflammatory glaucoma, younger age, and multiple topical medication use [5]. In cases with high risk for surgical failure, other procedures can provide an alternative option with a greater likelihood of success.

Tube shunts

Glaucoma tube shunt surgery commonly is used today in moderate to severe glaucoma and was originally designed to minimize the complications seen with trabeculectomy [2,6]. Similar to trabeculectomy, tube shunts create a new outflow track for aqueous humor to drain into the subconjunctival space. A tube is placed in the anterior chamber allowing flow through either a valved or non-valved implant secured approximately 10 mm from the limbus. Valved implants, such as the Ahmed Glaucoma Valve (New World Medical, Rancho Cucamonga, CA, USA) decrease the risk for post-operative hypotony. Non-valved implants such as the Baerveldt (Johnson & Johnson Vision, Jacksonville, FL, USA) have been shown to be superior in IOP reduction compared to valved implants, but maintain a higher risk of post-operative hypotony [7]. In tube shunts, the bleb is located more posterior than with trabeculectomy, which is thought to be advantageous from an infection risk and minimizing bleb complications. With the publication of the Tube versus Trabeculectomy (TVT) Study, tube shunts have been shown to be both safe and effective, with comparable results to trabeculectomy [6,8]. Efficacy has been further classified based on pre-operative IOP in primary surgery. Tube shunts are shown to have a higher success rate than trabeculectomy when pre-operative IOP is > 25 mm Hg. Trabeculectomy is more effective in patients with a pre-operative IOP of < 21 mm Hg [6,8].

MIGS is largely directed at enhancing the physiologic flow of aqueous humor. The main site of action is at Schlemm's canal, with various types of techniques to provide better drainage from the anterior chamber. The commonly used MIGS procedures can be sub-divided into overarching categories based on the type of procedure: stenting, trabeculotomy/goniotomy, suprachoroidal, and subconjunctival devices. MIGS is based on a minimally invasive approach, creating less post-surgical inflammation and reducing common post-operative complications seen in the more invasive trabeculectomy and tube shunts.

Stenting devices

Stenting devices such as the *iStent* (Glaukos Corporation, San Clemente, CA, USA) and *Hydrus* (Alcon, Fort Worth, TX, USA) enhance the physiologic flow of aqueous humor through the trabecular meshwork and into Schlemm's canal. *IStent* was the first FDA-approved MIGS device to be used in conjunction with cataract surgery [2]. Cataract removal alone has been shown to reduce IOP between 2 and 4 mm Hg, and with *iStent* can have a 20% decrease in IOP [9–11]. The original iStent was 360 um long and made of titanium. It was inserted through the trabecular meshwork and into Schlemm's canal through an injection device [2] (Video 1, Fig. 1). *Hydrus* is much larger, an 8 mm curved stent that was made to mimic the curvature in Schlemm's canal [2] (Video 2, Fig. 2). Although both Hydrus and iStent have been shown to effectively lower IOP with no significant differences between the two, *Hydrus* has been shown to be superior to *iStent* in reducing the amount of post-

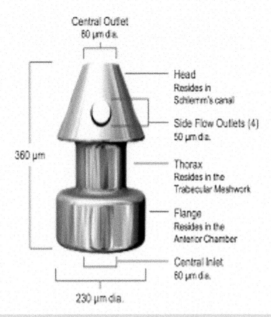

Fig. 1. Hydrus.

operative drops required for patients at 12 months [12]. Several modifications of the iStent have been brought to market, including the recently approved iStent infinite where three stents are placed into Schlemm's canal combined with cataract surgery or as a standalone procedure.

Trabeculotomy devices

Trabeculotomy devices involve opening up Schlemm's canal through either dilation and/or goniotomy of the trabecular meshwork. The gonioscopy-assisted transluminal trabeculotomy (GATT) involves using an iTrack catheter (Nova Eye Medical, Kent Town, SA) or a suture to dilate Schlemm's canal a full

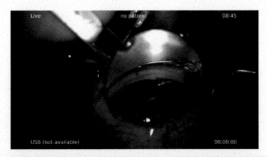

Fig. 2. GATT. (*From* Kim WI, Aref AA, Moore DB. Canaloplasty. American Academy of Ophthalmology EyeWiki. February 10, 2023. Accessed March 3, 2023. https://eyewiki.aao.org/Canaloplasty.)

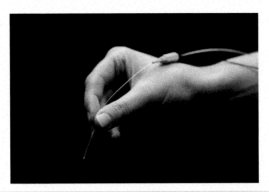

Fig. 3. iStent. (*Courtesy of* iStent inject® W, registered trademarks of Avedro, a Glaukos company.)

360° (Video 3, Fig. 3). In a 24-month follow-up study, *GATT* averaged a 9 mm Hg IOP decrease in primary-open angle glaucoma patients. *GATT* appeared more effective at IOP reduction in cases of secondary glaucoma, averaging a 14 mm Hg IOP reduction in those cases [13]. The Kahook Dual Blade (KDB, New World Medical, Rancho Cucamonga, CA, USA) is a two-blade device which is used to remove the trabecular meshwork (Video 4, Fig. 4). *KDB* alone can produce a 6 mm Hg IOP reduction on average. *OMNI* (Sight Sciences, Menlo Park, CA, USA) is a dual system which combines both approaches of dilation and goniotomy. During the *OMNI* procedure, a micro-catheter is placed in Schlemm's canal, but distinct from *GATT*, the trabecular meshwork is removed as the catheter is retracted. *OMNI* achieves a 10 to 12 mm Hg IOP reduction [14]. All of the trabeculotomy procedures carry the risk of significant hyphema [15].

Suprachoroidal devices

Although the majority of MIGS is focused on the trabecular meshwork, attempts also have been made to increase aqueous flow through stenting of the

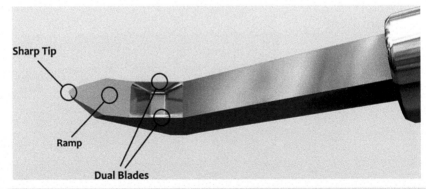

Fig. 4. KDB. (*From* Greenwood MD, Seibold LK, Radcliffe NM, et al. Goniotomy with a single-use dual blade: Short-term results. J Cataract Refract Surg. 2017;43(9):1197-1201.)

uveoscleral pathway. The *CyPass Micro-Stent* (Alcon, Fort Worth, TX, USA) is a 6.35 mm fenestrated stenting device which is placed ab interno in between the scleral spur and ciliary body into the supraciliary space [14,16]. Although early studies on the *CyPass Micro-Stent* did show IOP reduction, safety concerns led to the *CyPass* being taken off the market. Similar complications and adverse safety effects have been seen with other suprachoroidal devices such as the *SOLX gold shunt* (SOLX Inc, Waltham, MA, USA) and *STARflo* device (iSTAR Medical, Wavre, Belgium). The newest suprachoroidal device, the *MINIject* (iSTAR Medical, Wavre, Belgium) has shown short-term IOP reduction without fewer adverse effects [16]. Currently, no FDA-approved suprachoroidal device exists in the market.

Subconjunctival devices

Subconjunctival devices such as the *XEN gel stent* (Allergan Madison, NJ, USA) and *PreserFlo* (Glaukos Corporation, San Clemente, CA, USA) work similarly to traditional trabeculectomy surgery in that a new drainage system is created for aqueous to flow under the conjunctiva. Subconjunctival devices can be referred to as minimally invasive bleb surgery (MIBS), a subset of MIGS that involves creating a bleb with a minimally invasive technique. The *XEN gel stent* can be placed ab externo or ab interno into the anterior chamber while the *PreserFlo* device can be placed only from an ab externo approach. The *XEN stent* has a 45-um lumen that has been designed through fluid mechanics to achieve a steady flow rate and prevent hypotony [17](Video 5, Fig. 5). *XEN gel stent* has been shown to have an average IOP reduction of 7 mm Hg [18]. *PreserFlo* has a slightly larger lumen at 70 um, and is comprised of polystyrene material designed to prevent scarring and bleb encapsulation [19]. The *PreserFlo* lowers IOP by 50% to 55%. The PreserFlo is not FDA-approved for use in the United States.

DISCUSSION

The minimally invasive technique is the rapidly evolving present and future of glaucoma surgery. Since the first FDA-approved iStent device in 2012, MIGS

XEN® Gel Stent

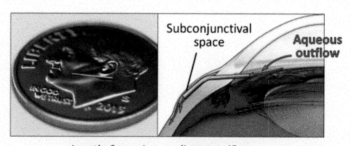

Length: 6 mm; Lumen diameter: 45 μm

Fig. 5. Xen gel stent. (*Courtesy of* XEN® GEL STENT, © 2021 AbbVie.)

treatments have rapidly increased in number and usage. Over the past 6 years, a two-fold increase in the use of MIGS, which has led to a relative decrease in traditional glaucoma surgeries, has been reported [20]. According to data from the Medicare database, MIGS currently accounts for 74% of all glaucoma surgeries, with trabeculectomy and tube shunts accounting for the remaining 26% [21]. Current trends of glaucoma surgery in the Medicare population are reflected in resident education and may predict the future physician tendency for MIGS and tube shunting procedures over trabeculectomy [22]. ACGME data show a stable number of glaucoma surgeries per resident but with an increasing trend toward shunting procedures. The decrease in trainee experience and comfort in trabeculectomy is an important consideration for education and trends in future practice patterns.

The *Trabeculectomy Ex-Press* device (Alcon, Fort Worth, TX, USA) is an implant that functions to enhance traditional trabeculectomy surgery. *EX-Press* surgery creates a subconjunctival bleb and scleral flap as seen in trabeculectomy, but the entrance into the anterior chamber is created by the stenting device instead of a surgically created opening. Using the *EX-Press* eliminates the need for a peripheral iridectomy, and has a relatively quicker post-operative recovery [23]. When compared to traditional trabeculectomy, *EX-Press* has comparable IOP results with no significant differences between the two. *EX- Press* typically lags behind trabeculectomy in IOP reduction in the early post-operative period, but by 3 months the IOP reduction is similar between the two procedures [23]. Devices such as the *EX- Press*, which enhance current effective procedures, provide an encouraging direction for improving the efficacy of MIGS-type devices.

One of the limitations of MIGS is the lack of consistent, randomized, and long-term study results available to us today. MIGS has been shown to be generally safe, with common complications including hyphema and device misplacement [14]. Stenting procedures such as iStent and Hydrus have the best safety profile, but with a mild degree of IOP lowering. Meanwhile, subconjunctival and bleb-forming MIGS procedures generally have a greater IOP reduction, but a relative increased risk of complications such as hypotony [14]. Although some MIGS devices show promising results, the inconsistencies in the current literature make these results difficult to analyze and compare. The current data on a majority of MIGS procedures consist of small, non-randomized, or retrospective studies with differences in definitions of treatment success [14]. To have more accurate and comparable evidence, larger randomized studies are needed, as well as long-term follow-up.

The 510(k) medical device clearance pathway is the process where the FDA is in agreement with the manufacturer that a medical device is similar to a previously approved product. This process requires no clinical trials and very little oversight, and while it leads to a quicker approval process, it is not without its detractors [24]. Over the past year, three new devices have been approved for angle glaucoma surgery. The iAccess Trephine (Glaukos Corporation, San Clemente, CA, USA), the Streamline Surgical System (New World Medical, Rancho

Cucamonga, CA, USA), and the SION Surgical Instrument (Sight Sciences, Menlo Park, CA, USA) were all approved by this process. Very little published information exists involving any of these new technologies, and it is doubtful that well-designed meaningful comparison studies will ever be conducted.

SUMMARY

Glaucoma management is a growing field that currently includes medical, laser, and surgical therapies. Surgical treatment usually is reserved for advanced cases with progressing visual field loss and/or optic nerve changes despite medical therapy. Although various risk factors such as age, race, previous eye surgery, and long-term medication use affect glaucoma risk, IOP currently is the only treatable risk factor. Lowering IOP to a sustainable threshold that prevents progression of disease is the target of surgical treatment. Various surgical procedures exist to choose from that will lower IOP, each with its risks and benefits. Traditional surgeries like trabeculectomy and glaucoma drainage devices remain the most effective surgical options in terms of lowering IOP, but the expanding field of MIGS procedures has allowed various new options available for patients who need minimal IOP control. Although MIGS is the current future of surgical glaucoma treatment, it is important to note that no "one size fits all" glaucoma surgical technique exists in terms of efficacy and safety; meaning each procedure must be considered by the clinician and chosen on a patient-by-patient basis.

CLINICS CARE POINTS

- Although MIGS is the current future of surgical glaucoma treatment, it is important to note that there is no "one size fits all" glaucoma surgical technique in terms of efficacy and safety. Therefore, each procedure must be considered by the clinician and chosen on a patient-by-patient basis.
- When considering trabeculectomy or tube shunt glaucoma surgery, take into consideration the pre-operative IOP. Tube shunts are shown to have a higher success rate in primary surgery when the pre-operative IOP is above 25 mm Hg compared with trabeculectomy.
- If cataract surgery is planned in a patient with mild to moderate glaucoma, consider concurrent MIGS procedures.
- When managing advanced glaucoma, remember that trabeculectomy and tube shunt procedures still provide the most significant IOP reduction.
- If a patient is a candidate for trabeculectomy surgery, consider the use of the Trabeculectomy Ex-Press shunt.

DISCLOSURE

Dr L.W. Herndon is a consultant to many companies in the glaucoma surgical market.

SUPPLEMENTARY DATA
Supplementary data related to this article can be found online at https://doi.org/10.1016/j.yaoo.2023.03.005.

References
[1] World report on vision. Geneva: World Health Organization; 2019. Licence: CC BY-NC-SA 3.0 IGO.
[2] Megevand G, Bron A. Personalizing surgical treatments for glaucoma patients. Prog Retin Eye Res 2021;81; https://doi.org/10.1016/j.preteyeres.2020.100879.
[3] Kirwin J, Lockwood A, Shah P, et al. Trabeculectomy in the 21st century: A multicenter analysis. Ophthalmology 2013;120(12):2532–9.
[4] Boland M, Corcoran K, Lee A. Changes in performance of glaucoma surgeries 1994 through 2017 based on claims and payment data for united states Medicare beneficiaries. Ophthalmology Glaucoma 2021;1(4); https://doi.org/10.1016/j.ogla.2021.01.004.
[5] Landers J, Martin K, Sarkies N, et al. A twenty-year follow-up study of trabeculectomy: Risk factors and outcomes. Ophthalmology 2012;119(4):694–702.
[6] Gedde S, Schiffman J, Feuer W, et al. Treatment outcomes in the tube versus trabeculectomy (TVT) study after five years of follow-up. Am J Ophthalmol 2012;153(5):789–803.
[7] Christakis P, Zhang D, Budenz D, et al. Five-year pooled data analysis of the Ahmed Baerveldt comparison study and the Ahmed versus Baerveldt study. Am J Ophthalmol 2017;176: 118–26.
[8] Gedde S, Chen P, Heuer D, et al. The primary tube versus trabeculectomy study: Methodology of a multicenter randomized clinical trial comparing tube shunt surgery and trabeculectomy with mitomycin C. Ophthalmology 2017;125(5):774–81.
[9] Lai J, Tham C, Chan J. The clinical outcomes of cataract extraction by phacoemulsification in eyes with primary angle-closure glaucoma (PACG) and co-existing cataractA prospective case series. J Glaucoma 2006;15(1):47–52.
[10] Chen P, Lin S, Junk A, et al. The effect of phacoemulsification on intraocular pressure in glaucoma patients. Ophthalmology 2015;122(7):1294–307.
[11] Samuelson T, Sarkisian S, Lubeck D, et al. Prospective, randomized, controlled pivotal trial of an ab interno implanted trabecular micro-bypass in primary open-angle glaucoma and cataract: Two-year results. Ophthalmology 2019;126(6):811–21.
[12] Ahmed I, Fea A, Au L, et al. A prospective randomized trial comparing Hydrus and iStent microinvasive glaucoma surgery implants for standalone treatment of open-angle glaucoma: The COMPARE study. Ophthalmology 2020;127(1):52–61.
[13] Grover D, Smith O, Fellman R, et al. Gonioscopy-assisted transluminal trabeculotomy: An ab interno circumferential trabeculotomy: 24 months follow-up. J Glaucoma 2018;27(5): 393–401.
[14] Vinod K, Gedde S. Clinical investigation of new glaucoma procedures. Curr Opin Ophthalmol 2017;28(2):187–93.
[15] Klabe K, Kaymak H. Standalone trabeculotomy and viscodilation of schlemm's canal and collector channels in open-angle glaucoma using the OMNI surgical system: 24-month outcomes. Clin Ophthalmol 2021;15:3121–9.
[16] Periera I, Wijdeven R, Wyss H, et al. Conventional glaucoma implants and the new MIGS devices: A comprehensive review of current options and future directions. Eye 2021;35: 3202–21. https://www.nature.com/articles/s41433-021-01595-x.
[17] Sheybani A, Reitsamer H, Ahmed I. Fluid dynamics of a novel micro-fistula implant for the surgical treatment of glaucoma. Glaucoma 2015;56:4789–95.
[18] Chen X, Liang Z, Yang K, et al. The outcomes of XEN gel stent implantation: A systematic review and meta-analysis. Front Med 2022;9; https://doi.org/10.3389/fmed.2022.804847.
[19] Pinchuk L, Riss I, Battle J, et al. The use of poly(styrene- block -isobutylene- block -styrene) as a microshunt to treat glaucoma. Regenerative Biomaterials 2016;3(2):137–42.

[20] Charters L. The use of MIGS trends and patterns in the US. Ophthalmol Times 2021;46(8). https://www.ophthalmologytimes.com/view/the-use-of-migs-trends-and-patterns-in-the-us.

[21] Ma A, Lee J, Warren J, et al. GlaucoMap – distribution of glaucoma surgical procedures in the United States. Clin Ophthalmol 2020;14:2551–60. https://www.ncbi.nlm.nih.gov/pmc/articles/PMC7473985/.

[22] Gedde S, Vinod K. Resident surgical training in glaucoma. Current Opines in Ophthalmology 2016;27(2):151–7. https://www.ncbi.nlm.nih.gov/pmc/articles/PMC5584582/.

[23] Chan J, Netland P. EX-PRESS glaucoma filtration device: Efficacy, safety, and predictability. Medical Devices 2015;8:381–8.

[24] Adashi EY, Robinson KM, Cohen IG. Deadly Legacy-The 510 (k) Path to Medical Device Clearance. JAMA Surgery 2022;157:185–6.

Neuro-ophthalmology

Advances in Ophthalmology and Optometry 8 (2023) 249–261

ADVANCES IN OPHTHALMOLOGY AND OPTOMETRY

Toxic Medications in Mitochondrial Optic Neuropathies

Henry Liu, MD[a,b,*], Alfredo A. Sadun, MD, PhD[a,b]

[a]Doheny Eye Center UCLA, 800 South Fairmount Avenue, Suite 215, Pasadena, CA 91105, USA;
[b]Department of Ophthalmology, David Geffen School of Medicine at University of California, Los Angeles, CA, USA

Keywords
- Mitochondrial optic neuropathy • Leber's hereditary optic neuropathy
- Autosomal dominant optic atrophy • Kjer's optic neuropathy
- Mitochondrial toxicity

Key points
- Mitochondrial optic neuropathies are a group of optic nerve disorders caused by mitochondrial dysfunction which may be congenital or acquired.
- The pathophysiology of mitochondrial optic neuropathies involves increased generation of reactive oxygen species.
- Inherited forms of mitochondrial optic neuropathies are delayed in onset with incomplete penetrance.
- Penetrance is highly variable and can be affected by certain medications or exposures that affect reactive oxygen species production.
- Avoiding certain medications or exposures can reduce the risk of vision loss.

INTRODUCTION

Mitochondrial optic neuropathy (MON) was first introduced as a term and a category of diseases in 2022 [1]. These are a group of optic nerve disorders caused by mitochondrial dysfunction. Whether congenital or acquired, the pathophysiology of these optic neuropathies involves the increased generation of reactive oxygen species (ROS). The retinal ganglion cells and their axons, which form the optic nerve, are highly energy-dependent and, therefore, are particularly sensitive to mitochondrial dysfunctions and more likely to produce

*Corresponding author. E-mail address: 1henryliu@gmail.com

https://doi.org/10.1016/j.yaoo.2023.03.003

more ROS from intense mitochondrial activity [2]. Leber hereditary optic neuropathy (LHON) often is considered the prototypical inherited mitochondrial disorder. The disease is caused by a mitochondria genome (mtDNA) mutation that codes for an ND subunit of complex I in the electron transport chain [3]. Point mutations at nucleotide positions 11,778, 14,484, and 3460 are responsible for over 95% of all LHON cases and encode for subunits ND-4 [4], ND-6 [3], and ND-1 [5], respectively. The most common point mutation is 11,778, accounting for 69% of cases, followed by 11,484 (14% of cases) and 3460 (13% of cases) [6].

All LHON mutations involve complex I, the beginning of the electron transport chain, which begins building the proton gradient through a series of oxidation-reduction reactions in the mitochondria [7]. Many studies suggest that the net decreases of adenosine triphosphate (ATP) and the chronic increase of ROS due to functional alterations of complex I play an important role in the pathogenesis of LHON [8], and subsequent cellular models have supported these findings [9,10]. The significance of these mechanisms was further evaluated by an important mouse mtDNA model harboring the ND-6 subunit mutation, which developed optic nerve pathology in conjunction with ROS accumulation but in the absence of neuronal ATP deficiency. This result demonstrated that chronic oxidative stress rather than ATP deficiency is the clinically relevant factor in LHON [11].

In addition to mtDNA mutations, nuclear gene mutations also have been identified to cause MONs. Autosomal dominant optic atrophy (ADOA), once known as Kjer optic neuropathy, involves the nuclear genes for OPA1, which encodes for a protein imported to the inner mitochondrial membrane that appears to control mitochondrial structure and movement [12]. ADOA follows a similar pathophysiology to LHON. Mutations to OPA1 lead to increased ROS production and may result in similar visual defects although the degree of vision loss generally is less severe than it is with LHON [13].

Both LHON and ADOA are disorders of optic atrophy beginning at the perimacular bundle. They differ in the age of presentation, with ADOA mostly affecting patients in their first decade of life [14] and LHON most commonly affecting patients in their second and third decades of life [6]. They are characterized by incomplete penetrance, as only a portion of LHON and ADOA carriers will go on to develop vision loss. Penetrance may vary substantially within the same mutation variants and branches of the same family [2,14,15]. Additionally, environmental factors have been shown to affect penetrance in LHON [16]. Observational studies have correlated exogenous ROS exposure to the conversion from an LHON carrier state to active disease. The exogenous exposures described include alcohol, cigarette smoke, and other types of organic fires that produce smoke [17–19]. Chronic increases in ROS burden are the likely trigger for these diseases, and reducing ROS may help prevent disease conversion. Alcohol and cigarette smoke are the most common sources of environmental ROS [17], but iatrogenic sources also should be considered.

Prior review articles have described medications with demonstrated and theoretical effects on mitochondrial function that may precipitate disease conversion [15,20]. The medications that should be avoided include hyperbaric oxygen, quaternary ammonium compounds, Ringer lactate solution, and antibiotics, such as erythromycin, ethambutol, linezolid, chloramphenicol, aminoglycosides, and tetracyclines [20]. Since the review of toxic medications in LHON by Kogachi and colleagues (2019) [20], new advancements have occurred in migraine treatment, and the COVID-19 pandemic has introduced widely used novel vaccines and antiviral therapies to the general population. Furthermore, the LHON online community (https://www.LHON.org) has raised concerns about the safety of cyanocobalamin supplementation, electronic cigarettes, and other medications. Understanding the implications of these agents on mitochondrial function may assist clinicians in providing optimal care for patients with inherited MONs such as LHON and ADOA. In this article, we will review these medications and exposures that have the potential to impair mitochondrial function and, hence, increase ROS generation. This article also will serve as an update to the review of toxic medications in LHON by Kogachi and colleagues (2019) [20]. Because LHON is the prototypical mitochondrial disorder and has been extensively studied, much of the literature reviewed in this article will focus on LHON. While other forms of inherited MONs in addition to LHON and ADOA exist, they are exceedingly rare and out of the scope of this discussion [2,14,15].

Cyanocobalamin

Vitamin B_{12}, also known as cobalamin, is a water-soluble vitamin essential for DNA synthesis and for cellular energy production by amino acid and fatty acid metabolism [21]. The vitamin in its methyl- or adenosyl-forms are cofactors for methionine synthase and L-methyl-malonyl-CoA mutase, and deficiencies of vitamin B_{12} can lead to hematologic, dermatologic, or neurological manifestations by impacting mitochondrial oxidative phosphorylation [22]. The causes of vitamin B_{12} deficiency typically stem from either inadequate dietary intake or malabsorption. Vitamin B_{12} is found in animal-based foods, and vegans or strict vegetarians may develop a deficiency of vitamin B_{12}, requiring supplementation [23].

Cyanocobalamin and hydroxocobalamin are two forms of vitamin B_{12} used for repletion in deficient patients. In the United States, cyanocobalamin is the most used form of vitamin B_{12}, due to the low cost of production and heat stability. Cyanocobalamin often is administered orally or parenterally and through a series of reactions within the body, converted to its bioactive form methylcobalamin or adenosylcobalamin [24]. The free cyanide group then is excreted renally as thiocyanate [25].

Cyanide is a potent mitochondrial toxin that disrupts oxidative phosphorylation by noncompetitively binding to complex IV, also known as cytochrome c oxidase [26]. The disruption of the electron transport chain by cyanide affects oxygen utilization and ATP production, leading to excess generation of ROS at complexes I and III, with resultant cardiovascular and neurological dysfunction [26,27]. In the case of LHON, patients are warned against the use of cyanocobalamin because of concerns about optic atrophy [28,29]. However, "it's not the poison, it's the dose," and the amount of cyanide in typical cyanocobalamin supplementation is minuscule. Limited literature exists regarding the toxicity of cyanocobalamin in LHON, and the warnings appear to have stemmed from a letter to the editor in *The Lancet* by Foulds and colleagues (1970) calling for withdrawal of cyanocobalamin. In their letter, Foulds and colleagues described four patients with early LHON who developed optic atrophy, which was unusually rapid and severe in the setting of cyanocobalamin administration [30].

The relationship between LHON and cyanide has been well studied, and it was postulated that LHON was in part due to defective cyanide metabolism [31–34]. These suspicions were based on early studies that found elevated levels of cyanocobalamin and elevated cyanocobalamin to hydroxocobalamin ratios in patients with LHON. Hydroxocobalamin is a form of cobalamin found in the body involved in cyanide detoxification by conversion of hydroxocobalamin to cyanocobalamin, and the cyanocobalamin to hydroxocobalamin ratio appeared to be used as an indirect measure of cyanide levels [31,33]. Based on the results of these studies, Wilson and colleagues (1971) suggested that hydroxocobalamin should be used in patients with LHON [33].

Few case reports have described improved visual acuity in patients with LHON following administration of hydroxocobalamin [35,36]. Two of the patients described received cyanocobalamin 1 mg intramuscularly 2 to 3 times weekly for months without changes in visual acuity before being treated with hydroxocobalamin 1 mg intramuscularly 1 to 2 times weekly. These patients demonstrated slowly improved visual acuity over 6 and 18 months [36]. Another case report described a patient with LHON during the acute phase and significantly elevated serum cyanide levels, and subsequent treatment with a cyanide antagonist reduced their cyanide levels, but it was not accompanied by vision improvement [34]. While elevated cyanocobalamin levels and ratios in LHON have been described in the literature, insufficient data exist to suggest causation.

Many patients with vitamin B_{12} deficiency due to malabsorption syndromes required lifelong replacement therapy administered orally (1000–2000 mcg daily) or parenterally (1000 mcg weekly) [37,38]. Despite the relatively high doses over time, no cases exist in the literature reporting cyanide toxicity due to cyanocobalamin supplementation. The oral bioavailability of cyanocobalamin is variable and inversely related to the dose administered [39]. Absorption of vitamin B_{12} relies on the binding of intrinsic factor and receptor-mediated endocytosis at the terminal ileum [40], suggesting that absorption may be limited by receptor saturation. Cyanocobalamin is water-soluble and renally excreted. Studies of radiolabeled cyanocobalamin have demonstrated that renal excretion is proportional to the administered dosage. Approximately 50% of cyanocobalamin is excreted 24 hours after administering 100 mcg of cyanocobalamin, and 70% excreted after administering 540 mcg [41].

Therefore, the risk of toxicity due to cyanocobalamin is likely to be low given its inverse dose-dependent bioavailability and high renal clearance.

Electronic Cigarettes

Cigarette smoke is a major environmental factor that has been strongly implicated as a trigger for conversion of LHON carriers, significantly increasing disease penetrance through observational studies [16,17]. Cytological studies examined fibroblast cell lines from affected LHON individuals, mutation carriers, and controls to better understand the mechanism of tobacco toxicity. Each cell line was exposed to cigarette smoke concentrate, and the results demonstrated a reduction of ATP levels in both affected individuals and carriers. Only affected individuals showed increased cellular damage due to oxidative stress [19]. Overwhelming evidence shows that cigarette smoke should be avoided in affected and LHON carriers.

Electronic cigarettes are an alternative to conventional cigarettes and are described as a noncombustible nicotine system that heat a solution of nicotine, flavoring, additives, propylene glycol, and glycerol to deliver vapor pseudo-smoke. These devices were invented by Lik Hon in Hong Kong in 2003 [42]. Electronic cigarettes were popularized in the mid-2010s and marketed as a safer alternative to their combustion counterparts [43]. However, the long-term effects of electronic cigarettes are largely unknown [43].

The use of electronic cigarettes has increased over time, particularly in teenagers and young adults [43,44]. While electronic cigarettes are not combustion operated, the potential exists that the pseudo-smoke vapor contains ROS. A cellular model studied the mechanisms of mitochondrial toxicity by electronic cigarette solutions and aerosols on neural stem cells. Both electronic cigarette solutions and aerosols altered mitochondrial dynamics and caused mitochondrial swelling and stress-induced mitochondrial hyperperfusion. Additionally, both toxicants increased mitochondrial superoxide levels and induced protein oxidation, suggesting that a significant increase occurs in ROS burden [45]. Another study using a cellular and novel acellular model measured ROS generation with different electronic cigarette brands, flavors, and voltages. The results showed ROS generation was highly dependent on each of the factors, and a positive correlation occurred for ROS production and voltage used [46]. While these cellular models demonstrate ROS production in electronic cigarettes, their clinical significance is not well understood and requires additional research in this area. It would be prudent to avoid any exogenous sources of ROS. However, a dearth of data exist regarding the use of electronic cigarettes in LHON.

COVID-19 Vaccines

In December 2020, the Food and Drug Administration (FDA) issued the first emergency use authorization for a vaccine for the prevention of COVID-19, a disease caused by severe acute respiratory syndrome coronavirus 2 (SARS-CoV-2) infection. Over 13 billion doses of the COVID-19 vaccine have been given to date [47]. Autoimmune or inflammatory sequela after COVID-19 vaccination have been described; however, this is not unique to COVID vaccines [48]. A case report of LHON triggered by Pfizer-BioNTech COVID-19 vaccine was described. This was in a previously healthy 15-year-old boy with a known family history (maternal cousin) of vision loss due a novel mutation m.14568 A > 6. The patient converted 1 week after the second dose of the mRNA vaccine [49]. This singular case report is insufficient to establish a definitive causative relation of LHON conversion and COVID-19 vaccines. The sheer number of COVID-19 vaccine doses given worldwide with only 1 described case of LHON conversion associated with the vaccine suggests that this is a statistical event and, hence, is reassuring regarding the danger of vaccines. No evidence exists that vaccinations for other disease such as influenza, herpes zoster, or monkeypox are triggers for LHON conversion.

Antiretroviral Medications

Highly active antiretroviral therapy (HAART) is a combination of different classes of medications used to treat human immunodeficiency virus (HIV) infection. The classes of medications include nucleoside/nucleotide reverse transcriptase inhibitors (NRTIs), nonnucleoside reverse transcriptase inhibitors (NNRTIs), protease inhibitors, integrase inhibitors, fusion inhibitors, and chemokine receptor antagonists [50]. Mitochondrial proteomic analysis of peripheral blood mononuclear cells from HIV patients receiving NRTIs, zidovudine or stavudine, exhibited decreased levels of mitochondrial enzymes, energy production, and mitochondrial chaperones [51]. Evidence exists that NRTIs can inhibit DNA gamma polymerase, which is involved in mtDNA replication and may lead to mitochondrial toxicity [52,53].

HIV protease inhibitors also have been implicated in mitochondrial dysfunction. An in vitro study demonstrated that the HIV protease inhibitors, indinavir, amprenavir, ritonavir, and saquinavir, have the potential to inhibit mitochondrial protease processing [54]. Other in vitro studies using mononuclear cell cultures exposed to ritonavir revealed changes in mitochondrial membrane potential, increased nicotinamide adenine dinucleotide phosphate (NADPH) oxidase subunits, and increased superoxide production [55]. Other cell culture studies of human endothelial cells treated with ritonavir in the therapeutic dose ranges demonstrated decreased cell viability, mtDNA damage, and increased cytotoxicity over time [56].

HAART therapy has been proposed to be a trigger for LHON conversion, and the potential clinical effect has been described through a number of case reports [57–60]. Each of the case reports described HIV patients on a multidrug regimen of NRTIs, NNRTIs, and/or protease inhibitors for several years, ranging from 3 to 8 years, followed by bilateral, sequential vision loss. These patients were either on a combination of NRTIs and a protease inhibitor or NRTIs and NNRTI. NRTIs were the common denominator among all treatment regimens, and there were no patients on monotherapy; therefore, it is challenging to discern a singular agent as the main culprit for disease conversion. While HAART therapy is a potential trigger for LHON conversion, suppressing viral loads in HIV patients is key in preventing HIV disease progression. Awareness of this possible side effect should be considered as part of the clinical decision-making process.

Nirmatrelvir/ritonavir (Paxlovid)

Paxlovid is an oral antiviral combination drug of nirmatrelvir/ritonavir used in the treatment of COVID-19. In addition to being an HIV protease inhibitor, ritonavir also is a potent CYP3A inhibitor and often is used as a pharmacokinetic enhancer [61]. By inhibiting CYP3A, ritonavir enhances the plasma concentration of nirmatrelvir, a novel SARS-CoV-2 main protease inhibitor. Unlike ritonavir, which has been demonstrated to cause mitochondrial dysfunction as described earlier, no in vitro or in vivo studies of nirmatrelvir on mitochondrial function exist to date. Although there is the potential for antiretroviral therapy to trigger LHON conversion, a typical course of Paxlovid is nirmatrelvir 300 mg with ritonavir 100 mg twice daily for 5 days [62]. This is significantly shorter in duration than HAART for the management of HIV, which is taken indefinitely to suppress viral loads.

Isotretinoin

Vitamin A derivatives, also known as retinoids, are a group of compounds involved in the regulation of cell growth and differentiation in multiple organ systems [63]. Isotretinoin is a retinoid often used systemically for the treatment of severe acne vulgaris, and while effective, it is a known teratogen [64] and has been associated with a broad range of adverse effects [65]. Ocular adverse effects secondary to isotretinoin are well described and most commonly involve the ocular surface. Neurological manifestations are less common and include pseudotumor cerebri, optic neuritis, and visual field defects [66].

Although low levels of retinoids regulate mitochondrial gene expression and are essential for mitochondrial function [67], retinoids at therapeutic doses may exert toxic effects regarding the redox environment and cause mitochondrial dysfunction [68]. Rigobello and colleagues demonstrated that isotretinoin decreased mitochondrial membrane potential and induced swelling of rat liver mitochondria [69]. Another study of rats given isotretinoin at human therapeutic doses demonstrated increased levels of oxidative stress markers at 3 months [70]. Similar findings occurred in patients undergoing treatment of cystic acne with isotretinoin, which also showed increased serum levels of 8-hydroxy-2-deoxyguanosine, a marker for DNA oxidative damage [71]. These studies suggest that isotretinoin may increase ROS production; however, it is unknown whether the medication will have an effect on LHON conversion rates.

Calcitonin Gene-Related Peptide Inhibitors

In 2018, the FDA approved the first calcitonin gene-related peptide (CGRP) receptor antagonist, erenumab, for the prevention of migraines [72]. Since its introduction, CGRP receptor antagonists have been widely prescribed, and several other monoclonal antibodies have also been approved. CGRP primarily is produced in the central and peripheral neurons [73,74]. It is a potent vasodilator and localized to C and Aδ sensory fibers for nociception [74]. Protective properties of CGRP to oxidative stress have been described in mice models of the vascular smooth muscle and cardiac myocyte. Luo and colleagues demonstrated that CGRP suppressed levels of ROS generated by NADPH oxidase in angiotensin-II-induced vascular smooth muscles [75]. A separate study showed that CGRP prevented apoptosis and oxidative stress levels in the setting of pressure-induced heart failure [76]. While these data show the potential protective properties of CGRP in the cardiovascular tissues, further studies are needed to determine the impact of CGRP antagonists on ROS generation.

Sulthiame
Sulthiame is a carbonic anhydrase inhibitor that was developed in the 1950s to treat focal seizures [77]. A recent case series described 2 patients, an 8-year-old girl (m.14484 T > C) and an 11-year-old boy (m.3460 G > A) with cryptogenic focal epilepsy who suffered vision loss in close temporal connection with the initiation of sulthiame therapy. Investigators went on to perform real-time spirometry on cell cultures of fibroblasts carrying the m.3460 G > A or m.14484 T > C mutation. The cells that were incubated in the presence of sulthiame demonstrated decreased oxygen consumption rates, suggesting that sulthiame impairs mitochondrial function. The authors concluded that sulthiame should be avoided in patients with known LHON mutations [78]. Anticonvulsants are a diverse class of drugs, and the theoretical effects of valproate on mitochondrial function also have been described [20].

Azithromycin
Erythromycin is an antibiotic agent that binds to the 50S bacterial ribosomal subunit and has been associated with LHON disease conversion [79]. Other antibiotics targeting the 50S bacterial ribosomal subunit such as chloramphenicol and linezolid have been identified to produce toxic optic neuropathies with similar clinical descriptions to LHON [80,81]. Therefore, it is recommended that these medications, particularly with prolonged courses, should be avoided in patients carrying LHON mutations [20]. Azithromycin is another macrolide antibiotic in the same class as erythromycin; however, no evidence exists that it is associated with LHON conversion. Interestingly, a mouse model of optic neuropathy showed reduced retinal ganglion cell loss and reduced inflammatory markers in mice treated with azithromycin, suggesting that azithromycin may be neuroprotective in oxidative stress–related acute optic neuropathies [82].

SUMMARY
We have reviewed the current understanding of commonly prescribed pharmacological agents and their potential to disrupt mitochondrial function and generate ROS. There are theoretic risks for certain agents with demonstrated effects on mitochondrial oxidative stress in vitro and in mice models. However, further research and investigation is necessary to better understand the clinical

significance of these findings. Severe vision loss, as in the case of LHON and ADOA, is debilitating for the affected patients and their family. Neuro-ophthalmologists must be vigilant in reducing the risk for conversion in carriers, and understanding the potential deleterious effects of the medications and exposures is key. However, important tradeoffs need to be understood with perspective. By weighing the risks and benefits of certain medications in the context of inherited MONs, personalized and optimal care can be delivered to patients with these rare diseases.

CLINICS CARE POINTS

- Avoiding agents that increase oxidative stress may reduce the risk of vision loss for carriers of mitochondrial optic neuropathy mutations.
- While some medication classes may increase oxidative stress, the dose and duration of therapy should be considered before prescribing.
- Understanding the potential risks is key when balancing the therapeutic benefits of these medications when treating this patient population.

DISCLOSURE

The authors have nothing to disclose.

References

[1] Sadun AA. Mitochondrial optic neuropathies. J Neurol Neurosurg Psychiatry 2002;72(4): 423.

[2] Carelli V, Ross-Cisneros FN, Sadun AA. Mitochondrial dysfunction as a cause of optic neuropathies. Prog Retin Eye Res 2004;23(1):53–89.

[3] Wallace DC, Singh G, Lott MT, et al. Mitochondrial DNA mutation associated with Leber's hereditary optic neuropathy. Science 1988;242(4884):1427–30.

[4] Huoponen K, Vilkki J, Aula P, et al. A new mtDNA mutation associated with Leber hereditary optic neuroretinopathy. Am J Hum Genet 1991;48(6):1147–53.

[5] Johns DR, Neufeld MJ, Park RD. An ND-6 mitochondrial DNA mutation associated with Leber hereditary optic neuropathy. Biochem Biophys Res Commun 1992;187(3):1551–7.

[6] Newman NJ. Hereditary optic neuropathies: from the mitochondria to the optic nerve. Am J Ophthalmol 2005;140(3):517–23.

[7] Hirst J. Towards the molecular mechanism of respiratory complex I. Biochem J 2009;425(2): 327–39.

[8] Degli Esposti M, Carelli V, Ghelli A, et al. Functional alterations of the mitochondrially encoded ND4 subunit associated with Leber's hereditary optic neuropathy. FEBS Lett 1994;352(3):375–9.

[9] Baracca A, Solaini G, Sgarbi G, et al. Severe impairment of complex I-driven adenosine triphosphate synthesis in leber hereditary optic neuropathy cybrids. Arch Neurol 2005;62(5):730–6.

[10] Floreani M, Napoli E, Martinuzzi A, et al. Antioxidant defences in cybrids harboring mtDNA mutations associated with Leber's hereditary optic neuropathy. Febs j 2005;272(5):1124–35.

[11] Lin CS, Sharpley MS, Fan W, et al. Mouse mtDNA mutant model of Leber hereditary optic neuropathy. Proc Natl Acad Sci USA 2012;109(49):20065–70.

[12] Delettre C, Lenaers G, Griffoin JM, et al. Nuclear gene OPA1, encoding a mitochondrial dynamin-related protein, is mutated in dominant optic atrophy. Nat Genet 2000;26(2): 207–10.

[13] Tang S, Le PK, Tse S, et al. Heterozygous mutation of Opa1 in Drosophila shortens lifespan mediated through increased reactive oxygen species production. PLoS One 2009;4(2): e4492.

[14] Carelli V, La Morgia C, Iommarini L, et al. Mitochondrial optic neuropathies: how two genomes may kill the same cell type? Biosci Rep 2007;27(1–3):173–84.

[15] Yu-Wai-Man P, Griffiths PG, Chinnery PF. Mitochondrial optic neuropathies - disease mechanisms and therapeutic strategies. Prog Retin Eye Res 2011;30(2):81–114.

[16] Kirkman MA, Yu-Wai-Man P, Korsten A, et al. Gene-environment interactions in Leber hereditary optic neuropathy. Brain 2009;132(Pt 9):2317–26.

[17] Sadun AA, Carelli V, Salomao SR, et al. Extensive investigation of a large Brazilian pedigree of 11778/haplogroup J Leber hereditary optic neuropathy. Am J Ophthalmol 2003;136(2):231–8.

[18] Sanchez RN, Smith AJ, Carelli V, et al. Leber hereditary optic neuropathy possibly triggered by exposure to tire fire. J Neuroophthalmol 2006;26(4):268–72.

[19] Giordano L, Deceglie S, d'Adamo P, et al. Cigarette toxicity triggers Leber's hereditary optic neuropathy by affecting mtDNA copy number, oxidative phosphorylation and ROS detoxification pathways. Cell Death Dis 2015;6(12):e2021.

[20] Kogachi K, Ter-Zakarian A, Asanad S, et al. Toxic medications in Leber's hereditary optic neuropathy. Mitochondrion 2019;46:270–7.

[21] Ankar A. and Kumar A., Vitamin B12 deficiency, 2022, StatPearls, Treasure Island, FL.

[22] Sadun AA. Metabolic optic neuropathies. Semin Ophthalmol 2002;17(1):29–32.

[23] Balcı YI, Ergin A, Karabulut A, et al. Serum vitamin B12 and folate concentrations and the effect of the Mediterranean diet on vulnerable populations. Pediatr Hematol Oncol 2014;31(1):62–7.

[24] Paul C, Brady DM. Comparative Bioavailability and Utilization of Particular Forms of B(12) Supplements With Potential to Mitigate B(12)-related Genetic Polymorphisms. Integr Med (Encinitas) 2017;16(1):42–9.

[25] Bhandari RK, Oda RP, Petrikovics I, et al. Cyanide toxicokinetics: the behavior of cyanide, thiocyanate and 2-amino-2-thiazoline-4-carboxylic acid in multiple animal models. J Anal Toxicol 2014;38(4):218–25.

[26] Way JL. Cyanide intoxication and its mechanism of antagonism. Annu Rev Pharmacol Toxicol 1984;24:451–81.

[27] Gunasekar PG, Borowitz JL, Isom GE. Cyanide-induced generation of oxidative species: involvement of nitric oxide synthase and cyclooxygenase-2. J Pharmacol Exp Ther 1998;285(1):236–41.

[28] Linnell JC, Matthews DM, England JM. Therapeutic misuse of cyanocobalamin. Lancet 1978;312(8098):1053–4.

[29] Vasavada A. and Sanghavi D., Cyanocobalamin, 2022, StatPearls, Treasure Island, FL.

[30] Foulds WS, Freeman AG, Phillips CI, et al. Cyanocobalamin: a case for withdrawal. Lancet 3 1970;1(7636):35.

[31] Wilson J. Leber's hereditary optic atrophy: a possible defect of cyanide metabolism. Clin Sci 1965;29(3):505–15.

[32] Wilson J. Leber's hereditary optic atrophy: some clinical and aetiological considerations. Brain 1963;86:347–62.

[33] Wilson J, Linnell JC, Matthews DM. Plasma-cobalamins in neuro-ophthalmological diseases. Lancet 1971;1(7693):259–61.

[34] Berninger TA, von Meyer L, Siess E, et al. Leber's hereditary optic atrophy: further evidence for a defect of cyanide metabolism? Br J Ophthalmol 1989;73(4):314–6.

[35] Chew SJ. Leber's hereditary optic atrophy: an atypical case with response to hydroxycobalamine therapy. Singapore Med J 1990;31(3):293–4.

[36] Foulds WSCJ, Chisholm IA, Bronte-Stewart J, et al. Hydroxocobalamin in the treatment of leber's hereditary optic atrophy. Lancet 1968;291(7548):896–7.

[37] Eussen SJ, de Groot LC, Clarke R, et al. Oral cyanocobalamin supplementation in older people with vitamin B12 deficiency: a dose-finding trial. Arch Intern Med 2005;165(10): 1167–72.

[38] Stover PJ. Vitamin B12 and older adults. Curr Opin Clin Nutr Metab Care 2010;13(1): 24–7.

[39] Berlin H, Berlin R, Brante G. Oral treatment of pernicious anemia with high doses of vitamin B12 without intrinsic factor. Acta Med Scand 1968;184(4):247–58.

[40] Kozyraki R, Cases O. Cubilin, the Intrinsic Factor-Vitamin B12 Receptor in Development and Disease. Curr Med Chem 2020;27(19):3123–50.

[41] Adams JF. The Urinary Excretion and Tissue Retention of Cyanocobalamin By Subjects Given Repeated Parenteral Doses. J Clin Pathol 1964;17(1):31–8.

[42] Hon L. Flameless electronic atomizing cigarette. U.S. Patent Application No. 10/547, 244; 2006.

[43] Hajek P, Etter JF, Benowitz N, et al. Electronic cigarettes: review of use, content, safety, effects on smokers and potential for harm and benefit. Addiction 2014;109(11):1801–10.

[44] Levy DT, Warner KE, Cummings KM, et al. Examining the relationship of vaping to smoking initiation among US youth and young adults: a reality check. Tob Control 2019;28(6): 629–35.

[45] Zahedi A, Phandthong R, Chaili A, et al. Mitochondrial Stress Response in Neural Stem Cells Exposed to Electronic Cigarettes. iScience 2019;16:250–69.

[46] Wan X, Pei H, Zhao MJ, et al. Efficacy and Safety of rAAV2-ND4 Treatment for Leber's Hereditary Optic Neuropathy. Sci Rep 2016;6:21587.

[47] Mathieu E RH, Rodés-Guirao L, Appel C, et al. Coronavirus Pandemic (COVID-19). OurWorldInData.org. Accessed 12 January, 2022. Available at: https://ourworldindata.org/coronavirus.

[48] Fagni F, Simon D, Tascilar K, et al. COVID-19 and immune-mediated inflammatory diseases: effect of disease and treatment on COVID-19 outcomes and vaccine responses. Lancet Rheumatol 2021;3(10):e724–36.

[49] Rizk M, Dunya I, Seif R, et al. A Case of Leber Hereditary Optic Neuropathy Triggered by Pfizer-BioNTech Vaccine: Evidence of Pathogenesis of a Novel Mutation. J Neuro Ophthalmol 2022; https://doi.org/10.1097/wno.0000000000001665.

[50] Eggleton JS, Nagalli S. Highly active antiretroviral therapy (HAART). Treasure Island, FL: StatPearls; 2022.

[51] Ciccosanti F, Corazzari M, Soldani F, et al. Proteomic analysis identifies prohibitin downregulation as a crucial event in the mitochondrial damage observed in HIV-infected patients. Antivir Ther 2009;15(3):377–90.

[52] Brinkman K, ter Hofstede HJ, Burger DM, et al. Adverse effects of reverse transcriptase inhibitors: mitochondrial toxicity as common pathway. Aids 1998;12(14):1735–44.

[53] Kakuda TN. Pharmacology of nucleoside and nucleotide reverse transcriptase inhibitor-induced mitochondrial toxicity. Clin Therapeut 2000;22(6):685–708.

[54] Mukhopadhyay A, Wei B, Zullo SJ, et al. In vitro evidence of inhibition of mitochondrial protease processing by HIV-1 protease inhibitors in yeast: a possible contribution to lipodystrophy syndrome. Mitochondrion 2002;1(6):511–8.

[55] Wang X, Mu H, Chai H, et al. Human Immunodeficiency Virus Protease Inhibitor Ritonavir Inhibits Cholesterol Efflux from Human Macrophage-Derived Foam Cells. Am J Pathol 2007;171(1):304–14.

[56] Zhong DS, Lu XH, Conklin BS, et al. HIV protease inhibitor ritonavir induces cytotoxicity of human endothelial cells. Arterioscler Thromb Vasc Biol 2002;22(10):1560–6.

[57] Shaikh S, Ta C, Basham AA, et al. Leber hereditary optic neuropathy associated with antiretroviral therapy for human immunodeficiency virus infection. Am J Ophthalmol 2001;131(1):143–5.

[58] Warner JEA, Ries KM. Optic Neuropathy in a Patient With AIDS. J Neuro Ophthalmol 2001;21(2):92–4.

[59] Mackey DA, Fingert JH, Luzhansky JZ, et al. Leber's hereditary optic neuropathy triggered by antiretroviral therapy for human immunodeficiency virus. Eye 2003/04/01 2003;17(3):312–7.

[60] Moura-Coelho N, Pinto Proença R, Tavares Ferreira J, et al. Late-onset Leber's hereditary optic neuropathy: the role of environmental factors in hereditary diseases. BMJ Case Rep 20 2019;12(3); https://doi.org/10.1136/bcr-2018-227977.

[61] Larson KB, Wang K, Delille C, et al. Pharmacokinetic enhancers in HIV therapeutics. Clin Pharmacokinet 2014;53(10):865–72.

[62] Fact sheet for healthcare providers: emergency authorization for Paxlovid. US Food and Drug Administration. Accessed 12 January, 2023. Available at: https://www.fda.gov/media/155050/download.

[63] Szymański L, Skopek R, Palusińska M, et al. Retinoic Acid and Its Derivatives in Skin. Cells 2020;9(12); https://doi.org/10.3390/cells9122660.

[64] Lammer EJ, Chen DT, Hoar RM, et al. Retinoic acid embryopathy. N Engl J Med 1985;313(14):837–41.

[65] Brzezinski P, Borowska K, Chiriac A, et al. Adverse effects of isotretinoin: A large, retrospective review. Dermatol Ther 2017;30(4); https://doi.org/10.1111/dth.12483.

[66] Fraunfelder FT, Fraunfelder FW, Edwards R. Ocular side effects possibly associated with isotretinoin usage. Am J Ophthalmol 2001;132(3):299–305.

[67] Everts HB, Berdanier CD. Regulation of mitochondrial gene expression by retinoids. IUBMB Life 2002;54(2):45–9.

[68] de Oliveira MR. Vitamin A and Retinoids as Mitochondrial Toxicants. Oxid Med Cell Longev 2015;2015:140267.

[69] Rigobello MP, Scutari G, Friso A, et al. Mitochondrial permeability transition and release of cytochrome c induced by retinoic acids. Biochem Pharmacol 1999;58(4):665–70.

[70] Daye M, Belviranli M, Okudan N, et al. The effect of isotretinoin therapy on oxidative damage in rats. Dermatol Ther 2020;33(6):e14111.

[71] Georgala S, Papassotiriou I, Georgala C, et al. Isotretinoin therapy induces DNA oxidative damage. Clin Chem Lab Med 2005;43(11):1178–82.

[72] Brauser D. FDA Approves First-in-Class Drug Erenumab (Aimovig) for Migraine Prevention. Medscape. Accessed 17 May, 2018. Available at: https://www.medscape.com/viewarticle/896851.

[73] Rosenfeld MG, Mermod JJ, Amara SG, et al. Production of a novel neuropeptide encoded by the calcitonin gene via tissue-specific RNA processing. Nature 1983;304(5922):129–35.

[74] Russell FA, King R, Smillie SJ, et al. Calcitonin gene-related peptide: physiology and pathophysiology. Physiol Rev. Oct 2014;94(4):1099–142.

[75] Luo HM, Wu X, Xian X, et al. Calcitonin gene-related peptide inhibits angiotensin II-induced NADPH oxidase-dependent ROS via the Src/STAT3 signalling pathway. J Cell Mol Med 2020;24(11):6426–37.

[76] Kumar A, Supowit S, Potts JD, et al. Alpha-calcitonin gene-related peptide prevents pressure-overload induced heart failure: role of apoptosis and oxidative stress. Physiol Rep 2019;7(21):e14269.

[77] May T, Korn-Merker E, Rambeck B, et al. Pharmacokinetics of sulthiame in epileptic patients. Ther Drug Monit 1994;16(3):251–7.

[78] Reinert M-C, Pacheu-Grau D, Catarino CB, et al. Sulthiame impairs mitochondrial function in vitro and may trigger onset of visual loss in Leber hereditary optic neuropathy. Orphanet J Rare Dis 2021;16(1):64.

[79] Luca CC, Lam BL, Moraes CT. Erythromycin as a potential precipitating agent in the onset of Leber's hereditary optic neuropathy. Mitochondrion 2004;4(1):31–6.

[80] Godel V, Nemet P, Lazar M. Chloramphenicol Optic Neuropathy. Arch Ophthalmol 1980;98(8):1417–21.

[81] Javaheri M, Khurana RN, O'Hearn TM, et al. Linezolid-induced optic neuropathy: a mitochondrial disorder? Br J Ophthalmol 2007;91(1):111.

[82] Zloto O, Zahavi A, Richard S, et al. Neuroprotective Effect of Azithromycin Following Induction of Optic Nerve Crush in Wild Type and Immunodeficient Mice. Int J Mol Sci 2022;23(19); https://doi.org/10.3390/ijms231911872.

Advances in Ophthalmology and Optometry 8 (2023) 263–279

"Zickzackbewegungen"
A Back-to-Basics Review of Square Wave Jerks

Ricarda M. Konder, BSc, MD[a],*, Daniel Lelli, MD, FRCPC[b,c]

[a]Department of Neurology, University of Ottawa, 1053 Carling Avenue, Ottawa, Ontario K1Y 4E9, Canada; [b]University of Ottawa, 1053 Carling Avenue, Ottawa, Ontario K1Y 4E9, Canada; [c]University of Ottawa Neurology Residency Program, Ottawa, Ontario, Canada

Keywords
• Square wave jerks • Macro square wave jerks • Saccadic intrusions

Key points

- The studies that established the current frequency cutoffs for "normal" versus "pathologic" square wave jerks (SWJs) are limited, and substantial discordance occurs between them.
- Based on the most reliable current evidence, an SWJ frequency cutoff of up to 16 SWJs per minute (in light and with fixation) and up to 25 SWJs per minute (in darkness) is reasonable.
- There is substantial discordance about accepted normal ranges for SWJ amplitude, ranging from as broad as 2° to 10° to as narrow as 0.5° to 5°.
- Pathologic SWJs occur across a broad range of neurologic disease, most notably neurodegenerative conditions such as Parkinson disease, multiple systems atrophy, and progressive supranuclear palsy.
- To our knowledge, no evidence exists that SWJ frequency increases with age in healthy persons.

INTRODUCTION

Square wave jerks (SWJs) are part of a group of oculomotor abnormalities termed "saccadic intrusions," where an abnormal involuntary saccade momentarily moves the eyes away from fixation. What defines SWJs is that they usually are purely horizontal movements (differentiating them from opsoclonus, which is multidirectional), and that they have an intersaccadic interval (differentiating

*Corresponding author. E-mail address: rkonder@toh.ca

https://doi.org/10.1016/j.yaoo.2023.03.006
2452-1760/23/

them from ocular flutter and opsoclonus). The intersaccadic interval has been standardized as a complete stillstand of 200 milliseconds or more [1]. A key feature of SWJs is that they occur with eyes open and closed, ultimately differentiating them from macrosaccadic oscillations, which occur only with the eyes open and are usually triggered by saccades to a target. For a comparison of the different types of saccadic intrusions, see Fig. 1. The first record of SWJs dates back to 1916, at which time they were termed "Zickzackbewegungen" ("zigzag movements") [2]. Other terms that have since been used to describe SWJs include "Gegenrücke" [3], "pathologic ocular fixation instability" [4], and "cerebellar nystagmus" [5]. In 1964, Jung and Kornhuber [6] first translated these movements from German into English as "square wave jerks," which remains standardized terminology until today. Usually, the amplitude of a SWJ is 2° to 10° [7], although other ranges, such as 0.5° to 5°, have been proposed [8]. Although SWJs usually are predominantly horizontal, reports exist of occasional vertical components [9]. Despite the sometimes rather striking amplitudes of SWJs, this phenomenon usually is asymptomatic to the patient, and oscillopsia is uncommon [8].

This review provides a comprehensive summary of the available literature about SWJs, focusing on their proposed neuroanatomic mechanisms and their known associated conditions to date. Our search of the literature revealed that the understanding of SWJs was strongly defined by a burst of research published in the 1980s, at which time multiple possible mechanisms were proposed and the thresholds for normal were established. However, there continues to be substantial discordance about what distinguishes "normal" from "pathologic" SWJs, and although multiple mechanistic theories exist, some key links have not yet been established into a unified neuroanatomic theory. This review summarizes and modernizes the state of the literature surrounding SWJs and exposes various gaps in understanding to serve as a basis for future research in this area.

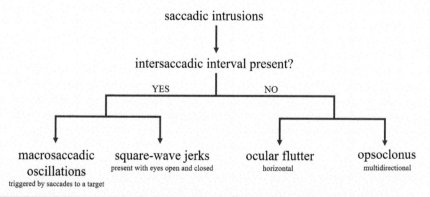

Fig. 1. Comparison among the most common saccadic intrusions.

SIGNIFICANCE
Proposed mechanisms of square wave jerks

Although the exact mechanism of SWJs still is not fully elucidated, several hypotheses exist. Multiple researchers have postulated that SWJs may simply represent a larger variation of microsaccades [7,10–14]. However, the two dominating current theories involve a "cerebellar hypothesis" and a "brainstem hypothesis," although increasing evidence supports that these are not mutually exclusive.

The cerebellar hypothesis was first proposed by researchers Dell'Osso and coworkers [15] and Daroff [16], and it has since been further reinforced by the high occurrence of SWJs in cerebellum-predominant conditions such as spinocerebellar ataxia (SCA) type 3 [17,18] and type 6 [19,20], ataxia with oculomotor apraxia type 2 [21], and Friedreich's ataxia [22–25]. Cerebellar oculomotor control is postulated to be a function of vermal structures [26], specifically the posterior cerebellar vermis [20] and the paramedian and deep cerebellar nuclei [27], all of which contribute to the overall role of the cerebellum as a saccade stabilizer.

More recently, the brainstem hypothesis has gained increasing traction, linking pathologic SWJs with targeted dysfunction in the pulse generator and the neural integrator [28,29], thereby implicating a wide array of structures including the midbrain, medulla oblongata, cerebellum, and even some cortical areas [30]. Further research eventually implicated the superior colliculi, postulating that increased activity in these areas (through a multitude of mechanisms) could lead to increased attentional shifts superimposed on a normal saccadic pathway [11,31,32]. The current state of the literature suggests that the initial saccade of an SWJ is likely involuntary in nature, possibly as a result of the temporary failure of inhibitory control of omnipause cells over saccadic pulse generators in the brainstem [33]. Saccadic pulse generators, especially the subclass of saccadic burst neurons that produce horizontal saccades, are unstable and, therefore, vulnerable to supranuclear noise [33]. Neurologic disease that affects cortical/subcortical centers, which usually inhibit descending trigger signals, therefore likely results in net overactivity in these burst neurons. A potential source of inhibitory control over the superior colliculi could be the frontal eye fields [34–36]. The basal ganglia are also likely implicated, because they exert tonic inhibition onto saccadic control cells in the superior colliculus via cells in the substantia nigra pars reticulata [37,38]. In a comparative study of SWJs in patients with various parkinsonian disorders, Otero-Millan and colleagues [39] provided evidence for this theory, implicating disease of the basal ganglia in the release of inhibitory control on the superior colliculus, thereby producing the initial saccade of the SWJ. O'Sullivan and colleagues [40] also discovered a possible contribution from the globus pallidus internus, noting that unilateral pallidotomy to the globus pallidus internus produced a significant increase in the number and the amplitude of SWJs. They note, however, that no known direct communication channels exist between the globus pallidus internus and the superior colliculus, nor with the pontine omnipause neurons of the substantia nigra pars reticulata. Another study by Fridley and colleagues [41] found that stimulation of the subthalamic nucleus strongly increased SWJ frequency in a population of patients with Parkinson disease (PD).

Overall, the two proposed mechanisms are not mutually exclusive and likely both play functional roles in the generation of SWJs. The details of these two proposed mechanisms are further explored in a subsequent section where studies in populations with specific neurologic conditions further reinforce both mechanisms.

Square wave jerks as a variant of normal

To use SWJs as a clue toward an underlying disease process, one first needs to understand how "normal" SWJs are quantified in the literature. The current thresholds are based on a small number of studies with significant discordance and significant differences in the mean age of their populations. The following paragraphs briefly outline and contrast the results of the seminal papers that have established the contemporary cutoffs for SWJ frequency and, where possible, amplitude.

The first study of 29 participants was conducted by Herishanu and Sharpe in 1981 [1]. In two groups of participants with mean ages 32 and 71, a significant difference occurred in SWJ frequency, namely 4.7 SWJs per minute in the younger group compared with 27 in the older group. SWJ amplitude did not differ between groups. The authors concluded that a frequency of nine SWJs or more per minute should be considered abnormal in young persons. No specific cutoff for the older age group was provided given that the sample size in this group was small (n = 2), which also implies extremely limited extrapolability.

In 1984, Elidan and colleagues [42] proposed a cutoff of 0.3 to 3 SWJs per minute based on his study of 38 patients who exhibited SWJs. An important note to make is that this study was not performed in healthy volunteers, but instead was a subsample of patients previously referred for dizziness or unsteadiness, meaning that results applied to a variety of pathologies (68% with no definite clinical diagnosis, 8% with central lesions, and 24% with peripheral vestibulopathy).

A subsequent study by Ohtsuka and colleagues [43] found means of 8 to 10 SWJs per minute in bright light with fixation on a target, and 20 SWJs per minute in darkness, in 6 out of 16 subjects (age range 18–74, no mean age given) who demonstrated SWJs. Note here that the purpose of this experiment was not to determine normal thresholds, but instead to demonstrate a direct transition from microsaccades to SWJs. For this reason, participants were not age-stratified, and this mean frequency, therefore, is based on a heterogeneous age group. They also noted that substantial individual variation occurred in their studied population, and that two participants did not demonstrate an increase in SWJ frequency between light and dark. This ultimately further limits the statistical power, and, thereby, the applicability to the general population.

Shallo-Hoffman and coworkers [44] first attempted the task of establishing quantifiable norms in light and in darkness. From a group of 50 participants, they concluded that a frequency of more than 16 SWJs per minute was abnormal during fixation (with participants' eyes open), and that more than 20 SWJs per minute were abnormal in darkness (with participants' eyes closed). The authors noted that, whereas SWJs occurred in all previously mentioned conditions, total darkness increased the amplitude of SWJs by 0.5° in half of the participants (no clear cutoffs were provided for a normal amplitude). Note here that this study tested fairly young participants (age range 21–37, mean age 25), which lowered their accepted SWJ frequency compared with studies of populations with a higher mean age.

A follow-up study by Shallo-Hoffman and coworkers [45] aimed to definitely address the age discrepancy by explicitly studying the characteristics of SWJs over a broad range of ages and in varying conditions (with eyes open and fixated, with eyes closed, and with lights off). In the condition of eyes open and fixated, they reported that the youngest age group (mean age 25) demonstrated a mean frequency of six SWJs per minute, whereas the highest age group (mean age 76) demonstrated 5.5 SWJs per minute. When the same population was studied in the dark, the youngest age group exhibited a mean frequency of 7.4 SWJs per minute, whereas the highest age group exhibited 8.8 SWJs per minute. This, therefore, was the first study that provided solid evidence that healthy subjects exhibit no age-related statistical difference in the mean frequency of SWJs, which was a striking difference from the previous results published by Herishanu and Sharpe [1]. Although no direct comparison was made between age groups for SWJ amplitude, the authors do note that "normal" SWJs did increase in amplitude in the eyes-closed and lights-off conditions across all age groups. They overall concluded that a mean frequency of more than 15 SWJ per minute (during fixation) and more than 25 SWJs per minute (in darkness and with eyes closed) should be considered abnormal.

The previously noted observation that SWJs changed their behavior in darkness and with eyes closed has been a source of discordance in the literature. During darkness, Herishanu and Sharpe [1] initially found that SWJs became replaced by saccades and drifts, a result not replicated by Shallo-Hoffman and coworkers [44] who found only increases in frequency and amplitude, but not morphology. A notable difference here is that in the Herishanu and Sharpe [1] study, participants were explicitly instructed to hold their eyes still, thereby potentially altering the character of these movements in the context of a voluntary inhibitory effort. Shaffer and colleagues [32] further demonstrated that increasing task demands during pursuit tasks significantly lowered the frequency of SWJs, further suggesting that a voluntary, suppressible component exists to these eye movements.

Only one study exists to date that explicitly investigates the characteristics of SWJs in children. Salman and colleagues [46] studied 38 participants aged 8 to 19 years and found a median frequency of three per minute (range 1–18), and median amplitude was 0.81°. No variation was again found with increasing age for all parameters. Note that this study was in light with eyes fixated, and no comparison was made with darkness.

In summary, the most robust evidence currently points to acceptable thresholds of up to 16 SWJs per minute in bright light with fixation and up to 25 SWJs in darkness, with no specific adjustments needed for advanced age [43–45]. Most studies do point to the likelihood that SWJ frequency does indeed increase in darkness [43–45] and does not change morphology as initially suggested by Herishanu and Sharpe [1]. Note that few studies explicitly establish norms for amplitude, but the currently accepted threshold seems to be 1° to 20° with eyes open and with eyes closed [42]. Given that some studies note that SWJ amplitude increases in darkness [44,45], a need exists for future research to replicate these studies to determine norms for amplitude under dark and light conditions.

Square wave jerks as a sign of neuropathology

Generally, an increase in the frequency or amplitude of SWJs should be seen as a potential biomarker of disease. Of note, the literature eventually separated SWJs from their counterparts of higher amplitude, usually termed macro-SWJs or square wave pulses [15,47]. Although macro-SWJs are nearly identical to SWJs in their morphology, they are differentiated from SWJs by the fact that they usually oscillate on one side of fixation [48] and usually have a higher amplitude, generally 20° to 50° [15,47]. They also may have a significantly shorter intersaccadic interval, usually around 80 milliseconds [8].

Among the best-studied entities relating to SWJs is Parkinson's Disease (PD) [49–52]. PD is characterized by the progressive loss of dopaminergic neurons in the substantia nigra pars compacta (of the basal ganglia), leading to a clinical phenotype of rigidity, resting tremor, generalized slowing of movement, and postural instability. In PD, SWJs are usually notable in their high amplitude (thereby often qualifying as macro-SWJs) and their frequency [52]. The pathophysiology of increased SWJs in those with PD is two-fold. First, given the usually inhibitory role of the substantia nigra over the superior colliculus (a critical area in the production of reflexive and voluntary saccades), it is hypothesized that a decrease in its output thereby results in a net increase of superior colliculus activity [53]. Second, as dopaminergic depletion progresses, frontal cortical areas (especially the frontal eye fields, which send projections via the substantia nigra pars reticulata to the superior colliculus) become implicated in an attempt to compensate for the loss of dopaminergic output from the basal ganglia [36,49,54]. This increased compensatory activity further exacerbates SWJs.

Atypical parkinsonisms, such as multiple systems atrophy (MSA), progressive supranuclear palsy (PSP), and corticobasal degeneration, also have been common areas of study because they relate to SWJs [51,55–61]. Although these disorders present with a similar parkinsonian phenotype to PD, they are distinctly different disorders characterized by the cerebral accumulation of different abnormal proteins. Some studies [50,61,62] suggest that the frequency of SWJs, whereas still higher in PD than in the general population, is overall much lower in PD compared with its atypical parkinsonian counterparts, most notably PSP and MSA. Prominent, frequent SWJs, therefore, may be helpful as a clinical differentiator between PD and atypical parkinsonisms. Aside from frequency as a potential differentiating factor, some evidence shows that SWJs in PSP are more horizontal and larger in amplitude compared with PD [39]. The finding of higher amplitude being an indicator of atypical parkinsonism over idiopathic PD has since been supported by a comparative study of patients with MSA [63]. Mechanistically, the presence of SWJs in multiple atypical parkinsonisms is interesting given that they are defined by different proteinopathies with different neuroanatomic preponderances for deposition. For example, SWJ emergence in PSP (a tauopathy characterized by impairment in vertical eye movements due to midbrain atrophy) is hypothesized to be caused by a compensatory coupling mechanism aimed at increasing vertical saccade burst [64]. Another proposed mechanism implicates atrophy of the middle and inferior temporal gyri, areas that have been identified as being atrophic in patients with PSP [65].

The hypothesis of the temporal lobe being a key driver in the generation of SWJs is further supported by the notable occurrence of SWJs in those with Alzheimer's dementia [66–68], a mixed amyloidopathy-tauopathy known to cause abnormal protein deposition in the temporal lobes. A direct comparison between patients with typical Alzheimer's dementia and those with posterior cortical atrophy (a subvariant featuring the same proteinopathy but with preferential deposition in the occipital and parietal lobes) showed that those with Alzheimer's dementia had a much higher rate of SWJs, whereas those with posterior cortical atrophy exhibited predominantly macrosaccadic oscillations [69]. This observation, therefore, also implicates the temporal lobes in the generation of SWJs. Although a potential mechanism could involve the presence of cortical projections to areas of the superior colliculi previously demonstrated in cats and macaque monkeys [61,70,71], the exact connective network in humans has not yet been identified and could represent an avenue for future research.

Another major class of SWJ-associated disorders is the cerebellar diseases, especially because they relate to the proposition of a cerebellar mechanism. The most well-studied disorders in their relation to SWJs are the spinocerebellar ataxias (SCAs). The early body of research confirmed the occurrence of SWJs in heterogeneous groups of patients with inherited SCA syndromes [72,73], which have now been progressively narrowed down to be SCA3 [17,18] and SCA6 [19,20]. In fact, evidence shows even presymptomatic individuals with the SCA6 gene exhibit an abnormally high frequency of SWJs [20]. The SCA literature supports that early eye movement abnormalities imply the level of the posterior cerebellar vermis and the flocculus [20]. An interesting mechanistic commonality is found between SCA6 and familial cortical myoclonic tremor with epilepsy which, despite their different clinical phenotypes, have been linked to changes in Purkinje cells in the cerebellar cortex [19]. Therefore, cerebellar cortical areas also could play a role in this potential pathway. Other cerebellum-predominant diseases that provide support for a cerebellar mechanism in SWJs include Friedreich's ataxia [22–25]; ataxia with oculomotor apraxia type 2 [21,74]; Joubert syndrome [75]; and structural cerebellar pathology, such as Langerhans cell histiocytosis [76,77], cerebellar hemorrhage [78], and anti–glutamic acid decarboxylase ataxia [79]. Spieker and colleagues [24] made an interesting observation in their study of patients with Friedreich's ataxia, namely that the frequency of SWJs did not correlate with the degree of floccular/parafloccular involvement. This led to the conclusion that the pathophysiology of SWJs in Friedreich's ataxia is not solely ascribable to the involvement of cerebellar structures.

Other conditions associated with pathologic SWJs are broad and include Huntington's disease [80], amyotrophic lateral sclerosis (ALS) [81–83], essential tremor [84], anorexia nervosa [85,86], chorea-acanthocytosis [87], organoarsenic poisoning [88], and acute head trauma [89,90]. The Huntington's disease literature links SWJ emergence to neurodegeneration of the superior colliculi, further reinforcing the brainstem hypothesis [80]. ALS studies also support the brainstem hypothesis, although for different reasons. Shaunak and colleagues [81] initially concluded that cortical involvement of the frontal eye fields in ALS overall results in the generation of SWJs by way of releasing inhibition on downstream brainstem centers, as previously described. SWJs occur at a higher rate in those with bulbar ALS than in those with other subtypes [83,91]. Guo and colleagues [91] therefore suggest that this finding further supports the brainstem hypothesis given that patients with bulbar involvement are more likely to have more extensive brainstem involvement than those with other subtypes. A study by Becker and colleagues [92] found an increase in amplitude, but no increase in frequency of SWJs between patients with ALS and healthy control subjects.

Although papers describing an SWJ association exist for X-linked ataxia [93], adult-onset Alexander disease [94], carbohydrate-deficient glycoprotein syndrome type Ia [95], Hermansky-Pudlak syndrome [96], pantothenate-kinase-associated neurodegeneration [97], mitochondrial encephalopathy with lactic acidosis and stroke-like episodes [98], PLA2G6-related neurodegeneration with brain iron accumulation [99], and neurosarcoidosis [100], the SWJ frequency was either not reported, not compared with healthy control subjects, or did not meet the frequency cutoff established previously. Therefore, a clear association between these diseases and a pathologic frequency of SWJs cannot be drawn. Of brief note, a strong research movement in the 1990s investigated the association between SWJs and schizophrenia. However, no clear conclusion exists to date, and although some studies suggest that the frequency of SWJs actually is lower in patients with schizophrenia [101], other studies found no significant difference in the number of SWJs between patients with schizophrenia and healthy control subjects [102–105].

PRESENT RELEVANCE AND FUTURE AVENUES TO INVESTIGATE

Ultimately, this review sheds light on multiple avenues that require further research in SWJs. First, as evidenced by our summary of the seminal work on SWJs in healthy subjects, a significant need exists to better define what qualifies SWJs as normal, especially given the limited number of studies in this area and the significant discordance between them. Ideally, the frequency cutoffs of up to 16 SWJ per minute (in light) and up to 25 SWJ per minute (in darkness) as established in the two studies by Shallo-Hoffman and colleagues [44,45] would require replication. Furthermore, normal amplitude also could be more rigorously defined, given that multiple amplitude cutoffs currently exist (previously suggested ranges include 2° to 10° [7] and 0.5° to 5° [8], which is a significant discordance). The question of whether an age-dependent difference occurs in SWJ frequency also needs to be further explored. Generally, the evidence proposing that the frequency of SWJs increases with age is limited and also defined by small sample sizes [1], thereby limiting applicability. The highest-quality study to date specifically quantifying age-stratified trends did not find a frequency difference [45].

Given some convincing evidence that points to SWJ variance with attention and effort, a standardized protocol should be used for future studies quantifying the behaviors of SWJs if they are ultimately to be used as a biomarker. We recommend that such a protocol would include specific cognitive controls (ie, frequent reminders to keep the eyes still), and the use of easily available equipment (eg, video goggles). In each study, SWJ behavior should be examined in light conditions (with fixation) and in darkness. Further studies relating to normal SWJs also could focus on why saccadic intrusions are almost invariably horizontal; this is different between humans and their macaque counterparts where microsaccades do not have a horizontal preference [106].

Further thinking is required in elucidating a final common mechanism for the generation of pathologic SWJs. Given that ample evidence exists to support the cerebellar hypothesis and the brainstem hypothesis as outlined previously, the final mechanism likely involves a combination of the two. However, exactly how these two pathways relate to one another has not yet been established. Additionally, an interesting phenomenon that emerged from examining specific conditions with pathologic SWJ frequencies is that of the likely role of the temporal lobes in their generation of SWJs, as demonstrated specifically in the Alzheimer's disease population with predominant temporal lobe atrophy. Both of these questions would require further basic science work in delineating potential connecting pathways, likely by way of postmortem examination and staining of animal and human brain tissues.

A surprising paucity of evidence exists for SWJ occurrence in autoimmune encephalitides, a disease class where brainstem and cerebellar involvement are a fairly frequent occurrence. With the exception of one case report outlining *de novo* SWJ emergence with anti–glutamic acid decarboxylase hypothyroidism [79], to our knowledge no other case reports exist. One study previously studied patients with anti-IgLON5 encephalitis, but did not find any associated SWJs [107]. Given the rapidly increasing body of research relating to autoimmune encephalitides and rhombencephalitides, we predict that some relationships with pathologic SWJs eventually will begin to emerge and may serve as a helpful differential diagnostic marker in some conditions.

Finally, further research in SWJs in the childhood population is needed. None of the seminal papers studying SWJs in healthy subjects studied patients younger

Table 1
Oculomotor findings suggestive of particular pathologies in patients with abnormal SWJs

	Smooth pursuit abnormality	Saccades	Gaze palsies	Alignment	Convergence insufficiency	Nystagmus	Eyelid opening apraxia
AD	Mild	Delayed	—	—	—	—	—
PD	Mild	Hypometric	—	—	Common	—	—
PSP	Severe	Slowed (vertical > horizontal)	Vertical > horizontal	Occasional	Common	—	Common
MSA [58,110]	Moderate	Hypometric or hypermetric	—	Esotropia, skew deviation	Rare	Gaze-evoked, positioning downbeat	—
CBD	Mild	Delayed	—	—	—	—	Common
Ataxias	Mild/moderate	Variable: hypermetric, slowed	Variable	Esotropia, skew deviation	Variable	Gaze-evoked, downbeat	—

Abbreviations: AD, Alzheimer disease; CBD, corticobasal degeneration.
Data from Refs [108,109].

than 18 years of age, and only one study specifically aimed to determine a normal frequency in children aged 8 to 19, approximately 20 years later [46]. Although the median frequency in children was three SWJs per minute, the reported range was 1 to 18 SWJs per minute, with most trending toward the lower end of the range and with no clearly discernible age-related upward trend. Given that their measure of up to 18 SWJs per minute is in approximate agreement with Shallo-Hoffman's reported 16 SWJs per minute (in light and during fixation), this again provides some evidence that there may not be an age-related frequency difference for a "normal" mean SWJ frequency. Further research in children younger than 8 years of age may help in elucidating whether this cutoff extends downward across the lifespan and potentially into infancy.

APPROACH TO SQUARE WAVE JERKS IN CLINICAL PRACTICE

When encountering a clearly pathologic frequency of SWJs in clinical practice, accompanying signs and symptoms are most important in elucidating any underlying pathology and determining if further work-up is required. The first step is taking a history focusing on common symptoms of neurodegenerative disease (eg, progressive memory/cognitive dysfunction) or cerebellar dysfunction (eg, imbalance, incoordination). Because parkinsonism is a common association, questions regarding motor symptoms of slowness of movement and speech, stiffness, softening of voice, and gait instability are important, in addition to screening for premotor manifestations, such as progressive hyposmia, symptoms of REM-sleep behavior disorder (acting out dreams, accidental injury during sleep, falling out of bed at night), depression, and constipation. A family history may reveal ataxia, prompting consideration of an inherited SCA syndrome. The neuro-ophthalmic examination should focus on the oculomotor examination and include tests of smooth pursuit, saccades, vestibulo-ocular reflex, optokinetic nystagmus, vergence, alignment, eyelid opening, and noting any nystagmus. Specific abnormalities suggest certain pathologies (Table 1). If feasible, a neurologic examination especially should focus on the cardinal "TRAP" features of parkinsonism, namely tremor (pure resting), rigidity (usually asymmetric), akinesia/bradykinesia, and postural instability in addition looking for cerebellar features such as truncal, appendicular, or gait ataxia. Although rarer, the presence of chorea may suggest underlying Huntington's disease, and the presence of asymmetric hand weakness, muscle atrophy, fasciculations, and/or progressive bulbar signs (dysarthria, dysphagia, hypophonia) may suggest potential ALS. In virtually all cases, if abnormalities are present on history or examination, brain imaging and referral for a neurologic consultation is recommended.

SUMMARY

This review provides an in-depth summary of the origins of SWJs along with their quantifiable thresholds, neuroanatomic underpinnings, and clinical associations in the context of neuropathology. By reviewing the initial studies that aimed to quantify a "normal" SWJ frequency, we conclude that, based on the most reliable current evidence, a cutoff of up to 16 SWJs per minute (in light and with fixation) and up to 25 SWJs per minute (in darkness) is appropriate. There does not seem to be an increase in SWJ frequency with age in healthy persons. Only one study so far has validated this interval in children, further suggesting that the role of age in SWJ frequency has previously been overestimated in the absence of underlying neurologic disease. We provide evidence that substantial discordance about accepted normal ranges for amplitude exists, and that further studies are needed to better quantify this.

In terms of clinical applications, pathologic SWJs occur across a wide range of neuropathology, most prominently in various parkinsonisms. A reasonable body of literature exists to support that the frequency and amplitude of SWJs are higher in those with PD than in healthy control subjects, and that frequency and amplitude are even higher (often qualifying as macro-SWJs) in atypical parkinsonisms, specifically in PSP and MSA. This allows for the presence of high-amplitude, high-frequency SWJs to be a helpful distinguishing marker for atypical parkinsonisms when evaluating patients with parkinsonian traits, which has significant implications for prognosis and treatment. In addition, multiple cerebellar conditions have been associated with SWJs, from neurodegenerative to structural causes. This is specifically helpful in the patient with a clinical phenotype of SCA, where the presence of pathologic SWJs can help narrow the differential diagnosis (most prevalent in SCA3 and SCA6).

From a mechanistic perspective, we conclude that ample evidence exists for pathologic SWJs emerging from dysfunction in the cerebellum and in the brainstem, as evidenced by numerous studies ranging from basic science to hypothetical models to correlation with clinical neurology. As previously remarked by the various authors who investigated these two mechanistic pathways, the cerebellar and brainstem hypotheses are highly unlikely to be mutually exclusive, but further study is needed to delineate exactly how these two pathways neuroanatomically relate to one another. Furthermore, we shed light on a previously neglected area of research that links the presence of pathologic SWJs to temporal lobe dysfunction, further implicating new cortical areas in the mechanism.

CLINICS CARE POINTS

- When evaluating SWJs in a patient, a frequency cutoff of up to 16 SWJs per minute (in light and with fixation) and up to 25 SWJs per minute (in darkness) should be used as normal.
- Numbers higher than these thresholds should be considered abnormal and are associated with a broad variety of neurologic disease spanning the brainstem, cerebellum, basal ganglia, frontal lobes, or potentially temporal lobes.
- An increase in SWJs higher than these thresholds is not a feature of normal aging and should cue the practitioner to look for underlying pathology.

CONFLICTS OF INTEREST

Dr R.M. Konder has no financial or commercial conflicts of interest to disclose.
Dr D. Lelli has no financial or commercial conflicts of interest to disclose.

References

[1] Herishanu YO, Sharpe JA. Normal square wave jerks. Invest Ophthalmol Vis Sci 1981;20: 268.

[2] Ohm J. Eine Registriervorrichtung für waagerechte Augen- und Lidbewegungen. Zeitschrift der Augenheilkunde 1916;36:198.

[3] Jung R. Nystagmographie: Zur Physiologie und Pathologie des optisch-vestibulären Systems beim Menschen. In: Bergmann GJ, Frey W, Schwiegk H, editors. Handbuch der inneren Medizin. Berlin: Springer; 1953. p. 1325–79.

[4] Vedel-Jensen N. Pathological ocular fixation instability. Acta Ophthalmol 1966;44: 481–93.

[5] Alpert JN, Coats AC, Perusquia E. Saccadic nystagmus in cerebellar cortical atrophy. Neurology 1975;25:676–80.

[6] Jung R, Kornhuber HH. Results of electronystagmography in man: the value of optokinetic vestibular and spontaneous nystagmus for neurologic diagnosis and research. In: Bender M, editor. The ocular motor system. New York: Harper and Row; 1964. p. 440–2.

[7] Feldon SE, Langston JW. Square-wave jerks: a disorder of microsaccades? Neurology 1977;27:278–81.

[8] Leigh RJ, Zee DS. The neurology of eye movements," vol. 70 in the Contemporary Neurology Series. New York: Oxford University Press; 2006. p. 762.

[9] Fukazawa T, Tashiro K, Hamada T, et al. Multisystem degeneration: drugs and square wave jerks. Neurology 1986;36:1230–3.

[10] Otero-Millan J, Macknik SL, Serra A, et al. Triggering mechanisms in microsaccade and saccade generation: a novel proposal. Ann N Y Acad Sci 2011;1233:107–16.

[11] Gowen E, Abadi RV, Poliakoff E, et al. Modulation of saccadic intrusions by exogenous and endogenous attention. Brain Res 2007;1141:154–67.

[12] Hafed ZM, Clark JJ. Microsaccades as an overt measure of covert attention shifts. Vision Res 2002;42:2533–45.

[13] Hafed ZM. Mechanisms for generating and compensating for the smallest possible saccades. Eur J Neurosci 2011;33:2101–13.

[14] Rolfs M, Laubrock J, Kliegl R. Shortening and prolongation of saccade latencies following microsaccades. Exp Brain Res 2006;169:369–76.

[15] Dell'Osso LF, Abel LA, Daroff RB. Inverse latent" macro square-wave jerks and macro saccadic oscillations. Ann Neurol 1977;2(1):57–60.

[16] Daroff RB. Ocular oscillations. Ann Otol 1977;86:102–7.

[17] Shimizu N, Takiyama Y, Mizuno Y, et al. Characteristics of oculomotor disorders of a family with Joseph's disease. J Neurol 1990;237:393–8.

[18] Bürk K, Fetter M, Abele M, et al. Autosomal dominant cerebellar ataxia type I: oculomotor abnormalities in families with SCA1, SCA2, and SCA3. J Neurol 1999;246:789–97.

[19] Bour LJ, van Rootselaar AF, Koelman JH, et al. Oculomotor abnormalities in myoclonic tremor: a comparison with spinocerebellar ataxia type 6. Brain 2008;131(9):2295–303.

[20] Christova P, Anderson JH, Gomez CM. Impaired eye movements in presymptomatic spinocerebellar ataxia type 6. Arch Neurol 2008;65(4):530–6.

[21] Clausi S, De Luca M, Chiricozzi FR, et al. Oculomotor deficits affect neuropsychological performance in oculomotor apraxia type 2. Cortex 2013;49:691–701.

[22] Dale RT, Kirby AW, Jampel RS. Square-wave jerks in Friedreich's ataxia. Am J Ophthalmol 1978;85(3):400–6.

[23] Kirkham TH, Guitton D, Katsarkas A, et al. Oculomotor abnormalities in Friedreich's ataxia. J Can Sci Neurol 1979;6(2):167–72.

[24] Spieker S, Schulz J, Petersen D, et al. Fixation instability and oculomotor abnormalities in Friedreich's ataxia. J Neurol 1995;242:517–21.

[25] Fahey MC, Cremer PD, Aw ST, et al. Vestibular, saccadic and fixation abnormalities in genetically confirmed Friedreich ataxia. Brain 2008;131:1035–45.

[26] Glickstein M, Sultan F, Voogd J. Functional localization in the cerebellum. Cortex 2011;47(1):59e80.

[27] Selhorst JB, Stark L, Ochs AL, et al. Disorders in cerebellar ocular motor control. Brain 1976;99:509–22.

[28] Dell'Osso LF. Ocular motor system control models and the cerebellum; hypothetical mechanisms. Cerebellum 2019;18(3):605–14.

[29] Suzuki Y, Kase M, Hashimoto M, et al. Leaky neural integration observed in square-wave jerks. Jpn J Ophthalmol 2003;47:535–6.

[30] Sanchez K, Rowe FJ. Role of neural integrators in oculomotor systems: a systematic narrative literature review. Acta Ophthalmol 2018;96:e111–8.

[31] Gowen E, Abadi RV. Saccadic instabilities and voluntary saccadic behaviour. Exp Brain Res 2005;164:29–40.

[32] Shaffer DM, Krisky CM, Sweeney JA. Frequency and metrics of square-wave jerks: influences of task-demand characteristics. Invest Ophthalmol Vis Sci 2003;44:1082–7.

[33] Zee DS, Robinson DA. A hypothetical explanation of saccadic oscillations. Ann Neurol 1979;5:405–14.

[34] Schlag-Ray M, Schlag J, Dassonville P. How the frontal eye field can impose a saccade goal on superior colliculus neurons. J Neurophysiol 1992;67:1003–5.

[35] Munoz DP, Wurtz RH. Fixation cells in monkey superior colliculus: characteristics of cell discharge. J Neurophysiol 1993;70:559–75.

[36] Shaikh AG, Xu-Wilson M, Grill S, et al. 'Staircase' square-wave jerks in early Parkinson's disease. Br J Ophthalmol 2011;95(5):705–9.

[37] Hikosaka O, Wurtz RH. Modification of saccadic eye movements by GABA-related substances. I. Effect of muscimol and bicuculline in monkey superior colliculus. J Neurophysiol 1985;53:266–91.

[38] Hikosaka O, Wurtz RH. Modification of saccadic eye movements by GABA-related substances. II. Effects of muscimol in monkey substantia nigra pars reticulata. J Neurophysiol 1985;53:292–308.

[39] Otero-Millan J, Schneider R, Leigh RJ, et al. Saccades during attempted fixation in parkinsonian disorders and recessive ataxia: from microsaccades to square-wave jerks. PLoS One 2013;8(3):e58535.

[40] O'Sullivan JD, Maruff P, Tyler P, et al. Unilateral pallidotomy for Parkinson's disease disrupts ocular fixation. J Clin Neurosci 2003;10(2):181–5.

[41] Fridley J, Adams G, Sun P, et al. Effect of subthalamic nucleus or globus pallidus interna stimulation on oculomotor function in patients with Parkinson's disease. Stereotact Funct Neurosurg 2013;91(2):113–21.

[42] Elidan J, Gay I, Lev S. Square wave jerks: incidence, characteristic, and significance. J Otolaryngol 1984;13(6):375–81.

[43] Ohtsuka K, Mukuno K, Ukai K, et al. The origin of square wave jerks: conditions of fixation and microsaccades. Jpn J Ophthalmol 1986;30(2):209–15.

[44] Shallo-Hoffman J, Petersen J, Mühlendyck H. How normal are "normal" square wave jerks? Investigative Ophthalmology and Visual Science 1989;30(5):1009–11.

[45] Shallo-Hoffman J, Sendler B, Mühlendyck H. Normal square wave jerks in differing age groups. Investigative Ophthalmology and Visual Science 1990;31(8):1650–2.

[46] Salman MS, Sharpe JA, Lillakas L, et al. Square wave jerks in children and adolescents. Pediatr Neurol 2008;38(1):16–9.

[47] Dell'Osso LF, Troost BT, Daroff RB. Macro square-wave jerks. Neurology 1975;25:975–9.

[48] Sharpe JA, Fletcher WA. Saccadic intrusions and oscillations. Can J Neurol Sci 1984;11:426–33.

[49] White OB, Saint-Cyr JA, Tomlinson RD, et al. Ocular motor deficits in Parkinson's disease. II. Control of the saccadic and smooth pursuit systems. Brain 1983;106(3):571–87.

[50] Rascol O, Sabatini U, Simonetta-Moreau M, et al. Square wave jerks in Parkinsonian syndromes. Journal of Neurology, Neurosurgery, and Psychiatry 1991;54:599–602.

[51] Gorges M, Pinkhardt EH, Kassubek J. Alteration of eye movement control in neurodegenerative movement disorders. Journal of Ophthalmology 2014;11, article ID 658243.

[52] Pretegiani E, Optican LM. Eye movements in Parkinson's disease and inherited parkinsonian syndromes. Front Neurol 2017;8:592.

[53] Hikosaka O, Wurtz RH. The basal ganglia. Rev Oculomot Res 1989;3:257–81.

[54] Nauta HJW. A proposed conceptual reorganization of the basal ganglia and telencephalon. Neuroscience 1979;4:1875–81.

[55] Anderson T, Luxon L, Quinn N, et al. Oculomotor function in multiple system atrophy: clinical and laboratory features in 30 patients. Movement Disorders 2008;23:977–84.

[56] Phokaewvarangkul O, Bhidayasiri R. How to spot ocular abnormalities in progressive supranuclear palsy? A practical review. Transl Neurodegener 2019;8:20.

[57] Troost BT, Daroff RB. The ocular motor defects in progressive supranuclear palsy. Ann Neurol 1977;2:397–403.

[58] Armstrong RA. Visual signs and symptoms of multiple system atrophy. Clin Exp Optom 2014;97:483–91.

[59] Rivaud-Péchoux S, Vidailhet M, Gallouedec G, et al. Longitudinal ocular motor study in corticobasal degeneration and progressive supranuclear palsy. Neurology 2000;54: 1029–32.

[60] Fisk JD, Goodale MA, Burkhart G, et al. Progressive supranuclear palsy: the relationship between ocular motor dysfunction and psychological test performance. Neurology 1982;32:698–705.

[61] Anagnostou E, Karavasilis E, Potiri I, et al. A cortical substrate for square-wave jerks in progressive supranuclear palsy. J Clin Neurol 2020;16(1):37–45.

[62] Gitchel GT, Wetzel PA, Baron MS. Pervasive ocular tremor in patients with Parkinson disease. Arch Neurol 2012;69(8):1011–7.

[63] Zhou H, Wang X, Ma D, et al. The differential diagnostic value of a battery of oculomotor evaluation in Parkinson's disease and multiple system atrophy. Brain and Behaviour 2021;11:e02184.

[64] Garbutt S, Matlin A, Hellmuth J, et al. Oculomotor function in frontotemporal lobar degeneration, related disorders and Alzheimer's disease. Brain 2008;131(5):1268–81.

[65] Josephs KA, Xia R, Mandrekar J, et al. Modeling trajectories of regional volume loss in progressive supranuclear palsy. Movement Disorders 2013;28:1117–24.

[66] Jones A, Friedland RP, Koss B, et al. Saccadic intrusions in Alzheimer-type dementia. J Neurol 1983;229:189–94.

[67] Parkinson J, Maxner C. Eye movement abnormalities in Alzheimer disease: case presentation and literature review. Am Orthopt J 2005;55:90–6.

[68] Kapoula Z, Yang Q, Otero-Millan J, et al. Distinctive features of microsaccades in Alzheimer's disease and in mild cognitive impairment. Age 2014;36:535–43.

[69] Shakespeare TJ, Kaski D, Yong KXX, et al. Abnormalities of fixation, saccade and pursuit in posterior cortical atrophy. Brain 2015;138:1976–91.

[70] Cranford JL, Ladner SJ, Campbell CB, et al. Efferent projections of the insular and temporal neocortex of the cat. Brain Res 1976;117:195–210.

[71] Maioli MG, Domeniconi R, Squatrito S, et al. Projections from cortical visual areas of the superior temporal sulcus to the superior colliculus, in macaque monkeys. Arch Ital Biol 1992;130:157–66.

[72] Zee DS, Yee RD, Cogan DG, et al. Ocular motor abnormalities in hereditary cerebellar ataxia. Brain 1976;99:207–34.

[73] Yamamoto H, Saito S, Sobue I. Bedside and electro-oculographic analysis of abnormal ocular movements in spinocerebellar degenerations: effects of thyrotropin-releasing hormone. Neurology 1988;38:110–4.

[74] Jordan JT, Samuel G, Vernino S, et al. Slowly progressive ataxia, neuropathy, and oculo-motor dysfunction. Arch Neurol 2012;69(10):1366–71.

[75] Rucker JC, Dell'Osso LF, Garbutt S, et al. 'Staircase' saccadic intrusions plus transient yoking and neural integrator failure associated with cerebellar hypoplasia: a model simu-lation. Semin Ophthalmol 2006;21:229–43.

[76] Anagnostou E, Papageorgiou SG, Potagas C, et al. Square-wave jerks and smooth pursuit impairment as subtle early signs of brain involvement in Langerhans' cell histiocytosis. Clin Neurol Neurosurg 2008;110:286–90.

[77] Autier L, Gaymard B, Bayen E, et al. Eye movement abnormalities in neurodegenerative Langerhans cell histiocytosis. Neurol Sci 2022;43:6539–46.

[78] Neshige R, Kuroda Y, Oda K, et al. A case of macro square wave jerks due to cerebellar hemorrhage'' [article in Japanese]. Rinsho Shinkeigaku 1984;24(9):912–5.

[79] Brokalaki C, Kararizou E, Dimitrakopoulos A, et al. Square-wave ocular oscillation and ataxia in an anti-GAD-positive individual with hypothyroidism. J Neuro Ophthalmol 2015;35:390–5.

[80] Bollen E, Reulen JPH, den Heyer JC, et al. Horizontal and vertical saccadic eye movement abnormalities in Huntington's chorea. J Neurol Sci 1986;74:11–22.

[81] Shaunak S, Orrell RW, O'Sullivan E, et al. Oculomotor function in amyotrophic lateral sclerosis: evidence for frontal impairment. Ann Neurol 1995;38:38–44.

[82] Donaghy C, Pinnock R, Abrahams S, et al. Ocular fixation instabilities in motor neurone disease. A marker of frontal lobe dysfunction? J Neurol 2009;256:420–6.

[83] Kang BH, Kim JI, Lim YM, et al. Abnormal oculomotor functions in amyotrophic lateral scle-rosis. J Clin Neurol 2018;14(4):464–71.

[84] Gitchel GT, Wetzel PA, Baron MS. Slowed saccades and increased square wave jerks in essential tremor. Tremor and Other Hyperkinetic Movements 2013;3:tre-03-178-4116-2.

[85] Phillipou A, Rossell S, Castle DJ, et al. Square wave jerks and anxiety as distinctive bio-markers for anorexia nervosa. Invest Ophthalmol Vis Sci 2014;55:8366–70.

[86] Phillipou A, Rossell SL, Gurvich C, et al. A biomarker and endophenotype for anorexia nervosa? Aust N Z J Psychiatry 2022;56(8):985–93.

[87] Gradstein L, Danek A, Grafman J, et al. Eye movements in chorea-acanthocytosis. Invest Ophthalmol Vis Sci 2005;46(6):1979–87.

[88] Nakamagoe K, Fujizuka N, Koganezawa T, et al. Residual central nervous system damage due to organoarsenic poisoning. Neurotoxicol Teratol 2013;37:33–8.

[89] Safran AB, Moody JF, Gauthier G. Sustained blepharoclonus upon eye closure. J Clin Neuro Ophthalmol 1983;3:133–6.

[90] Shinmei Y, Takahashi A, Nakamura K, et al. Cerebrospinal fluid hypovolemia syndrome after a traffic accident with abnormal eye movements: a case report. American Journal of Ophthalmology Case Reports 2020;20:100997.

[91] Guo X, Liu X, Ye S, et al. Eye movement abnormalities in amyotrophic lateral sclerosis. Brain Sci 2022;12:489.

[92] Becker W, Gorges M, Lulé D, et al. Saccadic intrusions in amyotrophic lateral sclerosis (ALS). Journal of Eye Movement Research 2019;12(6):8.

[93] Verhagen WIM, Huygen PLM, Arts WFM. Multi-system signs and symptoms in X-linked ataxia carriers. J Neurol Sci 1996;140:85–90.

[94] Martidis A, Yee RD, Azzarelli B, et al. Neuro-ophthalmic, radiographic, and pathologic manifestations of adult-onset Alexander disease. Arch Ophthalmol 1999;117(2):265–7.

[95] Stark KL, Gibson JB, Hertle RW, et al. Ocular motor signs in an infant with carbohydrate-deficient glycoprotein syndrome type Ia. Am J Ophthalmol 2000;130:533–5.

[96] Gradstein L, Fitzgibbon EJ, Tsilou ET, et al. Eye movement abnormalities in Hermansky-Pudlak syndrome. J AAPOS 2005;9:369–78.

[97] Egan RA, Weleber RG, Hogarth P, et al. Neuro-ophthalmologic and electroretinographic findings in pantothenate kinase-associated neurodegeneration (formerly Hallervorden-Spatz syndrome). Am J Ophthalmol 2005;140(2):267–74.

[98] Shinmei Y, Kase M, Suzuki Y, et al. Ocular motor disorders in mitochondrial encephalopathy with lactic acid and stroke-like episodes with the 3271 (T-C) point mutation in mitochondrial DNA. J Neuro Ophthalmol 2007;27(1):22–8.

[99] Khan AO, AlDrees A, Elmalik SA, et al. Ophthalmic features of PLA2G6-related paediatric neurodegeneration with brain iron accumulation. Br J Ophthalmol 2014;98:889–93.

[100] Freedman IG, Kohli AA. Tinnitus as a presenting symptom of neurosarcoidosis with ocular involvement. BMJ Case Rep 2021;14:e240254.

[101] Hutton SB, Carwford TJ, Kennard C, et al. Smooth pursuit eye tracking over a structured background in first-episode schizophrenic patients. Eur Arch Psychiatry Clin Neurosci 2000;250:221–5.

[102] Levin S, Luebke A, Zee DS, et al. Smooth pursuit eye movements in schizophrenics: quantitative measurements with the search-coil technique. J Psychiat Res 1988;22(3): 195–206.

[103] Friedman L, Abel LA, Jesberger JA, et al. Saccadic intrusions into smooth pursuit in patients with schizophrenia or affective disorder and normal controls. Biol Psychiatry 1992;31: 1110–8.

[104] Campion D, Thibaut F, Denise P, et al. SPEM impairment in drug-naïve schizophrenic patients: evidence for a trait marker. Biol Psychiatry 1992;32:891–902.

[105] Clementz BA, McDowell J. Smooth pursuit in schizophrenia: abnormalities of open- and closed-loop responses. Psychophysiology 1994;31:79–86.

[106] Weber H, Fischer B, Rogal L, et al. Macro square wave jerks in a rhesus monkey: physiological and anatomical findings in a case of selective impairment of attentive fixation. J Hirnforsch 1989;30:603–11.

[107] Macher S, Milenkovic I, Zrzavy T, et al. Ocular motor abnormalities in anti- IgLON5 disease. Front Immunol 2021;12:753856.

[108] Jung I, Kim JS. Abnormal eye movements in parkinsonism and movement disorders. J Mov Disord 2019;12(1):1–13.

[109] Kang SL, Shaikh AG, Ghasia FF. Vergence and strabismus in neurodegenerative disorders. Front Neurol 2018;9:299.

[110] Zhou H, Wang X, Ma D, et al. The differential diagnostic value of a battery of oculomotor evaluation in Parkinson's disease and multiple system atrophy. Brain Behav 2021;11: e02184.

Advances in Ophthalmology and Optometry 8 (2023) 281–298

ELSEVIER
MOSBY

ADVANCES IN OPHTHALMOLOGY AND OPTOMETRY

Neuro-Ophthalmic Complications of COVID-19 Infection and Vaccination

Kholoud Alotaibi, MD[a], Nooran Badeeb, MBBS[b],*,
Rustum Karanjia, MD, PhD[c,d,e,f]

[a]Department of Ophthalmology, McGill University, Ophthalmology & Visual Sciences, McGill Academic Eye Clinic 5252 Boulevard de Maisonneuve ouest, Montreal, Quebec/ H4A 3S5, Canada; [b]Department of Ophthalmology, University of Jeddah, Hamzah Ibn Al Qasim Street, Al Sharafeyah, Jeddah 23218, Saudi Arabia; [c]Department of Ophthalmology, University of Ottawa, Eye Institute-Ottawa Hospital, 501 Smyth Road, Ottawa, ON K1H 8M2, Canada; [d]Department of Ophthalmology, Doheny Eye Centers, David Geffen School of Medicine at UCLA, Doheny Eye Center UCLA Pasadena, 625 South Fair Oaks Avenue Suite 280/285/240/227, 227 South Fair Oaks Avenue Suite 280/285/240, Pasadena, CA 91105, USA; [e]Ottawa Hospital Research Institute, The Ottawa Hospital, 501 Smyth Road, Ottawa, ON K1H 8M2, Canada; [f]Doheny Eye Institute, 150 North Orange Grove Boulevard, Pasadena, CA 91103, USA

Keywords
- COVID-19 • Vaccine • SARS-CoV-2 • Severe acute respiratory syndrome
- Giant cell arteritis • Optic neuritis • Neuro-ophthalmology • Neuro-myelitis optica

Key points
- COVID-19 infection and vaccination have been associated with neuro-ophthalmic complications but causation has not been firmly established.
- Neuro-ophthalmic manifestations post-COVID-19 infection and vaccination are uncommon and have a good prognosis in most cases.
- Some of the proposed underlying mechanisms of COVID-19 infection-related neuro-ophthalmic complications are molecular mimicry, direct viral infection, hypoxemia, hypercoagulable status, and hyperviscosity.
- Similarly, the proposed underlying mechanisms of COVID-19 vaccine-related neuro-ophthalmic complications are molecular mimicry, autoimmune syndrome associated with vaccine adjuvant, hypercoagulable status, hyperviscosity, thrombosis, and vasculitis.

Continued

*Corresponding author. E-mail address: nooran.badeeb@gmail.com

https://doi.org/10.1016/j.yaoo.2023.03.004
2452-1760/23/Crown Copyright © 2023 Published by Elsevier Inc. All rights reserved.

Continued

- No guidelines are established for the management of neuro-ophthalmic associations post-COVID-19 infection and vaccination in the literature. Therefore, treatment should be tailored to the individual patient and follow established guidelines for the treatment of the clinical phenotype.

INTRODUCTION

Severe acute respiratory syndrome caused by corona virus 2 (SARS-CoV-2, COVID-19) is the novel viral infection responsible for the devastating and ongoing COVID-19 pandemic. Since the beginning of the pandemic, the World Health Organization (WHO) estimates more than a billion confirmed cases of COVID-19 infection, and more than 6 million deaths worldwide have occurred [1]. This devastating disease has had implications for all aspects of medicine with new disease phenotypes emerging, including in ophthalmology.

The scale of this pandemic has led to an unprecedented rapid creation of vaccines against COVID-19. Since becoming available to the public at the end of 2020, more than 12 billion COVID-19 vaccine doses have been administered worldwide. This has led to a marked reduction in the rate of infections, transmissions, hospitalizations, and death from COVID-19 infection and, hopefully, will lead to the end of this pandemic [2–4]. However, new presentations of autoimmune conditions have been associated with COVID-19 vaccination [5]. The postinfection and postvaccine manifestations of the COVID-19 pandemic are still emerging. Reports have demonstrated that SARS-CoV-2 infection and vaccination can affect multiple organ systems including the eyes, resulting in a spectrum of ocular manifestations such as conjunctivitis, episcleritis, uveitis, vascular occlusions, and retinitis. Moreover, neuro-ophthalmic manifestations exist, ranging from a simple headache to irreversible blindness from optic neuritis (ON) or giant cell arteritis (GCA).

Some of these new vaccines use novel technology, and long-term data on potential side effects are still pending. The WHO recommendation for reporting possible vaccine side effects is the presence of a temporal association between the administration of the vaccine and the onset of symptoms, with a suggested cutoff of 28 days between vaccination and symptoms. The exclusion exists of other triggers for the disease manifestation and the presence of published literature with an established possible relationship between the vaccination and disease onset or exacerbation [6].

This review aims to focus on, and summarize, the current state of knowledge of neuro-ophthalmic complications of COVID-19 infection and vaccination.

Methodology

The EMBASE, Ovid MEDLINE, and Cochrane central library were searched by a medical librarian from January 1, 2019, until September 28, 2022, using keywords to cover ocular and neuro-ophthalmological complications of

COVID-19 infection and vaccination. Manual selection was used to identify articles of interest. The search was restricted to English language.

DISCUSSION
Afferent neuro-ophthalmic complications
Optic neuritis
Post-COVID-19 infection. Generally, most cases of ON associated with COVID-19 infection have a remarkable improvement in vision after treatment with steroids, with only a few reported cases of irreversible vision loss [7,8]. Most of the cases were unilateral with variable onset ranging between 1 and 45 days postinfection [9–11]. All patients received (1 g/d) of intravenous methylprednisolone (IVMP) followed by oral prednisone taper [7]. Additionally, myelin oligodendrocyte glycoprotein (MOG)-related ON was found to have a favorable visual outcome following IVMP with vision better than 20/200 in all patients [11]. In a systematic review, only 3 cases of neuro-myelitis optica (NMO) Aquaporin 4 IgG-positive ON were identified [12]. Two were men, aged 70 years and 25 years, respectively, and one 7.5-year-old girl. They all presented within a month of their COVID-19 infection. Treatment with steroids, intravenous immunoglobulin (IVIG), plasma exchange (PLEX), and rituximab were administered, and gradual improvement was observed in 2 of the patients. Whereas the 70-year-old was treated only with antibiotics, fluids, and electrolytes, and eventually, the patient died from systemic complications of COVID-19 [12].

Post-COVID-19 vaccination. ON post-COVID-19 vaccination is the most commonly reported neuro-ophthalmic association [13], with 55 individual case reports published in the literature. Of these, two-thirds were vaccinated with the Oxford/AstraZeneca ChAdOx1, followed by BioNTech/Pfizer mRNA-vaccine BNT162b2 vaccine (26%) and Sinovac (7%). The onset of vision loss was within 3 weeks from the administration of the vaccine in most patients. This is 1 week after the antibodies from the vaccine are thought to be formed, which occurs on average at 2 weeks. Most cases were reported in Caucasians (44/55) women (38/55) with a median age of 45 years, which is higher than the typical cases of prepandemic ON. Unilateral involvement was more common than bilateral. MOG-positive ON was reported in 14 cases, followed by 7 cases of multiple sclerosis (MS)-associated ON. This contrasts with the existing literature where MS-ON accounts for the majority (57%) of cases [14,15]. Unlike, typical ON almost half of the patients presented with optic disc swelling (27/55). The treatment of choice was high-dose intravenous steroids in most patients, and a few patients received high doses of oral steroids, whereas 7 patients did not receive any steroids. PLEX was used in 6 patients either with or after the course of steroids. Median vision after treatment was 20/20. However, 5 cases occurred with vision worse than 20/200.

In a separate study of 14 cases of idiopathic ON post-COVID-19 vaccination [16–23], again most cases were in women (10 cases) half with unilateral involvement, and age ranged from 19 to 67 years. Vision changes were reported from hours to 3 weeks after BioNTech/Pfizer mRNA-vaccine BNT162b2, AstraZeneca ChAdOx1, Janssen (Johnson & Johnson), Covishield, CoronaVac-Sinovac Life, and Moderna mRNA-1273 vaccines. Optic disc swelling was noted in 8 patients on examination, and the presenting visual acuity of less than 20/200 was noted in 4 patients. Universally, there appears to be a good visual prognosis after receiving steroids. PLEX for 7 days was given only to 1 patient who failed to improve on IVMP and had a vision of counting fingers in both eyes [23].

MOG-ON was reported to comprise approximately 5% of ON cases prepandemic [15], with an increased rate of MOG-ON since the start of the pandemic [5,13,24–27]. There are 10 case reports of post-COVID-19 vaccine-associated MOG-ON in the literature. Most have been in men (7 cases) between the ages 28 and 66 years with most (7 cases) having unilateral involvement. Half had a visual acuity of less than 20/200 at presentation and the onset of vision loss was reported between 14 and 21 days and after the AstraZeneca ChAdOx1 vaccine. The treatment of choice was IVMP for 3 to 5 days, followed by oral steroids. In 4 patients, presenting with poor vision or bilateral involvement, PLEX was initiated. Only 1 patient had a spontaneous resolution of vision with no intervention.

NMO-ON was reported in (3%) of patients prepandemic, and it remained an uncommon cause of ON postvaccination [15]. Case reports of NMO-ON postvaccination exists and include cases after mRNA vaccination: a 43-year-old woman and a 31-year-old woman, both with unilateral involvement, one with complete recovery of her vision after receiving IVMP (1 g/d) for 10 days and the other with no visual recovery after receiving IVMP (1 g/d) for 5 days followed by 5 sessions of PLEX [28,29].

Giant cell arteritis
Post-COVID-19 infection. A noticeable increase in GCA cases occurred during the COVID-19 pandemic, a report by Lecler and colleagues, observed an increase of 70% from prepandemic [30]. Subsequently, higher rates of ocular involvement were seen with GCA during the pandemic [31,32]. This supports the notion of the role of viral infections as an underlying trigger for GCA. In the era of the pandemic, diagnosing GCA is challenging due to the similarities between COVID-19 infection manifestations and GCA. A study by Mehta and colleagues, found that they both share the clinical features of headache, fever, elevated C-reactive protein (CRP), and cough. Clinical manifestations that can aid in the differentiation of GCA would be jaw claudication, visual loss, platelet count, and lymphocyte count [33].

Post-COVID-19 vaccination. Three case reports exist of GCA presenting with arteritic anterior ischemic optic neuropathy after COVID-19 vaccination [34–36]: 2 in 87-year-old and 79-year-old women and 1 in a 68-year-old man. Two cases were after BioNTech/Pfizer mRNA-vaccine BNT162b2 vaccine and 1 after the AstraZeneca ChAdOx1 vaccine. They all presented within 5 days of receiving the vaccine and all had bilateral involvement. The visual acuity was less than 20/200 in at least 1 eye at the time of the presentation. Some had other symptoms of GCA including amaurosis fugax, headache, jaw claudication, scalp tenderness, and lethargy. At least 1 of the inflammatory markers was high, ESR in 2 cases and CRP in all 3 cases. A temporal artery biopsy was positive in 2 of the patients, and for one patient no information was provided about the biopsy. All patients were treated with high-dose IVMP (1 g/d) for 3–4 days followed by oral prednisolone [34–36], 1 patient subsequently received tocilizumab following a relapse 3 months after the initial presentation [34].

In both post-COVID-19 and postvaccination cases no proved causation exists and the time lapse for the postvaccination cases theoretically is too soon for the body to have mounted an immune response. Given the number of vaccinations administered to date, some overlap with GCA would be expected.

Nonarteritic anterior ischemic optic neuropathy
Post-COVID-19 infection. The relationship of COVID-19 and nonarteritic anterior ischemic optic neuropathy (NA-AION) is unknown [37]. NA-AION has been described in 6 case reports in association with COVID-19 infection [38–42]. Patients in these reports were aged older than 40 years and presented with acute painless unilateral or bilateral (2/6) altitudinal vision loss, which mainly was noted on awakening (4/6 patients). The onset of visual symptoms ranged from 1 to 4 weeks after COVID-19 infection except in 1 patient where visual symptoms preceded COVID-19 symptoms [41]. All cases demonstrated visual field defect on confrontational testing and Humphrey's visual field analysis [38,39].

Post-COVID-19 vaccination. NA-AION post-COVID-19 vaccination has rarely been reported [43–48]. All patients shared the clinical presentation of painless sudden vision changes either described as a blurring of vision or a visual field defect and all had unilateral involvement. The onset of visual symptoms was within 15 days from the vaccination (1–15 days). Most of the patients were aged older than 50 years and had 1 or more risk factors for developing NAION: small cup-to-disc ratio, hypertension, diabetes, or dyslipidemia.

Some of the cases underwent investigations to rule out GCA, along with brain and orbit imaging to rule out ON. IV or PO steroids were administered in some cases, either for the suspicion of ON or GCA. Some tried steroids as an intervention when the visual acuity was poor as a treatment of last resort to improve vision, and it was deemed successful in 1 case where vision improved from count fingers to 20/100 to 1 eccentrically after 6 weeks [48]. This case report does not demonstrate causation or bestow a treatment effect from steroids as up to a third of NAION cases will report some improvement in vision, especially once the disc edema resolves.

Papilledema
Post-COVID-19 infection. Headache is a prominent symptom of both elevated intracranial pressure (ICP) and COVID-19. In a cross-sectional study of 56

patients with COVID-19 infection, 13 had a new persistent headache prompting further clinical evaluation including lumbar puncture [49]. Of those, 85% (11/13) were found to have high opening pressure (>200mmH2O), and more than half (7/13) were greater than (250mmH2O) with normal composition and were diagnosed with idiopathic intracranial hypertension (IIH). Imaging of the brain was not significant except in 1 patient who had typical imaging features of increased intracranial pressure. All patients had normal fundoscopic examinations except for 2 who showed papilledema. Interestingly, blurred vision was reported by only 3 patients.

Cerebral venous sinus thrombosis (CVST) is a serious complication post-COVID-19 infection. Nearly all reported cases of papilledema related to CVST in the setting of COVID-19 had a favorable visual outcome except the case described by Omari and colleagues of a morbidly obese woman who presented with a bilateral progressive visual loss associated with severe headache and tinnitus. The patient recently was admitted to the hospital for bilateral pulmonary embolism and deep venous thrombosis, possibly due to COVID-19 infection [50]. CSF workup was remarkable only for an elevated opening pressure of more than (600 mmH2O). Despite maximum treatment, with acetazolamide and heparin, bilateral optic nerve sheath fenestration, and endovascular transverse sinus thrombectomy, her vision deteriorated to no light perception.

Post-COVID-19 vaccination. There have been 2 published case reports of papilledema in the setting of COVID-19 vaccination-associated IIH [51,52]. Both cases were young male patients with normal body mass index (BMI) and atypical demographics for IIH. One presented 7 days after the AstraZeneca ChAdOx1 vaccine, and the other 12 days after Sputnik V vaccine. Both had other symptoms of high ICP such as headache, pulsatile tinnitus, dizziness, and blurring of vision. MRI/MRV were normal except for signs of high ICP. Lumbar puncture with high opening pressure of (620mmH2O and 390mmH2O). One was treated with acetazolamide (750 mg) twice daily and torsemide (5 mg) once daily, and the other was given pulse IVMP (500 mg daily) for 5 days and oral acetazolamide (250 mg) 3 times a day. After 3 months, the symptoms and papilledema had completely resolved in both cases [51,52].

The above-mentioned cases did not involve CVST. However, coagulation problems that result in CVST have been reported post-COVID-19 vaccination, presenting with intracranial hypertension and papilledema. Other associated symptoms are headache, focal neurological deficit, seizures, and venous hemorrhage. Symptoms appear to happen approximately (10 days) from the day of the vaccination. Most cases were reported with the AstraZeneca ChAdOx1 vaccine [53,54]. The group most at risk was women aged under 60 years [54]. It is thought that CVST post-COVID-19 vaccine is secondary to vaccine-induced thrombotic thrombocytopenia (VITT), which is similar to heparin-induced thrombocytopenia (HIT) [53]. In a meta-analysis of 144 patients up to 80% had an accompanying thrombocytopenia and hypofibrinogenemia with a positive PF4 antibodies [54]. Most patients present to the emergency department and are treated with nonheparin anticoagulants. The mortality rate from CVST is as high as 40%, therefore, timely diagnosis is key [53].

Efferent neuro-ophthalmic complications
Ocular motility disorders
Diplopia is one of the more common symptoms reported post-COVID-19 infection and vaccination. Underlying pathologic conditions vary from cranial nerve palsy and Miller Fisher syndrome (MFS) to neuromuscular junction disorders such as myasthenia gravis (MG), and muscular pathologic conditions such as thyroid eye disease (TED) and idiopathic orbital inflammatory syndrome (IOIS).

Cranial neuropathies
Post-COVID-19 infection. In a systematic review, 56 patients with cranial neuropathy associated with COVID-19 were analyzed. Generally, COVID-19 infection was found associated with neuropathies of all cranial nerves (CN) with a predilection for CN VII, VI, and III [55]. Isolated cranial neuropathies were more prevalent than multiple cranial neuropathies. Unilateral involvement is more common than bilateral involvement, although bilateral involvement may be a sign of Guillain-Barré syndrome. Treatment included steroids, IVIG, acyclovir/valacyclovir, and rarely PLEX. Complete recovery was seen in 21 patients and partial recovery in 30 patients at discharge or last follow-up.

Post-COVID-19 vaccination. After the facial nerve, dysfunction of the abducens nerve is the most common reported neuropathy postvaccination from any vaccine, followed by the oculomotor and the trochlear nerves. A similar pattern was observed with COVID-19 vaccines. Several reports exist of patients presenting with new onset sixth and third nerve palsy [56–64]. The onset of diplopia usually was from 1 to 7 days; it has been reported postvaccination with BioNTech/Pfizer mRNA-vaccine BNT162b2, Moderna mRNA-1273, Covishield, AstraZeneca ChAdOx1, and Sinopharm. Age ranged from 23 to 88 years, with no obvious gender predominance. Almost all cases had unilateral involvement (8/9) and normal brain imaging (7/9), with one showing focal enlargement of the root exit zone and the cisternal portion of the left sixth nerve with post-gadolinium enhancement, and the other showing enhancement of both CN6 [63]. Two-thirds had full spontaneous recovery of symptoms after 2 months, including those with brain imaging abnormalities. Steroids were used in 2 out of 9 patients: 1 had no response and the other showed complete recovery after 5 days on low-dose steroids.

Multiple cranial neuropathies also have been reported post-COVID vaccination. One case reported by Manea and colleagues was of a 29-year-old man with left III, V, VI, and VII cranial nerve palsies 6 days after having his first dose of the Pfizer vaccine [65]. Another case by Shalabi and colleagues was a 41-year-old man with right IV, VI, VII, VIII, and X, associated with cervical lymphadenopathy 7 days after receiving his mRNA vaccine [66]. In both cases, an extensive workup was done, including brain imaging with contrast, infectious and inflammatory laboratory workup, a lumbar puncture to check for infections and malignant cells and even a full body computed tomography to rule out systemic malignancy were performed. In both cases, an enhancement occurred in post-gadolinium brain imaging of some of the involved cranial nerves, and a short-course of intravenous steroids was administered with subsequent clinical improvement [65,66]. As with NA-AION, improvement after steroids does not necessarily confirm a treatment affect because the natural history of isolated nerve palsies is for them to improve spontaneously.

Miller Fisher syndrome

Post-COVID-19 infection. MFS is variant of Guillain-Barré syndrome, which is characterized by a triad of ophthalmoplegia, loss of tendon reflexes, and acute onset of ataxia. MFS has been reported after COVID-19 infection and vaccination. Although the number of MFS cases in the context of COVID-19 infection is still increasing, no long-term sequelae were documented [67–69]. A proposed mechanism by which MFS develops is through an immune-mediated postinfectious process [70]. This is supported by the incubation period, the positive response to IVIG, and the presence of antiganglioside antibodies in 20% of reported cases [67,70].

Post-COVID-19 vaccination. The onset of symptoms in MFS postvaccination ranged from (7 to 18 days). It has been reported after administering Moderna vaccine, Oxford/AstraZeneca ChAdOx1, BioNTech/Pfizer mRNA-vaccine BNT162b2, tozinameran BNT162b2 mRNA, and CoronaVac-Sinovac Life. Different patterns of ophthalmoplegia were seen in these case reports [71–78]. In 5 out of 7 cases, evidence existed of albuminocytological dissociation in the cerebrospinal fluid sample analysis, which is defined as elevated proteins without pleocytosis. In 3 out of 7 antiganglioside antibodies such as anti-GQ1b antibody were positive [74,78]. Patients were treated with IVIG with recovery taking from weeks to months. One patient received physiotherapy only with reported full spontaneous recovery at 10-week follow-up [75].

Myasthenia gravis

Post-COVID-19 infection. Neuromuscular complications of COVID-19 pose a unique challenge for physicians worldwide. New onset ocular MG has been reported in patients with proven COVID-19 infection [79–83]. The incidence of MG was found to be marginally higher in patients with COVID-19 infection compared with general population (0.087% and 0.07%, respectively) [84]. Age has ranged from 6 to 65 years old. Patients complained mostly of diplopia and fatigable ptosis with limitations of ocular motility noted on examination. Treatment composed of standard dose of pyridostigmine, prednisone, and in some case IVIG. Some of the reported cases had a favorable outcome with complete recovery of their ocular MG, whereas others had only partial recovery [79,83]. All patients had elevated titers of antiacetylcholine receptor (AchR) antibodies. Two cases occurred following a complicated admission with multisystem inflammatory syndrome in children, which recently has been recognized by Centers for Disease Control and Prevention as a COVID-19 sequela [80,81].

Post-COVID-19 vaccination. New onset or exacerbation of ocular or generalized MG has been reported after administering BioNTech/Pfizer mRNA-vaccine BNT162b2, Moderna mRNA-1273, and AstraZeneca ChAdOx1 vaccines [85,86]. The age and gender of those patients mostly followed the demographic of the second peak of MG disease, which is commonly seen in men who are aged older than 60 years [87–94]. Exacerbation of preexisting MG postvaccine is thought to be from 1% to 15% [87]. Ocular MG cases presented with intermittent fatigable ptosis and diplopia [88,90,92,94]. In some of the cases, associated symptoms occurred such as fatigue and weakness, myalgia, dysarthria, dysphagia, and head drop [87,89,91,93]. In 8 of the 11 patients AchR antibodies was positive but none was positive for anti–muscle-specific kinase (MuSK) antibodies [85,87,88,90,91]. Electromyography was positive in 5 cases, showing either single-fiber electromyography (SFEMG) test of the orbicularis oculi identified with abnormal jitter or repetitive nerve stimulation providing diagnostic confirmatory for a postsynaptic neuromuscular junction disorder [85,93,94]. Computed tomography of the chest was negative except for 1 patient with mild thymic hyperplasia; interestingly, this case was double seronegative [93]. The treatment of choice was pyridostigmine alone [85,87,93,94] or combined with steroids [85,87–89,91,92] with complete or partial improvement of bulbomotor symptoms in most cases. PLEX was used for 5 days in a patient who showed no signs of improvement. The patient improved clinically after the second round of PLEX and was placed on azathioprine for maintenance [85].

Thyroid eye disease
TED is an autoimmune disease manifesting with enlargement of the extraocular muscles, proptosis, and eyelid retraction. It commonly is associated with Graves disease (GD). No case reports exist of TED related to COVID-19 infection.

Post-COVID-19 vaccination. In a study by Jafarzadeh and colleagues, subacute thyroiditis was found to be the most prevalent thyroid dysfunction after COVID-19 vaccination, followed by GD. TED was reported to be in 1.2% only [95]. TED post-COVID-19 vaccination was documented after BioNTech/Pfizer mRNA-vaccine BNT162b2 and Moderna mRNA-1273 vaccine, 2 were new onset, and 2 were reactivation [96,97]. Patients were middle-aged women with no history of smoking. Two were previously treated GD patients, 1 was a treated Hashimoto thyroiditis patient, and 1 patient had no history of underlying thyroid dysfunction [96,97]. Patients presented with different ocular manifestations of the TED as soon as 1 day and as far as 3 weeks from vaccine administration. Their ocular manifestations ranged from periorbital swelling, chemosis, proptosis, lid retraction, extraocular muscle restriction, and diplopia. Fortunately, none had any afferent issues on the examination such as compressive optic neuropathy. All showed evidence of thyroid dysfunction on laboratory workup except in 1 case [96,97]. A CT or MRI scan of the brain and orbit demonstrated enlargement of the EOM's in all of the individuals. Patients responded well to the treatment with Tepezza (Teprotumumab). Spontaneous improvement of symptoms after 4 months was noted in 1 patient [97].

IOIS can mimic the presentation of TED, and 1 case was reported after COVID-19 vaccination, presenting with diplopia, periorbital erythema, pain, and proptosis. Proper investigations and management are prompted in these cases to exclude other causes of orbital inflammation [98]. It is unclear if the association of TED and IOIS with COVID-19 vaccination is due to random chance alone, although it is interesting that most of the cases of TED were in patients who had an underlying predisposition for the disease including 2 reactivations of TED.

Pupillary defects
Adie's tonic pupil
Post-COVID-19 infection. Adie's pupil also has been identified as a potential long-term sequelae of COVID-19 infection. Only 2 cases are identified in the literature with long-term pupillary abnormalities following COVID-19 infection [99,100]. Both patients experienced visual dysfunction with evidence of anisocoria 3 weeks following COVID-19 infection, proven by a positive RT-PCR test or high titer of SARS-CoV-2 IgG antibodies. One patient had findings consistent with right trochlear nerve palsy including right hypertropia on an alternate cover test and right excyclotorsion [99]. Brain imaging using CT and MRI with contrast was unremarkable in both patients. The diagnosis of tonic pupil was confirmed in both cases using a diluted (0.125%) pilocarpine test. Treatment consisted of oral corticosteroids, remdesivir, IV antibiotics, dexamethasone, and deriphylline. However, the tonic pupil remained with difficulty focusing near objects despite medical therapy [100].

Post-COVID-19 vaccination. Only 1 case series exists of Adie's tonic pupil-associated post-COVID-19 vaccination. Gönültas and colleagues described 2 patients, 1 patient was a 27-year-old woman and another was a 48-year-old man, 10 and 12 days after receiving the Pfizer vaccine [101]. Both responded to the pharmacological testing using dilute pilocarpine (0.1%) with positive constriction of the affected pupil. One had absent deep tendon reflexes and, subsequently, was diagnosed with Holmes-Adie-syndrome [101].

Horner syndrome. One report exists of a transient isolated Horner syndrome (HS) in a 65-year-old woman 3 days after being infected with COVID-19 [102]. The patient had a normal workup including CT/CTA head, neck, and brain MRI with and without gadolinium. Complete resolution of her ptosis and miosis after 8 days of symptoms onset [102]. HS has not been reported yet in association with COVID-19 vaccination.

Proposed mechanisms of neuro-ophthalmic complications post-COVID-19 infection. Although the pathophysiology in the course of COVID-19 infection is not fully understood, several mechanisms have been proposed to explain neuro-ophthalmic manifestations from COVID-19 infection, most favoring an immune-mediated background. The SARS-CoV-2 virus may be implicated through molecular mimicry, inducing an autoimmune response, and causing disorders such as ON and MG [9,10,82,103,104].

The SARS-CoV-2 virus also has been reported to have a neurotoxic effect through binding to the angiotensin enzyme 2 (ACE2) receptor, which is an important entry receptor for the virus to vital organs such as the brain. Direct viral infection could explain some of the autoimmune disorders occurring in patients post-COVID-19 infection such as ON, cranial neuropathies, and Adie's tonic pupils [8,55,105,106]. Retrograde transport of the virus particles to the central nervous system is thought to underlie some of these disorders and is supported by a postmortem case series that found that SARS-CoV-2 viral proteins in the cranial nerves of (53%) of the investigated patients [107]. Moreover, viral particles are thought to travel from the lungs to the autonomic center in the brain stem causing disorders such as HS [102]. Moreover, in cases such as GCA, the virus is thought to have an affinity to the vascular endothelium causing direct damage [31,108]. The SARS-CoV-2 virus can cause a disruption the blood–brain barrier by proinflammatory cytokines and result in increased permeability of the blood–brain barrier, which gives access for antibodies such as MOG antibodies to the central nervous system [109].

Reports also have suggested that COVID-19-induced hypoxemia and hypercoagulability can increase the risk of circulatory insufficiency and NA-AION [110,111]. Moreover, hypercoagulability and hyperviscosity can lead to venous congestion and IIH or CVST [49,54].

Proposed mechanism of neuro-ophthalmic complications post-COVID-19 vaccination. Multiple mechanisms have been proposed for post–vaccine-related complications, some are very similar to those proposed for post-COVID-19 infection. One is the molecular mimicry theory, where the vaccine introduces proteins to the host that mimic self-antigens or similar conformational structures. In the case of ON, the molecular mimicry between the virus and central nervous system (CNS) myelin, where they share the same amino acid sequence, leads to the formation of antibodies that attack myelin and cause demyelination [24].This theory also has been proposed for cranial neuropathies postvaccination where autoimmune inflammatory demyelinating peripheral neuropathy occurs [56,57,62]. A similar mechanism is well established in MFS where molecular mimicry may induce GQ1b or GT1a ganglioside antibody production and cause a secondary, acute, demyelinating, inflammatory polyneuropathy affecting the peripheral nervous system [72,73]. Similarly in MG, the host immune system perceives the vaccine antigen as similar to host AChRs and attacks those receptors [87,88,90,92,94].

The other theory is the presence of adjuvant material in some of the vaccines, which are added to the vaccine to enhance immune response but may also produce an unwanted exaggerated immune reaction. This material is thought to play a role in the pathogenesis of an autoimmune syndrome associated with adjuvants ASIA that can possibly explain ON, GCA, and MG postvaccination [22,92,112].

Similarly, the vaccine could work to trigger and unmask the disease in individuals who were genetically predisposed to develop autoimmune diseases such as in patients with ON, GCA, TED, and MG [24,93,96]. Especially in those with symptoms occurring within a few days after receiving the vaccine [113].The presence of the human leukocyte antigen DRB1*16:02 genotype in patients with GCA also supports the genetic predisposition theory.

It is thought that endothelial cell dysfunction secondary to neuroinflammation from the vaccine can lead to hypercoagulopathy, hyperviscosity, thrombosis, and venous stasis. Subsequently, this might lead to cranial neuropathies [64]: NA-AION and IIH [40,51,52].

SUMMARY

To date, COVID-19 infection and vaccines have been associated with neuro-ophthalmic complications but causation remains to be proven. At the moment, most of our information comes from case reports and case series yet the literature is still growing with the continuation of the global pandemic and vaccination programs. It is important to remember that these neuro-ophthalmic conditions still occurred in the absence of COVID-19 and given the billions of cases of COVID-19 infection and vaccines, which have been administered worldwide, overlap is inevitable due to random chance alone. It also is important to note that while COVID-19 vaccines may be associated with neuro-ophthalmic sequela, COVID-19 is a deadly disease with its own long-term sequela, and the sequela postvaccination are treatable with almost universally good outcomes if recognized and treated early. Insufficient evidence exists to justify the deferment of vaccination based on these very rare neuro-ophthalmic associations, some of which are highly likely due to random chance alone. Both the SARS-CoV-2 virus and all the vaccines that have been produced to combat this global pandemic may have the potential to cause or exacerbate neuro-ophthalmic conditions, and ophthalmologists should be mindful of this potential and treat accordingly.

CLINICS CARE POINTS

- Consider SARS-CoV-2 infection and ask about COVID-19 symptoms when presented with an otherwise unexplained cranial neuropathy.
- Treat patients in accordance with best practices for the clinical neuro-ophthalmic phenotype with which they present irrespective of any COVID-19 association.
- Understand that post-COVID-19 conditions can occur months after the COVID-19 infection.

CONFLICT OF INTEREST
None.

SOURCE OF SUPPORT
None.

Acknowledgments
We would like to acknowledge Ms Risa Shorr our medical librarian for her collaboration and help in the literature review process.

References
[1] World Health Organization, Novel Coronavirus (2019-nCoV): situation report, 11, 2020, World Health Organization, [Internet]. Available at: https://apps.who.int/iris/handle/ 10665/330776. Accessed May 20, 2022.

[2] Ranzani OT, Hitchings MDT, Dorion M, et al. Effectiveness of the CoronaVac vaccine in older adults during a gamma variant associated epidemic of covid-19 in Brazil: Test negative case-control study. BMJ 2021;374:n2015.

[3] Chung H, He S, Nasreen S, et al. Effectiveness of BNT162b2 and mRNA-1273 covid-19 vaccines against symptomatic SARS-CoV-2 infection and severe covid-19 outcomes in Ontario, Canada: Test negative design study. BMJ 2021;374:n1943.

[4] Bernal J.L., Andrews N., Gower C., et al., Effectiveness of the Pfizer-BioNTech and Oxford-AstraZeneca vaccines on covid-19 related symptoms, hospital admissions, and mortality in older adults in England: test negative case-control study, BMJ, 373, 2021, Available at: https://www.bmj.com/content/373/bmj.n1088. Accessed September 27, 2022.

[5] Netravathi M, Dhamija K, Gupta M, et al. COVID-19 vaccine associated demyelination & its association with MOG antibody. Mult Scler Relat Disord 2022;60:103739.

[6] World Health Organization. COVID-19 vaccines :safety surveillance manual module : responding to adverse events. Geneva: World Health Organization; 2020.

[7] Jossy A, Jacob N, Sarkar S, et al. COVID-19-associated optic neuritis - A case series and review of literature. Indian J Ophthalmol 2022;70:310–6, Wolters Kluwer Medknow Publications.

[8] Mabrouki FZ, Sekhsoukh R, Aziouaz F, et al. Acute Blindness as a Complication of Severe Acute Respiratory Syndrome Coronavirus-2, Cureus 2021;13(8):e16857.

[9] Rojas-Correa DX, Reche-Sainz JA, Insausti-García A, et al. Post COVID-19 Myelin Oligodendrocyte Glycoprotein Antibody-Associated Optic Neuritis. Neuro Ophthalmol 2021;13(8):e16857.

[10] Rodríguez-Rodríguez MS, Romero-Castro RM, Alvarado-de la Barrera C, et al. Optic neuritis following SARS-CoV-2 infection. J Neurovirol 2021;27(2):359–63.

[11] Assavapongpaiboon B, Apinyawasisuk S, Jariyakosol S. Myelin oligodendrocyte glycoprotein antibody-associated optic neuritis with COVID-19 infection: A case report and literature review. Am J Ophthalmol Case Rep 2022;26:101491.

[12] Mirmosayyeb O, Ghaffary EM, Bagherieh S, et al. Post COVID-19 infection neuromyelitis optica spectrum disorder (NMOSD): A case report-based systematic review. Multiple Sclerosis and Related Disorders 2022;60:103697, Elsevier B.V.

[13] Martinez-Alvarez L, Ning Neo Y, Davagnanam BMedSci FRCR I, et al. Title suggestion: Post vaccination optic neuritis: observations from the SARS-CoV-2 pandemic. Available at: https://ssrn.com/abstract=3889990. Accessed June 11, 2022.

[14] Hassan MB, Stern C, Flanagan EP, et al. Population-Based Incidence of Optic Neuritis in the Era of Aquaporin-4 and Myelin Oligodendrocyte Glycoprotein Antibodies. Am J Ophthalmol 2020;220:110–4.

[15] Chen JJ, Pittock SJ, Flanagan EP, et al. Optic neuritis in the era of biomarkers. Surv Ophthalmol 2020;65:12–7, Elsevier USA.

[16] Leber HM, Sant'Ana L, Konichi da Silva NR, et al. Acute Thyroiditis and Bilateral Optic Neuritis following SARS-CoV-2 Vaccination with CoronaVac: A Case Report. Ocul Immunol Inflamm 2021;29:1200–6, Taylor and Francis Ltd.

[17] Roy M, Chandra A, Roy S, et al. Optic neuritis following COVID-19 vaccination: Coincidence or side-effect? - A case series. Indian J Ophthalmol 2022;70(2):679–83.

[18] Assiri SA, Althaqafi RMM, Alswat K, et al. Post COVID-19 Vaccination-Associated Neurological Complications. Neuropsychiatr Dis Treat 2022;18:137–54.

[19] Arnao V, Maimone MB, Perini V, et al. Bilateral optic neuritis after COVID vaccination. Neurol Sci 2022;43:2965–6, Springer-Verlag Italia s.r.l.

[20] Elnahry AG, Asal ZB, Shaikh N, et al. Optic neuropathy after COVID-19 vaccination: a report of two cases. Int J Neurosci 2021;1–7.

[21] Katayama H, Itoh K, Hashimoto M. Bilateral Optic Neuritis after COVID-19 mRNA Vaccination. Case Rep Ophthalmol 2022;13(2):578–83.

[22] García-Estrada C, Gómez-Figueroa E, Alban L, et al. Optic neuritis after COVID-19 vaccine application. Clin Exp Neuroimmunol 2022;13(2):72–4.

[23] Bhatti M.T., Gilbert A.L., Watson G., et al., Shot in the dark. Surv Ophthalmol. Available at: https://linkinghub.elsevier.com/retrieve/pii/S0039625722001230. Accessed June 11, 2022.

[24] Badeeb N., Torres C. and Albreiki D., Case of Bilateral Optic Neuritis With Positive Myelin Oligodendrocyte Glycoprotein Antibody Testing Post-COVID-19 Vaccination, J Neuro Ophthalmol, 2022, Available at: http://journals.lww.com/jneuro-ophthalmology. Accessed June 11, 2022.

[25] Donaldson LC, Margolin EA. Myelin Oligodendrocyte Glycoprotein Antibody-Mediated Optic Neuritis Following COVID-19 Vaccination. J Neuro Ophthalmol 2022; https://doi.org/10.1097/WNO.0000000000001482.

[26] Wang J, Huang S, Yu Z, et al. Unilateral optic neuritis after vaccination against the coronavirus disease: two case reports. Doc Ophthalmol 2022;145(1):65–70.

[27] Morena J, Gyang TV. Myelin Oligodendrocyte Glycoprotein Antibody-Associated Disease and Transverse Myelitis Probably Associated With SARS-CoV-2 mRNA Vaccines: Two Case Reports. Neurohospitalist 2022;12(3):536–40.

[28] Caliskan I, Bulus E, Afsar N, et al. A Case With New-onset Neuromyelitis Optica Spectrum Disorder Following COVID-19 mRNA BNT162b2 Vaccination. Neurol 2022;27(3):147–50.

[29] Shirah B, Mulla I, Aladdin Y. Optic Neuritis Following the BNT162b2 mRNA COVID-19 Vaccine in a Patient with Systemic Lupus Erythematosus Uncovering the Diagnosis of Neuromyelitis Optica Spectrum Disorders. Ocul Immunol Inflamm 2022;1–3, Taylor and Francis Ltd.

[30] Lecler A, Villeneuve D, Vignal C, et al. Increased rather than decreased incidence of giant-cell arteritis during the COVID-19 pandemic. Ann Rheum Dis 2021;80(6):e89.

[31] Szydełko-Paśko U, Przeździecka-Dołyk J, Kręcicka J, et al. Arteritic Anterior Ischemic Optic Neuropathy in the Course of Giant Cell Arteritis After COVID-19. American Journal of Case Reports 2022;23(1):e933471.

[32] Luther R, Skeoch S, Pauling JD, et al. Increased number of cases of giant cell arteritis and higher rates of ophthalmic involvement during the era of COVID-19. Rheumatol Adv Pract 2021;4(2):rkaa067.

[33] Mehta PK, Sebastian S, van der Geest SM, et al. Giant Cell Arteritis and COVID-19: Similarities and Discriminators. A Systematic Literature Review. J Rheumatol 2021;48(7):1053–9.

[34] Maleki A, Look-Why S, Manhapra A, et al. COVID-19 recombinant mRNA vaccines and serious ocular inflammatory side effects: Real or coincidence? J Ophthalmic Vis Res 2021;16(3):490–501.

[35] Xia C, Edwards R, Omidvar B. A Case of Giant Cell Arteritis With a Normal Erythrocyte Sedimentation Rate (ESR) Post ChAdOx1 nCoV-19 Vaccination. Cureus 2022;14(5): e25388.

[36] Che SA, Lee Y, Yoo YJ. Bilateral Ischemic Optic Neuropathy From Giant Cell Arteritis Following COVID-19 Vaccination. J Neuro Ophthalmol 2022; https://doi.org/10.1097/WNO.0000000000001570.

[37] Clarke KM, Riga V, Shirodkar AL, et al. Proning related bilateral anterior ischaemic optic neuropathy in a patient with COVID-19 related acute respiratory distress syndrome. BMC Ophthalmol 2021;21(1):276.

[38] Yüksel B, Bıçak F, Gümüş F, et al. Non-Arteritic Anterior Ischaemic Optic Neuropathy with Progressive Macular Ganglion Cell Atrophy due to COVID-19. Neuro Ophthalmol 2022;46(2):104–8.

[39] Sanoria A, Jain P, Arora R, et al. Bilateral sequential non-arteritic optic neuropathy post-COVID-19. Indian J Ophthalmol 2022 Feb 1;70(2):676–9.

[40] Sitaula S, Poudel A, Gajurel BP. Non-arteritic anterior ischemic optic neuropathy in COVID-19 infection – A case report. Am J Ophthalmol Case Rep 2022;27:101684.

[41] Babazadeh A, Barary M, Ebrahimpour S, et al. Non-arteritic anterior ischemic optic neuropathy as an atypical feature of COVID-19: A case report. J Fr Ophtalmol 2022;45: e171–3, Elsevier Masson s.r.l.

[42] Rho J, Dryden SC, McGuffey CD, et al. A Case of Non-Arteritic Anterior Ischemic Optic Neuropathy with COVID-19. Cureus 2020;12(12):e11950.

[43] Lin WY, Wang JJ, Lai CH. Non-Arteritic Anterior Ischemic Optic Neuropathy Following COVID-19 Vaccination. Vaccines (Basel) 2022;10(6):e5126254.

[44] Tsukii R, Kasuya Y, Makino S. Nonarteritic Anterior Ischemic Optic Neuropathy following COVID-19 Vaccination: Consequence or Coincidence. Case Rep Ophthalmol Med 2021;2021:1–4.

[45] Franco SV, Fonollosa A. Ischemic Optic Neuropathy After Administration of a SARS-CoV-2 Vaccine: A Report of 2 Cases. American Journal of Case Reports 2022;23(1):e935095.

[46] Elhusseiny AM, Sanders RN, Siddiqui MZ, et al. Non-arteritic Anterior Ischemic Optic Neuropathy with Macular Star following COVID-19 Vaccination. Ocul Immunol Inflamm 2022;30:1274–7, Taylor and Francis Ltd.

[47] Chung SA, Yeo S, Sohn SY. Nonarteritic Anterior Ischemic Optic Neuropathy Following COVID-19 Vaccination: A Case Report. Kor J Ophthalmol 2022;36:168–70, Korean Ophthalmological Society (KOS).

[48] Nachbor KM, Naravane AV, Adams OE, et al. Nonarteritic Anterior Ischemic Optic Neuropathy Associated With COVID-19 Vaccination. Available at: http://links.lww.com/WNO/A525. Accessed April 12, 2022.

[49] Silva MTT, Lima MA, Torezani G, et al. Isolated intracranial hypertension associated with COVID-19. Cephalalgia 2020;40(13):1452–8.

[50] Omari A, Kally P, Schimmel O, et al. Vision Loss Secondary to COVID-19 Associated Bilateral Cerebral Venous Sinus Thromboses. Ophthalmic Plast Reconstr Surg 2022;38(3): e65–7.

[51] Farahani AA, Shahali H. Intracranial Hypertension and Papilledema: An Unusual Complication After the Adenoviral DNA Vector–Based Coronavirus Disease 2019 Vaccination in an Air Medical Transportation Pilot. Air Med J 2022;41(6):560–5.

[52] Thunstedt DC, Straube A, Schöberl F. Isolated intracranial hypertension following COVID-19 vaccination: A case report. Cephalalgia Rep 2021;4.

[53] Jaiswal V, Nepal G, Dijamco P, et al. Cerebral Venous Sinus Thrombosis Following COVID-19 Vaccination: A Systematic Review. J Prim Care Community Health 2022;13:21501319221074450.

[54] Matar RH, Than CA, Nakanishi H, et al. Outcomes of patients with thromboembolic events following coronavirus disease 2019 AstraZeneca vaccination: a systematic review and meta-analysis. Blood Coagul Fibrinolysis 2022;33(2):90–112.

[55] Finsterer J, Scorza FA, Scorza CA, et al. COVID-19 associated cranial nerve neuropathy: A systematic review. Bosn J Basic Med Sci 2022;22:39–45, Association of Basic Medical Sciences of FBIH.

[56] Cicalese M.P., Ferrua F., Barzaghi F., et al., Third cranial nerve palsy in an 88-year-old man after SARS-CoV-2 mRNA vaccination: Change of injection site and type of vaccine resulted in an uneventful second dose with humoral immune response, BMJ Case Rep, 15 (2), 2022,e246485.

[57] Kerbage A, Haddad SF, Haddad F. Presumed oculomotor nerve palsy following COVID-19 vaccination. SAGE Open Med Case Rep 2022;10:2050313X221074454.

[58] Veisi A, Najafi M, Hassanpour K, et al. Facial and Abducens Nerve Palsies Following COVID-19 Vaccination: Report of Two Cases. Neuro Ophthalmol 2022;46(3):203–6.

[59] Pawar N, Ravindran M, Padmavathy S, et al. Acute abducens nerve palsy after COVID-19 vaccination in a young adult. Indian J Ophthalmol 2021;69(12):3764–6.

[60] Reyes-Capo DP, Stevens SM, Cavuoto KM. Acute abducens nerve palsy following COVID-19 vaccination. Journal of AAPOS 2021;25(5):302–3.

[61] Basnet K, Bhandari R, Basnet K, et al. Isolated abducens nerve palsy following AstraZeneca vaccine: A case report. Annals of Medicine and Surgery 2022;81:104434.

[62] Karam EZ, Ríos Macias P, Chahin G, et al. Inflammatory Sixth Nerve Palsy Post-COVID-19 Vaccination: Magnetic Resonance Imaging Findings. Neuro Ophthalmol 2022;46(5):314–8.

[63] Mahgerefteh JS, Oppenheimer AG, Kay MD. Binocular Horizontal Diplopia Following mRNA-1273 Vaccine. J Neuro Ophthalmol 2022; https://doi.org/10.1097/WNO.0000000000001545.

[64] Pappaterra MC, Rivera EJ, Oliver AL. Transient Oculomotor Palsy Following the Administration of the Messenger RNA-1273 Vaccine for SARS-CoV-2 Diplopia Following the COVID-19 Vaccine. J Neuro Ophthalmol 2023;43(1):e14–5.

[65] Manea MM, Dragoş D, Enache I, et al. Multiple cranial nerve palsies following COVID-19 vaccination—Case report. Acta Neurol Scand 2022;145:257–9, John Wiley and Sons Inc.

[66] Shalabi F, Lossos A, Karussis D. A case report of unilateral cervical lymphadenopathy and multiple cranial neuropathies following mRNA-COVID-19 vaccination. BMC Neurol 2022;22(1):369.

[67] Dinkin M, Sathi S. Efferent neuro-ophthalmic complications of coronavirus disease 2019. Curr Opin Ophthalmol 2022;33:471–84, Lippincott Williams and Wilkins.

[68] Li Z, Li X, Shen J, et al. Miller Fisher syndrome associated with COVID-19: an up-to-date systematic review. Environ Sci Pollut Res Int 2021;28(17):20939–44.

[69] Kuang W, Desai P, Voloshko A, et al. COVID-19-Associated Miller Fisher Syndrome With Long Latency Period: A Case Report. Cureus 2022;14(5):e24638.

[70] Guilmot A, Maldonado Slootjes S, Bissay V, et al. SARS-CoV-2-associated Guillain–Barré syndrome in four patients: what do we know about pathophysiology? Acta Neurol Belg 2022;122(3):703–7.

[71] Nanatsue K, Takahashi M, Itaya S, et al. A case of Miller Fisher syndrome with delayed onset peripheral facial nerve palsy after COVID-19 vaccination: a case report. BMC Neurol 2022;22(1):309.

[72] Dang YL, Bryson A. Miller-Fisher Syndrome and Guillain-Barre Syndrome overlap syndrome in a patient post Oxford-AstraZeneca SARS-CoV-2 vaccination. BMJ Case Rep 2021;14(11):e246701.

[73] Nishiguchi Y, Matsuyama H, Maeda K, et al. Miller Fisher syndrome following BNT162b2 mRNA coronavirus 2019 vaccination. BMC Neurol 2021;21(1):452.

[74] Yamakawa M, Nakahara K, Nakanishi T, et al. Miller Fisher Syndrome Following Vaccination against SARS-CoV-2. Internal Medicine 2022;61(7):1067–9.

[75] Siddiqi AR, Khan T, Tahir MJ, et al. Miller Fisher syndrome after COVID-19 vaccination: Case report and review of literature. Medicine (United States) 2022;101(20):e29333.

[76] Michaelson NM, Lam T, Malhotra A, et al. Miller Fisher Syndrome Presenting After a Second Dose of Pfizer-BioNTech Vaccination in a Patient With Resolved COVID-19_ A Case Report. J Clin Neuromuscl Dis 2021;23(2):113–5.

[77] Kim JE, Yoon BA, Kim YH, et al. Miller Fisher syndrome following COVID-19 vaccines: A scoping review. Acta Neurol Scand 2022;146(5):604–9.

[78] Abičić A, Adamec I, Habek M. Miller Fisher syndrome following Pfizer COVID-19 vaccine. Neurol Sci 2022;43(3):1495–7.

[79] Brossard-Barbosa N., Donaldson L., Margolin E., et al., Seropositive Ocular Myasthenia Gravis Developing Shortly After COVID-19 Infection: Report and Review of the Literature Clinical Correspondence, J Neuro Ophthalmol, 2022, Available at: http://links.lww. Accessed June 27, 2023.

[80] Essajee F, Lishman J, Solomons R, et al. Transient acetylcholine receptor-related myasthenia gravis, post multisystem inflammatory syndrome in children (MIS-C) temporally associated with COVID-19 infection. BMJ Case Rep 2021;14(8):e244102.

[81] Yavuz P, Demir OO, Ozsurekci Y, et al. New-Onset Ocular Myasthenia after Multisystem Inflammatory Syndrome in Children. J Pediatr 2022;245:213–6.

[82] Huber M, Rogozinski S, Puppe W, et al. Postinfectious Onset of Myasthenia Gravis in a COVID-19 Patient. Front Neurol 2020;11:576153.

[83] Sriwastava S, Tandon M, Kataria S, et al. New onset of ocular myasthenia gravis in a patient with COVID-19: a novel case report and literature review. J Neurol 2021;268: 2690–6, Springer Science and Business Media Deutschland GmbH.

[84] Patlolla R, Thepmankorn P, Heshmati K, et al. Myasthenia Gravis After SARS-CoV-2 Infection: A Cerner Real-World COVID-19 De-identified Dataset Analysis. Neurology 2021;96(15):4382.

[85] Fanella G, Baiata C, Candeloro E, et al. New-onset myasthenia gravis after mRNA SARS-CoV-2 vaccination: a case series. Neurol Sci 2022;43(10):5799–802.

[86] Ishizuchi K, Takizawa T, Sekiguchi K, et al. Flare of myasthenia gravis induced by COVID-19 vaccines. J Neurol Sci 2022;436:120225, Elsevier B.V.

[87] Ramdas S, Hum RM, Price A, et al. SARS-CoV-2 vaccination and new-onset myasthenia gravis: A report of 7 cases and review of the literature. Neuromuscul Disord 2022;32(10):785–9.

[88] Abicic A, Sitas B, Adamec I, et al. New-Onset Ocular Myasthenia Gravis After Booster Dose of COVID-19 Vaccine. Cureus 2022;14(7):e27213.

[89] Slavin E., Fitzig J., Neubert C., et al., New-Onset Myasthenia Gravis Confirmed by Electrodiagnostic Studies After a Third Dose of SARS-CoV-2 mRNA-1273 Vaccine, Am J Phys Med Rehabil, 101 (12), 2022, e176–e179, Available at: https://journals.lww.com/10.1097/PHM.0000000000002076. Accessed May 12, 2022.

[90] Kang MC, Park KA, Min JH, et al. Myasthenia gravis with ocular symptoms following a ChAdOx1 nCoV-19 vaccination: A case report. Am J Ophthalmol Case Rep 2022;27: 101620.

[91] Hoshina Y, Sowers C, Baker V. Myasthenia Gravis Presenting after Administration of the mRNA-1273 Vaccine. Eur J Case Rep Intern Med 2022;9(8):003439.

[92] Huang BD, Hsueh HW, Yang SH, et al. New-Onset Myasthenia Gravis After ChAdOx1 nCOV-19 Vaccine Inoculation. J Neuro Ophthalmol 2022; https://doi.org/10.1097/WNO.0000000000001548.

[93] Lee MA, Lee C, Park JH, et al. Early-Onset Myasthenia Gravis Following COVID-19 Vaccination. J Korean Med Sci 2022;37(7).

[94] Maher DI, Hogarty D, ben Artsi E. Acute onset ocular myasthenia gravis after vaccination with the Oxford-AstraZeneca COVID-19 vaccine. Orbit 2022;1–5.

[95] Jafarzadeh A, Nemati M, Jafarzadeh S, et al. Thyroid dysfunction following vaccination with COVID-19 vaccines: a basic review of the preliminary evidence. J Endocrinol Invest 2022;45:1835–63, Springer Science and Business Media Deutschland GmbH.

[96] Rubinstein TJ. Thyroid Eye Disease Following COVID-19 Vaccine in a Patient With a History Graves' Disease: A Case Report. Ophthalmic Plast Reconstr Surg 2021;37(6): e221-3.

[97] Park K, Fung S, Ting M, et al. Thyroid eye disease reactivation associated with COVID-19 vaccination. Taiwan J Ophthalmol 2022;12(1):93-6.

[98] Yucel Gencoglu A, Mangan MS. Orbital Inflammatory Pseudotumor following mRNA COVID-19 Vaccination. Ocul Immunol Inflamm 2022;1-4.

[99] Ordás CM, Villacieros-Álvarez J, Pastor-Vivas AI, et al. Concurrent tonic pupil and trochlear nerve palsy in COVID-19. J Neurovirol 2022;6:970-2.

[100] Gopal M, Ambika S, Padmalakshmi K. Tonic Pupil Following COVID-19. J Neuro Ophthalmol 2021;41(4):e764-6.

[101] Gönültaş EN, Gönültaş G, Can GD. Adie Pupil After BNT162b2 mRNA COVID-19 Vaccine. J Neuro Ophthalmol 2022; https://doi.org/10.1097/WNO.0000000000001670.

[102] Naor MS, Mathew PG, Sharon R. Transient Horner syndrome associated with COVID-19: A case report. eNeurologicalSci 2021;25:100349, Elsevier B.V.

[103] Peters J, Alhasan S, Vogels CBF, et al. MOG-associated encephalitis following SARS-COV-2 infection. Multiple Sclerosis and Related Disorders 2021;50:102857, Elsevier B.V.

[104] Lucchese G, Flöel A. Molecular mimicry between SARS-CoV-2 and respiratory pacemaker neurons. Autoimmun Rev 2020;19(7):102556, Elsevier B.V.

[105] Kahloun R, Abroug N, Ksiaa I, et al. Infectious optic neuropathies: a clinical update. Eye and Brain. Dove Medical Press Ltd.; 2015. p. 59-81.

[106] Kaya Tutar N, Kale N, Tugcu B. Adie-Holmes syndrome associated with COVID-19 infection: A case report. Indian J Ophthalmol 2021;69(3):773-4.

[107] Matschke J, Lütgehetmann M, Hagel C, et al. Neuropathology of patients with COVID-19 in Germany: a post-mortem case series. Lancet Neurol 2020;19(11):919-29.

[108] Riera-Marti N, Romani J, Calvet J. SARS-CoV-2 infection triggering a giant cell arteritis. Med Clin 2021;156(5):253-4.

[109] Zhou S, Jones-Lopez EC, Soneji DJ, et al. Myelin Oligodendrocyte Glycoprotein Antibody-Associated Optic Neuritis and Myelitis in COVID-19. J Neuro Ophthalmol 2020;40(3): 398-402.

[110] Dhont S, Derom E, van Braeckel E, et al. The pathophysiology of "happy" hypoxemia in COVID-19. Respir Res 2020;21(1):198, BioMed Central Ltd.

[111] Tang N, Li D, Wang X, et al. Abnormal coagulation parameters are associated with poor prognosis in patients with novel coronavirus pneumonia. J Thromb Haemostasis 2020;18(4):844-7.

[112] Nichani P, Micieli JA. Granuloma Annulare, Scalp Necrosis, and Ischemic Optic Neuropathy From Giant Cell Arteritis After Varicella-Zoster Virus Vaccination. J Neuro Ophthalmol 2021;41(2):e145-8.

[113] Stübgen JP. A literature review on optic neuritis following vaccination against virus infections. Autoimmun Rev 2013;12:990-7.

Cornea and External Diseases

ELSEVIER
MOSBY

Advances in Ophthalmology and Optometry 8 (2023) 299–312

ADVANCES IN OPHTHALMOLOGY AND OPTOMETRY

Diagnosis and Management of Ocular Surface Neoplasia

Tianyu Liu, MD*, Devin Cohen, MD, Sabhyta Sabharwal, MD

Scheie Eye Institute, University of Pennsylvania, 51 North 39th Street, Philadelphia, PA 19104, USA

Keywords
- Ocular surface squamous neoplasm • Conjunctival intraepithelial neoplasia
- Squamous cell carcinoma • Primary acquired melanosis • Conjunctival melanoma
- Conjunctival lymphoma

Key points
- Ocular surface neoplasms include ocular surface squamous neoplasms (OSSNs), melanocytic neoplasms, and lymphoproliferative neoplasms.
- Histopathology remains the gold standard for diagnosis of ocular surface neoplasms but novel imaging modalities including in vivo confocal microscopy, anterior segment optical coherence tomography, and ultrasound biomicroscopy may aid in diagnosis.
- Traditional treatment entails surgical excision for OSSN and conjunctival melanoma and radiotherapy or systemic chemotherapy for conjunctival lymphoma but adjuvant therapies including local chemotherapy, immunotherapy, targeted genetic therapies, and novel radiotherapy regimens may play an increasing role.

INTRODUCTION

Ocular tumors can develop in any structure of the eye, from the retina to the eyelid. The ocular surface, consisting of the cornea and conjunctiva, also is vulnerable to neoplastic growth. From benign nevi to conjunctival lymphoma and ocular surface squamous cell carcinomas (SCCs), a variety of neoplastic pathologic conditions can present on the ocular surface. Although relatively rare compared with other ocular tumors, ocular surface tumors require prompt recognition, given their potential associated morbidity and mortality. Ocular surface tumors may be more readily observed during routine eye examination given their superficial location, and their detection can shed light on the

*Corresponding author. E-mail address: tianyu.tom.liu@gmail.com

https://doi.org/10.1016/j.yaoo.2023.02.013
2452-1760/23/© 2023 Elsevier Inc. All rights reserved.

underlying immune status of some patients. Given the influence of ultraviolet (UV) light in the progression of many ocular surface tumors, the prevalence of these conditions varies geographically. Ocular surface tumors are commonly seen by comprehensive ophthalmologists, cornea specialists, or ocular oncologists. Every ophthalmologist should be prepared to recognize these tumors, which are often subtle in presentation.

In this review, we will cover the presentation and management of ocular surface squamous neoplasms (OSSNs), melanocytic neoplasms, and lymphoproliferative neoplasms while highlighting key advances in diagnostic modalities and treatment strategies.

SIGNIFICANCE AND IN-DEPTH ANALYSIS
Epithelial neoplasms
Epidemiology, clinical presentation, and histopathology
Affecting the eye's squamous epithelium, OSSNs include conjunctival intraepithelial neoplasia (CIN), corneal intraepithelial neoplasia, SCC, and its variant mucoepidermoid carcinoma. They are the most common nonpigmented malignancy of the ocular surface [1]. The incidence of OSSNs varies regionally, with an increased incidence of OSSNs among those living closer to the equator with greater UV radiation exposure [2,3]. Although the average age of occurrence of OSSNs is in the sixth decade of life, the age of onset is younger among those living within 30° of the equator [4].

In addition to UV exposure and age, other risk factors for OSSNs include ocular surface trauma, human immunodeficiency virus (HIV), human papillomavirus (HPV), hepatitis B and C, cigarette smoking, xeroderma pigmentosa, lightly pigmented hair and eyes, xerophthalmia (vitamin A deficiency), and exposure to petroleum products, arsenic, and beryllium [5,6]. Given the strong association between HIV and ocular surface tumors, HIV testing is recommended in patients aged younger than 50 years diagnosed with CIN [7].

Clinically, OSSNs can be isolated to the conjunctiva or rarely to the cornea but most commonly originate in the interpalpebral limbal zone, presenting initially as a unilateral, vascularized, gelatinous-appearing gray mass [4,8]. Some may develop overlying leukoplakia or corkscrew feeder vessels. CIN is the most common tumor of the ocular surface (Fig. 1) [7]. These lesions contain disorganized spindle and epidermoid cells; on pathology, a sharp transition occurs between healthy and dysplastic epithelium. CIN is graded similarly to gynecologic cancers, with CIN I, II, and III representing mild, moderate, and severe epithelial involvement and cellular atypia, respectively [5,6]. Conjunctival carcinoma in situ involves dysplasia spanning the entire epithelium. These lesions can be visualized with fluorescein, lissamine green, toluidine blue, methylene blue, or Rose Bengal staining [5].

Less common than conjunctival neoplasia, corneal epithelial neoplasia often results from adjacent dysplastic limbal spread, presenting with abnormal squamous epithelium that appears gray or frosted, often developing a fimbriated border appearance [5]. These lesions often are nourished by a neighboring

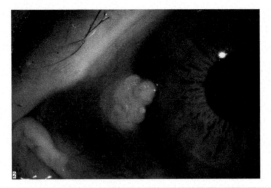

Fig. 1. Conjunctival intraepithelial neoplasia.

neoplastic pannus. The lesions can be noted on corneal retro-illumination during slit-lamp examination [9].

In comparison to corneal and conjunctival intraepithelial neoplasms, SCC invades the epithelial basement membrane. Often preceded by CIN and presenting similarly to CIN, SCC is the most common conjunctival malignancy (Fig. 2) [7]. SCC may rarely present bilaterally with a papillary and keratinized appearance, sometimes with an adjacent feeder vessel [6]. Mucoepidermoid carcinoma is an aggressive subtype of SCC, characterized by mucin-staining dysplastic squamous cells and neoplastic goblet cells. In comparison to CIN and SCC, which predominantly develop in the interpalpebral limbal zone, mucoepidermoid carcinoma can present anywhere on the ocular surface, with a relatively worse prognosis compared with other forms of OSSNs [6,8].

Diagnosis and treatment
Some patients with OSSNs may present with irritation of the ocular surface, a noticeable mass, large feeder vessels, or reduced visual acuity prompting examination. However, many patients remain asymptomatic from OSSN lesions,

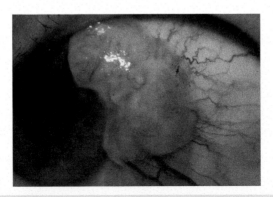

Fig. 2. Conjunctival squamous cell carcinoma.

which are detected incidentally during slit-lamp examination. Diagnosis depends on histopathology. Between exfoliative and impression cytology, which are both used, impression cytology is the more commonly used noninvasive procedure to biopsy the conjunctiva [5].

Treatment of OSSNs traditionally entailed surgical excision with a "no-touch" technique to avoid seeding tumor, with a standard goal of 2 to 4 mm of clean conjunctival margins. Corneal epitheliectomy is performed using absolute alcohol, followed by tumor resection and double freeze–thaw cycles of cryotherapy before wound closure. An increasing trend exists toward treatment with topical chemotherapies, which have been found to have comparable efficacy to surgical resection and cryotherapy, and will be described in detail in a later section [8].

Melanocytic neoplasms
Epidemiology, clinical presentation, and histopathology
Conjunctival melanocytic tumors include conjunctival nevi, complexion-related melanosis (CAM), primary acquired melanosis (PAM), and conjunctival melanoma. They constituted 52% of conjunctival tumors seen at a single large tertiary referral center [10].

Conjunctival nevi are the most common conjunctival melanocytic tumor [10]. They typically present in the first or second decade of life as slightly elevated, variably pigmented lesions located on the interpalpebral bulbar conjunctiva [11]. They predominantly are found in White patients with an equal or slight female-predominant gender distribution [12,13]. They can be pigmented, partially pigmented, or amelanotic (Fig. 3) [12,13]. They are located most frequently on the bulbar conjunctiva, caruncle, or plica semilunaris, and rarely in the fornix or palpebral conjunctiva [12,13]. Associated features include intralesional cysts, intrinsic vessels, and feeder vessels [12,13]. On histopathology, conjunctival nevi consist of nests of benign melanocytes and can be classified as junctional (in basal layer of epithelium), compound (in epithelium and subepithelium), or

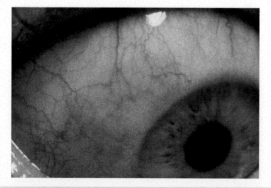

Fig. 3. Amelanotic conjunctival nevus.

subepithelial (in subepithelium only) [12,14]. Conjunctival nevi have a less than 1% risk of transformation into malignant melanoma [12,14].

CAM, also known as racial melanosis, is a benign conjunctival hyperpigmentation more commonly found in darkly pigmented individuals and presents early in life as bilateral, possibly asymmetric patchy flat pigmentation along the limbus that may extend onto the cornea or bulbar conjunctiva and may increase in size with age [10,11,15]. On histopathology, CAM consists of hyperpigmentation at the basal layer of epithelium usually without melanocytic proliferation [15]. No reported cases exist of CAM transforming into conjunctival melanoma but conjunctival melanoma rarely can develop in darkly pigmented individuals [15].

PAM is characterized by unilateral patchy flat noncystic pigmentation that typically develops in middle-aged lightly pigmented individuals and is the second most common conjunctival melanocytic tumor (Fig. 4) [10,11,15]. PAM presents primarily in White patients with a slight female predominance and most commonly is located on the bulbar conjunctiva, limbal conjunctiva, or cornea [16]. On histopathology, PAM consists of abnormal melanocytes near the basal layer of the epithelium with varying degrees of atypia based on nuclear features and growth pattern (Fig. 5) [11]. PAM without atypia has essentially no potential for malignant transformation, whereas PAM with atypia has a 13% to 46% risk of transformation into melanoma [16].

Conjunctival melanoma is a malignant proliferation of atypical melanocytes into the subepithelial space and represents the most common conjunctival malignancy (Fig. 6) [10]. The incidence of conjunctival melanoma seems to be increasing worldwide, including in the United States, Finland, and Sweden, potentially due to increased exposure to UV light [17]. Conjunctival melanoma can originate from PAM (53%–74%; Fig. 7), from conjunctival nevi (4%–7%), or de novo (19%–37%) [18]. It typically presents in White individuals in the fifth to sixth decades as a variably pigmented, elevated conjunctival lesion with possible vascularity [11,15]. Compared with PAM, melanoma more likely affects older individuals, is located on the tarsus; lacks pigmentation; be greater

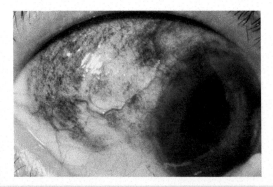

Fig. 4. Primary acquired melanosis.

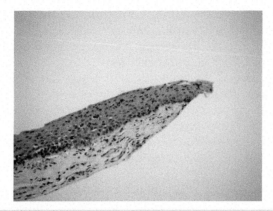

Fig. 5. Hematoxylin and eosin stain of primary acquired melanosis with mild atypia.

than 1-mm thick; and has feeder vessels, cysts, intrinsic vessels, or hemorrhage [10]. Conjunctival melanoma carries a risk of recurrence or new melanoma growth after excision, local invasion to the eyelid, orbit, or globe, and distant metastases most commonly to the lymph nodes, brain, lung, and liver, with a 5% to 13% risk of melanoma-related death [11,15,18,19].

Diagnosis and treatment
The diagnosis of conjunctival melanocytic tumors begins with careful external examination and slit-lamp biomicroscopy. Benign appearing lesions such as nevi, CAM, and limited PAM can be periodically observed and photographed. Suspicious appearing lesions should be sampled, ideally by excisional biopsy to reduce the risk of tumor seeding. The lesion should be completely excised using a no-touch technique, with double freeze–thaw cryotherapy applied to the

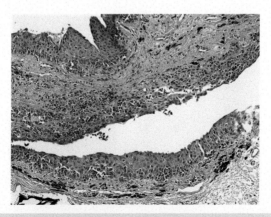

Fig. 6. Hematoxylin and eosin stain of primary acquired melanosis and conjunctival melanoma.

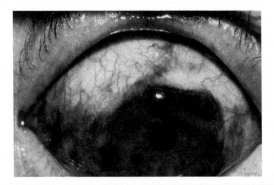

Fig. 7. Conjunctival melanoma originating from primary acquired melanosis.

remaining conjunctival margins. Incisional biopsy generally is avoided for melanocytic tumors, especially lesions concerning for melanoma, as incisional biopsy has been associated with increased risk of recurrence, metastasis, and death [19]. Extensive PAM occupying more than 3 clock hours of conjunctiva can be managed with incisional map biopsy of all 4 quadrants followed by double freeze–thaw cryotherapy to affected sites [11,15].

The gold standard treatment of conjunctival melanoma involves excision with wide (4–6 mm) margins using a no-touch technique, partial lamellar sclerectomy, absolute alcohol epitheliectomy for areas of corneal involvement, double freeze–thaw cryotherapy to the remaining conjunctival margins, and conjunctival closure with direct closure, conjunctival autograft, mucous membrane graft, or amniotic membrane transplantation [11,19]. This approach has not been studied in a randomized trial but it was shown in an observational study to be potentially important for preventing metastasis and death in univariate but not multivariate analysis [19]. Some authors advocate for a less-invasive surgical approach with smaller conjunctival margins and more judicious use of sclerectomy but evidence comparing different treatment approaches remains limited [20]. Lesions extending into the globe may require enucleation, and lesions extending into the orbit may require exenteration [11,15]. Patients at high risk of regional spread may benefit from sentinel lymph node biopsy, which has been shown to be positive in 11% to 17% of high-risk patients [20].

Lymphoproliferative neoplasms

Epidemiology, clinical presentation, and histopathology

Lymphomas are clonal proliferations of B-lymphocytes or T-lymphocytes, or less frequently natural killer cells. In the conjunctiva, they can occur as primary tumors or secondarily from systemic lymphoma. Conjunctival lymphoma, a subset of ocular adnexal lymphoma, is the third most prevalent primary malignancy of the ocular surface, although it only accounts for 5% to 10% of all extranodal lymphomas (Fig. 8). Exact triggers for its development remain poorly understood [21].

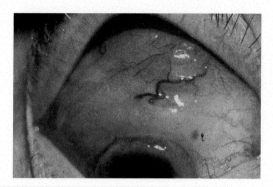

Fig. 8. Conjunctival lymphoma.

B-cell non-Hodgkin lymphomas (NHLs) account for the large majority (98%) of cases. The 4 major categories of B-cell NHLs are extranodal marginal zone lymphoma (EMZL, 81%), follicular lymphoma (FL, 8%), diffuse large B-cell lymphoma (DLBCL, 3%), and mantle cell lymphoma (MCL, 3%). EMZL and FL generally are considered low grade while DLBCL and MCL are considered high grade [22].

EMZL typically presents in patients in their late 60s with a slight female predominance. These neoplasms classically are preceded by a benign, chronic inflammatory process, and some postulate that they originate because of prolonged stimulation of B-lymphocytes from infectious antigens such as *Helicobacter pylori* or *Chlamydia psittaci*, although this remains controversial [22]. EMZL usually is unilateral and typically appears as a salmon-colored, fleshy, mobile, nonlobulated patch. Roughly half of cases occur in the fornix, with a significantly smaller percentage occurring in the bulbar conjunctiva and even fewer occurring in tarsal or limbal locations. One large review demonstrated that 92% of conjunctival EMZL were primary tumors [23]. Microscopically, common findings include heterogeneous aggregates of centrocytes, monocytoid cells, and small lymphocytes, often with intranuclear inclusions termed Dutcher bodies, and intact or disrupted reactive follicles in a subepithelial location [23].

FL also typically presents in patients in their late 60s. It most often occurs as a primary unilateral malignancy, which presents in the fornices or bulbar conjunctiva. It appears similarly to EMZL on examination with a salmon-pinkish color, although it typically is multinodular [24]. It is important to differentiate FL from reactive lymphoid hyperplasia (RLH), a benign condition, which can be indistinguishable clinically from FL. Histologically, RLH follicles are a polymorphic population of lymphocytes, dendritic cells, and tingible body macrophages that provide a classic "starry sky" appearance. In contrast, the follicles of FL are usually monomorphic, containing mostly centrocytes and occasional centroblasts [25].

DLBCL presents most frequently in men in their 70s. DLBCL also resembles EMZL but with a color closer to gray than salmon pink [24]. More aggressive tumors occur that often demonstrate rapid growth, ulceration, invasion of surrounding tissues, feeder vessels, and lymph node enlargement from regional spread [21]. DLBCL may develop de novo or transform from a less aggressive subtype, most commonly FL. A larger percentage of these tumors are secondary lymphomas than is seen with EMZL or FL, with one series showing up to 42% of patients having a secondary DLBCL [26]. Histologically, they are composed of large noncohesive cells with vesicular nuclei, multiple irregular eosinophilic nucleoli, and demonstrate diffusely disrupted architecture [27].

MCL presents approximately 5 times more frequently in men than in women. It is a high-grade lymphoma; more than half of patients have bilateral disease and 50% 90% of patients have systemic lymphoma at the time of diagnosis. Lesions often are large at presentation, with variable coloration, from salmon-pink to dark red [24]. Its cellular composition is similar to EMZL with a monomorphous B-cell population closely resembling centrocytes. Abnormal CD5 coexpression and cyclin D1 nuclear staining are 2 important markers to help differentiate these malignancies from EMZL [21].

Diagnosis and treatment
The diagnosis of conjunctival lymphoma includes a complete ophthalmic examination, as well as systemic examination if there is concern for a lymphoproliferative process. The gold standard for diagnosis remains incisional biopsy for histopathological and cytological examination [21].

External beam radiation therapy (EBRT) is the predominant treatment of choice when managing low-grade tumors such as EMZL and FL, with one study showing that 80% of patients remained progression-free and recurrence-free during a 5-year follow-up period [28]. Chemotherapy is the treatment of choice for high-grade tumors, and it has shown to eliminate approximately two-thirds of aggressive conjunctival lymphoma subtypes [24]. Chlorambucil is the most frequently used single-agent chemotherapy treatment; combination chemotherapy regimens include cyclophosphamide, vincristine, prednisolone and cyclophosphamide, hydroxydaunorubicin, vincristine, and prednisolone (CHOP), which often is used in conjunction with rituximab.

Complete excision with no other treatment may be considered in cases of well-encapsulated low-grade lesions. However, this treatment course has been associated with high-recurrence rates, likely due to tumor microinfiltration into the surrounding tissue, and has not been shown to impact survival rates [24]. Observation alone may be appropriate in some cases of low-grade, asymptomatic, unilateral tumors, especially in the elderly or those at high risk for treatment complications. However, one of the above treatment options typically is recommended to prevent progression [21].

CURRENT RELEVANCE AND FUTURE AVENUES TO INVESTIGATE
Noninvasive imaging modalities
Although histopathology remains the gold standard for diagnosis of ocular surface neoplasms, growing interest exists in using noninvasive imaging modalities

to aid in diagnosis. These modalities include in vivo confocal microscopy (IVCM), anterior segment optical coherence tomography (AS-OCT), and ultrasound biomicroscopy (UBM).

Epithelial neoplasms
AS-OCT can be used for cross-sectional evaluation of OSSNs to appreciate lesion depth, which represents an advantage over impression cytology. On AS-OCT, OSSN displays hyperreflective and thickened epithelium. IVCM is helpful in early diagnosis and monitoring treatment response. However, it is used less frequently than AS-OCT for OSSN because it is unable to provide the same detail of corneal layers in multiple views as OCT [5]. UBM can be a useful adjunctive diagnostic tool to assess possible deeper involvement of the tumor [29]. Finally, the advent of autofluorescence imaging in cancer imaging has exciting application potential in OSSN, with the ability to differentiate tumor cells from healthy cells [30]. Multispectral autofluorescence imaging is capable of precise tumor localization, which is particularly useful in delineating OSSN margins.

Melanocytic neoplasms
Studies on use of these novel imaging modalities for melanocytic conjunctival tumors remain limited, and none has been validated as a replacement for histopathologic diagnosis. IVCM, both stationary and handheld, have been shown to have 89% to 100% sensitivity and 74% to 100% specificity for diagnosing conjunctival melanoma, although in very small-scale studies [31,32]. AS-OCT may help differentiate nevi from melanoma due to the presence of intralesional cysts in nevi [33]. To date limited studies of UBM exist for conjunctival melanoma. One study of 3 cases of conjunctival melanoma found that UBM measurements of tumor thickness correlated with histopathologic tumor thickness [34].

Lymphoproliferative neoplasms
With AS-OCT, conjunctival lymphoma is characterized by an unaffected epithelial layer overlying a hyporeflective, homogenous subepithelial mass with smooth borders containing a monomorphic stippled pattern of hyporeflective dots likely corresponding to the infiltration of monoclonal lymphocytes on histopathology. AS-OCT cannot differentiate between benign RLH and lymphoma. AS-OCT may be helpful in monitoring lesion resolution or detecting residual disease after treatment [33]. Limited literature exists on the use of IVCM or UBM for the diagnosis of conjunctival lymphoma.

Evolving roles of adjuvant therapies
Epithelial neoplasms
The efficacy of topical chemotherapies including interferon-α2b (INF-α2b), mitomycin C (MMC), and 5-fluorouracil (5-FU) has been found to be comparable to surgical resection and cryotherapy for OSSN [8]. Subconjunctival and topical antivascular endothelial growth factor agents such as bevacizumab also have been found to decrease the size and vascularity of OSSN limited to the conjunctiva [35].

Recently, radiotherapy has been gaining traction as an adjuvant therapy for OSSN. Plaque brachytherapy offers targeted treatment while limiting radiation elsewhere. Early reports utilized strontium-90, which is notably limited in availability. Rao and colleagues [36] recently published their study of ruthenium-106, an accessible source of beta-radiation, as both an efficacious and safe adjuvant therapy for OSSN with stromal and/or scleral invasion.

Melanocytic neoplasms
Topical chemotherapy, including INF-α2b, MMC, and 5-FU, is used more often for epithelial malignancies such as SCC but also has been used for PAM and conjunctival melanoma in small case series with mixed results. These agents have limited penetration into the subepithelium and may be less effective for deeper disease [11,20].

Radiotherapy can be delivered as EBRT or plaque brachytherapy with strontium, ruthenium, or iodine [11,20]. No randomized controlled trials of adjuvant radiotherapy for conjunctival melanoma exist but case series report decreased rates of local recurrence [20].

Finally, a greater understanding of the genetic pathways underlying conjunctival melanoma biology has led to increasing interest in targeted therapies for conjunctival melanoma. B-Raf proto-oncogene serine/threonine-protein kinase (BRAF) and mitogen-activated protein kinase kinase (MEK) inhibitors, which target the Ras-Raf-MEK-ERK (MAPK) pathway, have been used in a limited number of cases for primary or metastatic conjunctival melanoma with varying results [37,38]. Furthermore, checkpoint inhibitors including ipilimumab, nivolumab, and pembrolizumab have been used as monotherapy and combination therapies for primary and metastatic conjunctival melanoma in a limited number of cases with promising early outcomes [37,38].

Lymphoproliferative neoplasms
Subconjunctival intralesional INF-α2b may aid in the treatment of lymphoproliferative ocular surface neoplasms by bolstering the immune response and amplifying the transcription of tumor suppressor gene p53, leading to apoptosis [39]. Intralesional rituximab has been studied for the treatment of conjunctival EMZL, with a lower response rate than EBRT but with potentially fewer adverse effects [40]. The addition of systemic rituximab has been shown to prolong event-free and progression-free survival compared with rituximab or chlorambucil monotherapy for EMZL in a randomized trial [41].

In recent years, "ultra-low dose" radiation therapy has been used for low-grade systemic lymphomas. This regimen consists of two 2-Gy fractions administered on 2 consecutive days, and it has shown promising results in small scale studies [42,43].

SUMMARY
An array of benign and malignant neoplasms can present on the ocular surface, and it is essential for the ophthalmic provider to appropriately evaluate, diagnose, and manage these lesions. Ocular surface neoplasms can be categorized

into squamous, melanocytic, and lymphoproliferative neoplasms, all of which encompass both benign and malignant conditions that must be accurately differentiated. Making the correct diagnosis begins with a thorough understanding of pertinent risk factors and requires performing a detailed ocular and systemic evaluation, especially early in the disease course when patients may not actively endorse any symptoms suggestive of malignancy. Novel imaging modalities including IVCM, AS-OCT, and UBM may play a growing role in the diagnosis of ocular surface neoplasms, although to date the gold standard for diagnosis remains histopathological evaluation.

The treatment paradigm for ocular surface neoplasms is shifting as well. Traditionally, the treatment of malignant OSSNs and conjunctival melanomas required surgical excision with cryotherapy to surgical margins, whereas the treatment of conjunctival lymphoma involved radiotherapy for low-grade lymphomas and chemotherapy for high-grade lymphomas. More recently, adjuvant therapies including local chemotherapy, immunotherapy, and novel radiotherapy regimens have shown promise in achieving comparable efficacy with less treatment-related morbidity. Furthermore, a growing understanding of the genetic mechanisms underlying various ocular surface neoplasms may lead to novel targeted therapies in the future.

CLINICS CARE POINTS

- Perform a careful ophthalmic and systemic examination when suspecting ocular surface neoplasm, especially if concern exists for metastasis or underlying systemic malignancy.
- Consider using imaging modalities such as IVCM, AS-OCT, or ultrasound biomicroscopy to aid in diagnosis.
- Consider using adjuvant therapies for the treatment of ocular surface neoplasms to reduce treatment-related morbidity.

DISCLOSURE

The authors have nothing to disclose.

References

[1] Cicinelli MV, Marchese A, Bandello F, et al. Clinical management of ocular surface squamous neoplasia: a review of the current evidence. Ophthalmol Ther 2018;7:247–62.
[2] Sun EC, Fears TR, Goedert JJ. Epidemiology of squamous cell conjunctival cancer. Cancer Epidemiol Biomarkers Prev 1997;6:73–7.
[3] Newton R. A review of the aetiology of squamous cell carcinoma of the conjunctiva. Br J Cancer 1996;74:1511–3.
[4] Basti S, Macsai MS. Ocular surface squamous neoplasia: a review. Cornea 2003;22:687–704.

[5] Gurnani B, Kaur K. Ocular surface squamous neoplasia. In: StatPearls. Treasure Island (FL: StatPearls Publishing; 2022. Available at: http://www.ncbi.nlm.nih.gov/books/NBK573 082/. Accessed November 30, 2022.

[6] Chang V, Bunya VY, Gurnani B. Ocular Surface Squamous Neoplasia, EyeWiki. (2022). Available at: https://eyewiki.aao.org/Ocular_Surface_Squamous_Neoplasia. Accessed November 30, 2022.

[7] Karp CL, Scott IU, Chang TS, et al. Conjunctival intraepithelial neoplasia. A possible marker for human immunodeficiency virus infection? Arch Ophthalmol 1996;114:257–61.

[8] Syed NA, Berry JL, Heegaard S, et al. 2022-2023 Basic and Clinical Science Course, Section 04: Ophthalmic Pathology and Intraocular Tumors, 2022. Available at: https://store.aao.org/2022-2023-basic-and-clinical-science-course-section-04-ophthalmic-pathology-and-intraocular-tumors.html. Accessed November 30, 2022.

[9] Bajracharya L, Sapkota J. An unusual presentation of corneal intraepithelial neoplasia: a case report. Nepal J Ophthalmol 2022;14:178–82.

[10] Shields CL, Alset AE, Boal NS, et al. Conjunctival tumors in 5002 cases. Comparative analysis of benign versus malignant counterparts. The 2016 James D. Allen Lecture. Am J Ophthalmol 2017;173:106–33.

[11] Shields CL, Shields JA. Tumors of the conjunctiva and cornea. Indian J Ophthalmol 2019;67:1930–48.

[12] Shields CL, Fasiuddin AF, Fasiudden A, et al. Conjunctival nevi: clinical features and natural course in 410 consecutive patients. Arch Ophthalmol 2004;122:167–75.

[13] Levecq L, De Potter P, Jamart J. Conjunctival nevi clinical features and therapeutic outcomes. Ophthalmology 2010;117:35–40.

[14] Gerner N, Nørregaard JC, Jensen OA, et al. Conjunctival naevi in Denmark 1960-1980. A 21-year follow-up study. Acta Ophthalmol Scand 1996;74:334–7.

[15] Oellers P, Karp CL. Management of pigmented conjunctival lesions. Ocul Surf 2012;10: 251–63.

[16] Shields JA, Shields CL, Mashayekhi A, et al. Primary acquired melanosis of the conjunctiva: experience with 311 eyes. Trans Am Ophthalmol Soc 2007;105:61–71 [discussion: 71-72].

[17] Triay E, Bergman L, Nilsson B, et al. Time trends in the incidence of conjunctival melanoma in Sweden. Br J Ophthalmol 2009;93:1524–8.

[18] Shields CL, Markowitz JS, Belinsky I, et al. Conjunctival melanoma: outcomes based on tumor origin in 382 consecutive cases. Ophthalmology 2011;118:389–95, e1–2.

[19] Shields CL, Shields JA, Gündüz K, et al. Conjunctival melanoma: risk factors for recurrence, exenteration, metastasis, and death in 150 consecutive patients. Arch Ophthalmol 2000;118:1497–507.

[20] Cohen VML, O'Day RF. Management issues in conjunctival tumours: conjunctival melanoma and primary acquired melanosis. Ophthalmol Ther 2019;8:501–10.

[21] McGrath LA, Ryan DA, Warrier SK, et al. Conjunctival lymphoma. Eye 2022;1–12; https://doi.org/10.1038/s41433-022-02176-2.

[22] Shields CL, Chien JL, Surakiatchanukul T, et al. Conjunctival tumors: review of clinical features, risks, biomarkers, and outcomes–The 2017 J. Donald M. Gass Lecture, Asia. Pac J Ophthalmol (Phila). 2017;6:109–20.

[23] Ferry JA, Fung CY, Zukerberg L, et al. Lymphoma of the ocular adnexa: a study of 353 cases. Am J Surg Pathol 2007;31:170–84.

[24] Kirkegaard MM, Coupland SE, Prause JU, et al. Malignant lymphoma of the conjunctiva. Surv Ophthalmol 2015;60:444–58.

[25] Stacy RC, Jakobiec FA, Schoenfield L, et al. Unifocal and multifocal reactive lymphoid hyperplasia vs follicular lymphoma of the ocular adnexa. Am J Ophthalmol 2010;150: 412–26.e1.

[26] Kirkegaard MM, Rasmussen PK, Coupland SE, et al. Conjunctival lymphoma–an international multicenter retrospective study. JAMA Ophthalmol 2016;134:406–14.

[27] Munch-Petersen HD, Rasmussen PK, Coupland SE, et al. Ocular adnexal diffuse large B-cell lymphoma: a multicenter international study. JAMA Ophthalmol 2015;133:165–73.

[28] Baldini L, Blini M, Guffanti A, et al. Treatment and prognosis in a series of primary extranodal lymphomas of the ocular adnexa. Ann Oncol 1998;9:779–81.

[29] Char DH, Kundert G, Bove R, et al. 20 MHz high frequency ultrasound assessment of scleral and intraocular conjunctival squamous cell carcinoma. Br J Ophthalmol 2002;86:632–5.

[30] Habibalahi A, Bala C, Allende A, et al. Novel automated non invasive detection of ocular surface squamous neoplasia using multispectral autofluorescence imaging. Ocul Surf 2019;17:540–50.

[31] Messmer EM, Mackert MJ, Zapp DM, et al. In vivo confocal microscopy of pigmented conjunctival tumors. Graefes Arch Clin Exp Ophthalmol 2006;244:1437–45.

[32] Cinotti E, Singer A, Labeille B, et al. Handheld in vivo reflectance confocal microscopy for the diagnosis of eyelid margin and conjunctival tumors. JAMA Ophthalmol 2017;135: 845–51.

[33] Nanji AA, Sayyad FE, Galor A, et al. High-resolution optical coherence tomography as an adjunctive tool in the diagnosis of corneal and conjunctival pathology. Ocul Surf 2015;13: 226–35.

[34] Ho VH, Prager TC, Diwan H, et al. Ultrasound biomicroscopy for estimation of tumor thickness for conjunctival melanoma. J Clin Ultrasound 2007;35:533–7.

[35] Faramarzi A, Feizi S. Subconjunctival bevacizumab injection for ocular surface squamous neoplasia. Cornea 2013;32:998–1001.

[36] Rao R, Honavar SG, Lahane S, et al. Histopathology-guided management of ocular surface squamous neoplasia with corneal stromal or scleral invasion using ruthenium-106 plaque brachytherapy. Br J Ophthalmol 2021; https://doi.org/10.1136/bjophthalmol-2021-319201 bjophthalmol-2021-319201.

[37] Brouwer NJ, Verdijk RM, Heegaard S, et al. Conjunctival melanoma: new insights in tumour genetics and immunology, leading to new therapeutic options. Prog Retin Eye Res 2022;86: 100971.

[38] Grimes JM, Shah NV, Samie FH, et al. Conjunctival melanoma: current treatments and future options. Am J Clin Dermatol 2020;21:371–81.

[39] Blasi MA, Tiberti AC, Valente P, et al. Intralesional interferon-α for conjunctival mucosa-associated lymphoid tissue lymphoma: long-term results. Ophthalmology 2012;119: 494–500.

[40] Demirci H, Ozgonul C, Diniz Grisolia AB, et al. Intralesional rituximab injection for low-grade conjunctival lymphoma management. Ophthalmology 2020;127:1270–3.

[41] Zucca E, Conconi A, Martinelli G, et al. Final results of the IELSG-19 randomized trial of mucosa-associated lymphoid tissue lymphoma: improved event-free and progression-free survival with rituximab plus chlorambucil versus either chlorambucil or rituximab monotherapy. J Clin Oncol 2017;35:1905–12.

[42] Fasola CE, Jones JC, Huang DD, et al. Low-dose radiation therapy (2 Gy × 2) in the treatment of orbital lymphoma. Int J Radiat Oncol Biol Phys 2013;86:930–5.

[43] Pinnix CC, Dabaja BS, Milgrom SA, et al. Ultra-low-dose radiotherapy for definitive management of ocular adnexal B-cell lymphoma. Head Neck 2017;39:1095–100.

Advances in Ophthalmology and Optometry 8 (2023) 313–328

ADVANCES IN OPHTHALMOLOGY AND OPTOMETRY

Approach to the Diagnosis and Management of the Cloudy Cornea in Neonates and Infants

Tomas Andersen, MD, MPH*, Vivian Qin, MD, Tejus Pradeep, MD

Scheie Eye Institute, Perelman School of Medicine, University of Pennsylvania, 51 North 39th Street, Philadelphia, PA 19104, USA

Keywords
- Cloudy cornea • Corneal clouding • Corneal opacification
- Neonatal and infantile corneal anomalies

Key points
- Treat corneal opacification to prevent amblyopia and vision loss.
- The differential diagnosis of causes is broad.
- Interventions range from observation to topical medications to surgery.
- Phenotyping and genotyping guide prognosis and treatment.

INTRODUCTION

Congenital corneal opacification represents loss of corneal clarity before 4 weeks of age [1]. These children are at risk of deprivation amblyopia and permanent visual impairment [1]. Some causes are furthermore associated with systemic disease with attendant morbidity and mortality [2]. Despite a low incidence of 2.2 to 3.11 per 100,000 births, congenital corneal opacification is devastating, and management is challenging [2].

One mnemonic for causes of corneal clouding is S.T.U.M.P.E.D., referring to sclerocornea, trauma, ulcer, metabolic, Peters anomaly, edema (endothelial dystrophy and glaucoma), and dermoid [3]. This mnemonic is useful, as it helps generate a differential diagnosis [3]. One limitation is that S.T.U.M.P.E.D. mixes causes such as trauma, metabolic errors, endothelial dystrophy, and dermoid with signs such as sclerocornea, ulcer, and Peters

*Corresponding author. E-mail address: Tomas.Andersen@pennmedicine.upenn.edu

https://doi.org/10.1016/j.yaoo.2023.02.014

anomaly [4]. Another limitation is that it does not provide an organizational framework for the diseases [5].

One classification system organizes these diseases as primary or congenital versus secondary or acquired [3]. Primary disease is subdivided based on localization to the cornea or association with systemic or metabolic disorders [3]. Secondary disease is subdivided into traumatic or nontraumatic causes [3]. This classification of the diseases offers a broader differential diagnosis and increased organization relative to S.T.U.M.P.E.D.

Another framework organizes the diseases as primary versus secondary [4–6]. Primary disease is always developmental and is subdivided into isolated corneal disease or corneal disease with systemic associations [4]. Secondary disease is either developmental or acquired [4]. All causes are classified as whether they improve with keratoplasty [4]. This system provides a better framework for characterizing diseases by phenotype, genotype, and therapeutic options [4–6]. This framework also emphasizes consistency and clarity with terminology such as sclerocornea and Peters anomaly [4–6].

With an understanding of these frameworks, the authors now review the specific diseases per the latter framework and discuss advances in the field.

SIGNIFICANCE/IN-DEPTH ANALYSIS
Primary disease
Congenital hereditary endothelial dystrophy
In congenital hereditary endothelial dystrophy (CHED), an autosomal recessive disease, patients harbor an SLC4A11 gene mutation, which codes for a transmembrane protein on corneal endothelial cells [7]. Patients present at birth with dense bilateral corneal haze and thickening, and histology shows diffuse edema with a thickened Descemet membrane (DM) [7] (Fig. 1). Treatment is primarily surgical [5]. Penetrating keratoplasty (PK) has demonstrated good outcomes. Recently, CHED was the commonest reason for Descemet stripping automated endothelial keratoplasty (DSAEK) in children [8–10].

Posterior polymorphous corneal dystrophy
Posterior polymorphous corneal dystrophy (PPCD) is autosomal dominant with locus heterogeneity and, rarely, can present at birth [5,7]. Histology shows a multilayered endothelium with epitheliumlike cells staining positively for cytokeratin. Clinical examination shows polymorphous endothelial opacities [5]. Treatment is primarily surgical [5]. Although Descemet membrane endothelial keratoplasty (DMEK) has been attempted without success, DSAEK has shown good outcomes [11]. Despite limited data, PK is thought to have good outcomes [5].

Congenital hereditary stromal dystrophy
Congenital hereditary stromal dystrophy is an extremely rare, autosomal dominant condition, caused by a mutation in the DCN (decorin) gene [7]. Patients present with diffuse, limbus-to-limbus corneal clouding, with whitish flakelike stromal opacities and a smooth normal epithelial surface [5].

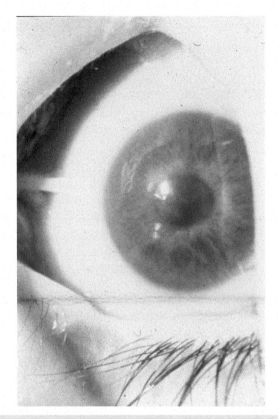

Fig. 1. Diffuse corneal clouding in CHED. (*Courtesy of* Stephen E. Orlin, MD, Philadelphia, PA.)

Treatment can be surgical, with deep anterior lamellar keratoplasty (DALK) having achieved good graft clarity [12].

X-linked endothelial dystrophy
X-linked endothelial dystrophy (XECD) is an extremely rare X-linked dominant condition, presenting at birth, due to an unknown gene [7]. Girls are asymptomatic with craterlike endothelial changes seen, whereas boys can show the same endothelial changes and a variable degree of clouding [7]. Despite limited reports, PK has shown good outcomes [5].

Isolated peripheral sclerocornea-cornea plana 1 and 2
Sclerocornea should refer exclusively to isolated peripheral sclerocornea with cornea plana (Fig. 2) [4]. In cornea plana 1, reduced corneal curvature, hyperopia, replacement of peripheral cornea with scleral tissue, and arcus senilis occur. No genetic cause is known [4]. Cornea plana 2 is due to KERA gene mutations and presents similarly to cornea plana 1 with the addition of variable central haze and iridocorneal adhesions that can cause angle closure [4].

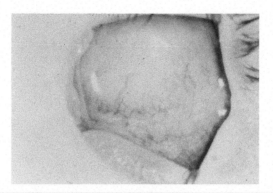

Fig. 2. Sclerocornea. (*Courtesy of* Stephen E. Orlin, MD, Philadelphia, PA.)

Sclerocornea is thought to be caused by defective neural crest cell migration between the corneal epithelium and endothelium [13]. In contrast to Peters anomaly, the central visual axis tends to be less involved than the periphery [14]. Cases tend to be bilateral, and approximately 50% are inherited with autosomal dominant more severe than recessive [14,15]. Management involves amblyopia treatment and corneal transplantation [14]. Successful PK has been reported, although it tends to be unfavorable with complications including corneoscleral adhesions [16].

Dermoid
Corneal dermoid is a congenital choristoma or histologically normal tissue located in an abnormal location (Fig. 3) [17]. Dermoids are classified as grade I (superficial, <5 mm), grade II (extension to DM), and grade III (cover the entirety of the cornea, extension into anterior chamber) [18]. Important systemic associations include Goldenhar syndrome and trisomy 8 [4].

Although benign, dermoids should be treated if they cause visual impairment, astigmatism, discomfort, or poor cosmesis [19]. For grade I and II

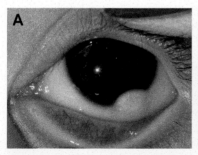
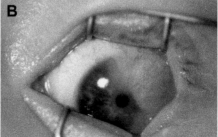

Fig. 3. (**A**) Inferotemporal limbal dermoid with hair growth. (**B**) Superotemporal limbal dermoid with vascularity. (*Courtesy of* Stephen E. Orlin, MD, Philadelphia, PA.)

dermoids, simple excision with or without lamellar sclerokeratoplasty has been effective [18,19]. For patients with dermoids extending into the anterior chamber, PK may be necessary [4]. Advances in surgical treatment include intraoperative optical coherence tomography (iOCT) [20] and femtosecond laser techniques [21]. As postoperative astigmatism after dermoid removal can induce amblyopia, patients must be followed-up postoperatively [4].

Microphthalmia with linear skin defects

Microphthalmia with linear skin defects, also called microcornea, dermal aplasia, and sclerocornea, is a rare X-linked dominant disorder [22,23]. The cornea seems keratinized [4]. The remainder of anterior segment development is often normal, but glaucoma is common [4].

Secondary disease

Peters anomaly. Peters anomaly is an anterior segment dysgenesis due to defective neural crest-derived cell migration causing posterior corneal defects, central corneal opacity, and variable kerato-irido-lenticular adhesions (Fig. 4) [24]. Fetal alcohol syndrome and mutations in PAX6, PITX2, and FOXC1 genes have been implicated [3,25].

Peters type 1 involves central corneal opacification often associated with iridocorneal adhesions, whereas Peters type 2 describes central corneal opacification associated with keratolenticular adhesions [24]. Peters-plus syndrome entails bilateral corneal opacification, height restriction, characteristic facies, and delayed development [26].

Anterior segment imaging advances have improved diagnostic accuracy, as high-resolution ultrasound biomicroscopy (UBM) and anterior segment OCT (asOCT) can evaluate for kerato-irido-lenticular adhesions obscured by corneal opacification [24]. Keratoplasty can help Peters type 1 but not Peters type 2 [4]. For patients at high risk of graft failure, keratoprosthesis may be pursued instead [27,28].

Congenital anterior staphyloma. Congenital anterior staphyloma is an uncommon anterior segment dysgenesis [29]. The cornea is ectatic with a protrusion of central opacified tissue (Fig. 5) [3]. Histologically, stromal thickening, vascularization, and fibrosis occur, and DM may be absent [3]. Patients tend not to do well with corneal transplantation [3].

Primary congenital glaucoma

Primary congenital glaucoma (PCG) is caused by dysgenesis of the iridotrabecular system [30]. Various genetic loci have been implicated, and inheritance patterns can be sporadic or autosomal recessive [31]. The commonest gene mutation is in *CYP1B1*, which produces a steroid metabolism protein important for trabecular meshwork development [31].

The classic symptomatic triad is photophobia, blepharospasm, and epiphora. Corneal findings are secondary to elevated intraocular pressure (IOP), which causes corneal edema as well as corneal stretching, resulting in buphthalmos,

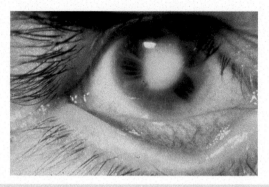

Fig. 4. Central leukoma in Peters anomaly. (*Courtesy of* Stephen E. Orlin, MD, Philadelphia, PA.)

enlarged corneal diameter, and horizontal breaks in DM called Haab striae (Fig. 6) [30].

Treatment of IOP elevation can clear corneal edema [5]. However, if IOP is left untreated, permanent stromal scarring can occur [5]. The definitive treatment is surgical, with adjuvant IOP-lowering medical treatment [31]. Surgical options include goniotomy, trabeculectomy, trabeculotomy, glaucoma drainage implant, and cyclophotocoagulation [31]. iOCT is one recent innovation [32]. Although goniotomy is an excellent option, it cannot be performed in patients with corneal opacification [31]. PK may be indicated for visually significant scarring [30].

Axenfeld-rieger syndrome
Axenfeld-Rieger syndrome also is associated with iridotrabecular dysgenesis [4]. It is associated with mutations in PITX2 or FOXC1 and tends to be autosomal dominant, although it may be sporadic [4,33]. Patients tend not to have

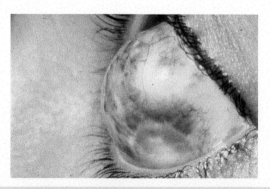

Fig. 5. Congenital anterior staphyloma. (*Courtesy of* Stephen E. Orlin, MD, Philadelphia, PA.)

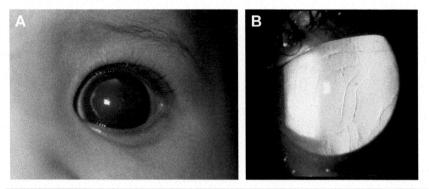

Fig. 6. (**A**) Buphthalmic eye in PCG. (**B**) Haab striae in PCG. (*Courtesy of* Stephen E. Orlin, MD, Philadelphia, PA.)

central corneal opacification but commonly have a posterior embryotoxon and iris strands adherent to an anteriorly displaced Schwalbe line (Fig. 7) [4]. Glaucoma is common, and management is similar to that of PCG [31,32].

Aniridia
Aniridia is a genetic condition featuring partial or complete absence of the iris (Fig. 8) [34]. It occurs in approximately 1.8 in 100,000 live births [35]. Isolated aniridia is most frequently due to PAX6 gene mutations [36]. Aniridia also may be associated with Wilms tumor [36]. The lens may become adherent to the cornea, causing a central corneal opacification [4]. Management may involve medical and surgical glaucoma care, cataract surgery, and/or keratoplasty [34,37,38].

Mucolipidosis IV
Mucolipidosis IV is the one metabolic syndrome that causes corneal clouding within a few weeks of birth [4,39]. It is extremely rare and is associated with systemic findings such as severe psychomotor disturbances sometimes requiring hospitalization [4,5,39].

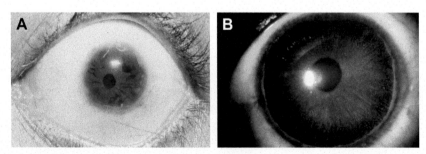

Fig. 7. (**A**) ARS with polycoria. (**B**) ARS with prominent embryotoxon. ARS, Axenfeld-Rieger syndrome. (*Courtesy of* Stephen E. Orlin, MD, Philadelphia, PA.)

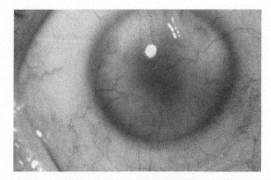

Fig. 8. Aniridia with pannus. (*Courtesy of* Stephen E. Orlin, MD, Philadelphia, PA.)

Mucopolysaccharidoses
The mucopolysaccharidoses comprise rare lysosomal storage disorders that cause ocular accumulation of glycosaminoglycans [40]. The glycosaminoglycans disrupt the regular distribution of collagen fibrils and cause a yellowish-grey appearance [40]. Although 13 subtypes of mucopolysaccharidoses exist, the 3 most relevant that cause corneal opacification are Hurler syndrome (by 6 months), Scheie syndrome (by 12–24 months), and Morquio syndrome (by 6 weeks) [3]. Patients require systemic therapies for their lysosomal storage disorders [41]. For corneal disease, DALK is the preferred surgical intervention, because glycosaminoglycan accumulation mostly is in the corneal stroma [2]. PK also has demonstrated success [2].

Cystinosis
In cystinosis, cystine crystals deposit in various body tissues [3]. It often presents in infants as Fanconi syndrome, characterized by failure to thrive, rickets, and renal failure [3]. When the eye is involved, peripheral anterior stromal corneal crystals are noted [3]. Systemic cysteamine may help nonocular crystals, whereas topical cysteamine can decrease corneal crystal burden [3].

Forceps- and amniocentesis-related injuries
Forceps injuries are associated with challenging labor and periorbital trauma [6,42]. Amniocentesis injuries may be mistaken for developmental causes. Approximately one-third of these patients have corneal edema at birth [6,43,44].

Forceps compression of the globe against the orbital roof causes horizontal corneal expansion and subsequent vertical or oblique DM folds and tears (Fig. 9) [45]. The left eye frequently is affected due to high rates of left occiput anterior presentation [46]. Type 1 forceps-related injury involves DM scroll formation at one edge of the break, type 2 represents scrolling at both edges, type 3 has a fibrous and retrocorneal membrane, and type 4 describes discontinuous DM with minimal fibrosis [46,47]. DM tears can progress to detachment or rupture [48,49].

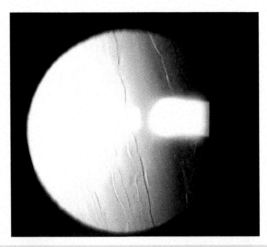

Fig. 9. Vertically oriented DM disruptions from birth trauma. (*Courtesy of* Stephen E. Orlin, MD, Philadelphia, PA.)

The natural history usually is biphasic [46,49]. First, corneal opacification occurs within a week of life and may spontaneously resolve, as the endothelium synthesizes thicker basement membrane covering the defect within the first 6 weeks, occasionally with permanent DM tears [46,49]. Second, endothelial decompensation may occur from age 25 to greater than 60 years [46,49]. Slit lamp diagnosis can be supported by asOCT, UBM, and in vivo confocal microscopy [45].

Cycloplegic refraction and patching are critical in addressing anisometropic amblyopia from myopic astigmatism [45,50]. Medical management with topical hyperosmotic agents and steroids may be beneficial [45,50]. Surgical intervention may include injection of air into the anterior chamber and corneal puncture to release viscous fluid [48]. DSAEK can help cases of late endothelial decompensation [49]. PK may be pursued for anterior stromal scarring [46].

Ulcer

Neonatal keratitis may present more subtly than infectious keratitis in older patients, therefore delaying diagnosis [51]. Yellow-white ulcer, discharge, and tearing are the commonest presenting signs [51]. The commonest microbial cause based on studies in tropical climates is bacterial, with pseudomonas and gram-positive organisms most frequently cultured [51]. Gonococcal, herpes simplex, and fungal causes also are common [51]. Prematurity, extended intensive care unit stay, vaginal delivery, maternal infection, and comorbid ocular malformations are risk factors [51]. Maintaining a high index of suspicion, obtaining cultures, and starting appropriate fortified antibiotics helps resolve most infections with resultant scar formation [51].

Entropion, in isolation or with dermatologic conditions such as ichthyosis, can cause corneal exposure and ulceration [52,53]. Corneal anesthesia and congenital insensitivity to pain with anhidrosis may lead to ulceration [54–56]. Neurotrophic keratopathy can be caused by hypoplasia of the trigeminal nuclei, Riley-Day syndrome, Moebius syndrome, Goldenhar syndrome, or focal brainstem pathology [54–56]. Treatment includes lubrication, bandage contact lenses, autologous serum tears, and cenegermin [54]. Surgical options include tarsorrhaphy, amniotic membrane grafts, and corneal neurotization [57–59].

RELEVANCE AND FUTURE AVENUES
Classification of disease
Past limitations
Historically, the lack of consistently used nomenclature has hindered advances in the field of neonatal and congenital corneal clouding [4]. For example, some investigators have used the term sclerocornea to describe isolated peripheral sclerocornea and cornea plana, whereas others have used the term generically to describe corneal opacification regardless of the underlying cause [4,60]. Similarly, some investigators have described cases of Peters anomaly without anterior segment imaging, confirming kerato-irido-lenticular adhesions [4,60].

Future improvements
The development of classification systems, however, allows for increased clarity regarding causes of pediatric corneal opacification [3,4]. Diseases once described by terms that have historically been vague or used with different meanings can now be more clearly categorized [4]. The overall goal of improved precision in nomenclature and classification is to know which patients will benefit most from medical or surgical interventions [4]. Future improvement within the field could involve consistency in categorization among the different classification systems. For example, in one classification system [3], metabolic causes are considered primary or congenital, whereas in another classification system they are deemed secondary and acquired [4]. Clarifying these inconsistencies among frameworks will further help the field.

Understanding of phenotype and genotype
Past limitations
Existing research in the field has sometimes lacked clarity regarding phenotype [4]. Investigators who studied clinicopathologic correlation of pediatric corneal opacification discovered that 2 in 5 clinical diagnoses were incorrect when evaluated with UBM [61]. For instance, cases that clinically seemed to be suitable to diagnose as sclerocornea actually demonstrated iridocorneal or keratolenticular adhesions by UBM [61]. In other cases, patients were diagnosed with Peters anomaly without sonographic or histologic confirmation [60]. It, therefore, is not surprising that the existing literature reveals contradictory phenotype-genotype correlations for cases clinically diagnosed as Peters anomaly without anterior segment imaging [4].

Future improvements
The pathway to accurate phenotyping and genotyping lies in advances in ancillary ophthalmic imaging to aid in accurate diagnosis [4]. The use of UBM, asOCT, and histology is essential in the complete evaluation of pediatric corneal opacification [4,6]. These imaging modalities can resolve ambiguity, for example in sclerocornea and Peters anomaly [4]. As future research within the field more definitively clarifies genotypes for specific phenotypes, gene therapy may eventually have a role. Just as CRISPR/Cas9 has preliminarily been studied in TGFB-1 corneal dystrophies [62], so too could it potentially be studied in the future in conditions such as PPCD.

Prospects for prognosis and treatment
Mainstays of treatment
Treatment modalities for pediatric corneal opacification are varied [4]. Approaches range from topical medications for infectious ulcers, to surgical excisions for dermoids, to PK and endothelial keratoplasty (EK), keratoprosthesis, and optical iridectomy for some cases of kerato-irido-lenticular adhesions [4]. In all cases, expedient evaluation is essential to determine the cause of corneal opacification, because the risks of delayed treatment are deprivation amblyopia and permanent vision loss [1]. Even after surgical intervention, close follow-up remains essential to monitor for postoperative astigmatism and graft survival [4,11].

Innovations and future directions in treatment
Intraoperative anterior segment imaging (iOCT) plays an increasingly important role in surgical management [20,63,64]. In cases with extensive corneal opacification, iOCT can guide surgical planning by revealing, for example, the presence of cataracts that could not be evaluated clinically [20]. During surgical dermoid excision, iOCT can help determine the depth of dermoid penetration into the cornea, sclera, and/or anterior chamber [20]. During surgery for a patient with corneal opacification due to mucopolysaccharidosis, for example, iOCT can help determine whether DALK can be pursued rather than a PK, thus avoiding risks of endothelial graft rejection and decreasing the risk of wound dehiscence [11,20]. In PK in cases with synechiae, iOCT can help visualize structures to avoid trauma to the iris during trephination [64]. It furthermore can provide real-time indication of graft-host override or underride to assure optimal transplantation during PK [64], as well as real-time assessment of endothelial graft position during EK [20]. In the future, iOCT will become more commonplace during surgery for these conditions.

Given that corneal transplantation carries the risk of graft rejection [20], future advances may involve interventions that do not rely on donor grafts [65]. For cases of neonatal and infantile corneal opacification due exclusively to endothelial dysfunction, future avenues of therapy may include human corneal endothelial cell (HCEC) injection [65]. Five-year data on coinjection of cultured HCECs and Rho-kinase inhibitors (ROCKi), which may aid in corneal endothelial cell repopulation, revealed outcomes on par with DSAEK and DMEK without the side effects of donor tissue [65,66]. In the future, coinjection of HCECs with ROCKi may play a role in caring for pediatric patients with such conditions as CHED, PPCD, and XECD.

Although innovations such as iOCT and future advances in HCEC injection and gene therapy will benefit patients in developed countries, the disproportionate burden of pediatric corneal opacification continues to exist in low-resource settings [67]. For every 70 corneas needed, there is only one cornea available [68]. A minority of countries have well-established eye banking systems [69]. In these low-resource settings where either donor tissue is unavailable or where graft follow-up cannot be assured, optical iridectomy remains a promising therapeutic modality [5]. In other scenarios where opacification is too extensive for optical iridectomy and/or corneal transplantation is neither available nor reasonable, surgical placement of a keratoprosthesis has many benefits [70]. Keratoprosthesis allows for a clear visual axis without the rejection risk associated with corneal transplantation, although life-long postoperative care is required [70].

SUMMARY

Neonatal and infantile corneal opacification occurs in the setting of a heterogeneous group of diseases [1]. Early detection and diagnosis are paramount, because these conditions can quickly lead to vision loss and amblyopia [1]. Even with appropriate and expedient treatment, patients must be monitored closely to ensure appropriate visual development and eye health [4,11]. In some cases, evaluation of corneal clouding can contribute to the diagnosis of systemic illness [2].

One of the most significant advances in the field of neonatal and infantile corneal opacification has been the development of classification systems for the implicated diseases [4–6]. Although the commonly accepted S.T.U.M.P.E.D. mnemonic generates an excellent initial differential diagnosis, other classification systems offer greater organizational structure [3,4]. The principal benefit of classifying the diseases accurately is that proper phenotype and genotype correlation ultimately helps determine appropriate therapeutic modalities to achieve the best possible outcomes [4]. The field will continue to benefit from further clarification of the existing classification systems, as one framework [3] describes metabolic diseases as primary or congenital, whereas another framework [4] categorizes them as secondary and acquired.

Advances in anterior segment ophthalmic imaging such as UBM and asOCT have had a profound impact on the field [4,20,63,64]. When Peters anomaly was first described over 100 years ago, such imaging modalities were unavailable [6]. As a result, Peters anomaly has commonly—and sometimes incorrectly—described a variety of phenotypic manifestations even without evidence of kerato-irido-lenticular adhesions [4]. Consequently, contradictory phenotypic and genotypic understanding of these diseases exist and, therefore, also a lack of clarity on the role of surgical intervention [4]. The trend toward including anterior segment imaging and histology in the diagnosis of Peters anomaly will help to define the various forms of kerato-irido-lenticular dysgenesis more precisely, and more specific genotyping for each possible phenotype will ultimately help contribute to future disease-specific therapies and treatments [4].

Treatments for these diseases will continue to benefit from such advances such as iOCT, which guides surgeons in real time, helping them to determine whether a DALK can be pursued rather than a PK, or whether a dermoid extends into the anterior chamber, or whether synechiae may complicate trephination during a PK, or whether there is graft override during a PK, or whether an endothelial graft is well positioned [20,64]. Future nonsurgical interventions may eventually potentially include HCEC and ROCKi injection for endothelial dysfunction and gene therapy for endothelial dystrophies. In low-resource settings where grafts are less available, optical iridectomy and keratoprosthesis may continue to play an important role.

In conclusion, the field of pediatric corneal opacification has advanced and will continue to advance through improved nomenclature, classification, imaging, phenotyping, genotyping, and therapeutics [4].

CLINICS CARE POINTS

- Careful ophthalmic history taking and examination are necessary to correctly diagnose corneal opacification in neonates and infants.
- Immediate diagnosis and management are necessary for imminently sight-threatening causes such as infectious keratitis and corneal ulceration.
- Other causes of corneal opacification also are time-sensitive, but care should be taken for thorough workup including UBM and asOCT when indicated to ensure optimal medical and surgical planning.
- Timely and disease-specific intervention is crucial for preventing loss of vision and in some cases loss of life.

DISCLOSURE

The authors have nothing to disclose.

References

[1] Karadag R, Rapuano CJ, Hammersmith KM, et al. Causes of congenital corneal opacities and their management in a tertiary care center. Arq Bras Oftalmol 2020;83(2):98–102.

[2] Nagpal R, Goyal RB, Priyadarshini K, et al. Mucopolysaccharidosis: a broad review. Indian J Ophthalmol 2022;70(7):2249–61.

[3] Katzman LR, Reiser BJ. Pediatric Corneal Opacities. American Academy of Ophthalmology. Published June 21, 2016. Available at: https://www.aao.org/disease-review/pediatric-corneal-opacities. Accessed December 28, 2022.

[4] Nischal KK. Genetics of congenital corneal opacification–impact on diagnosis and treatment. Cornea 2015;34(Suppl 10):S24–34.

[5] Nischal KK. A new approach to the classification of neonatal corneal opacities. Curr Opin Ophthalmol 2012;23(5):344–54.

[6] Nischal KK. Congenital corneal opacities - a surgical approach to nomenclature and classification. Eye (Lond) 2007;21(10):1326–37.

[7] Weiss JS, Møller HU, Aldave AJ, et al. IC3D classification of corneal dystrophies–edition 2. Cornea 2015;34(2):117–59, published correction appears in Cornea. 2015 Oct;34(10): e32] [published correction appears in Cornea. 2022 Dec 1;41(12):e23.

[8] Javadi MA, Baradaran-Rafii AR, Zamani M, et al. Penetrating keratoplasty in young children with congenital hereditary endothelial dystrophy. Cornea 2003;22(5):420–3.

[9] Medsinge A, Nischal KK. Paediatric keratoplasty: choices and conundrums. Br J Ophthalmol 2013;97(10):1225–7.

[10] Ashar JN, Ramappa M, Chaurasia S. Endothelial keratoplasty without Descemet's stripping in congenital hereditary endothelial dystrophy. J AAPOS 2013;17(1):22–4.

[11] Sharma N, Agarwal R, Jhanji V, et al. Lamellar keratoplasty in children. Surv Ophthalmol 2020;65(6):675–90.

[12] Kim JH, Ko JM, Lee I, et al. A novel mutation of the decorin gene identified in a Korean family with congenital hereditary stromal dystrophy. Cornea 2011;30(12):1473–7.

[13] Quiroz-Casian N, Chacon-Camacho OF, Barragan-Arevalo T, et al. Sclerocornea-microphthalmia-aphakia complex: description of two additional cases associated with novel FOXE3 mutations and review of the literature. Cornea 2018;37(9):1178–81.

[14] Binenbaum G, McDonald-McGinn DM, Zackai EH, et al. Sclerocornea associated with the chromosome 22q11.2 deletion syndrome. Am J Med Genet A 2008;146A(7):904–9.

[15] Harissi-Dagher M, Colby K. Anterior segment dysgenesis: peters anomaly and sclerocornea. Int Ophthalmol Clin 2008;48(2):35–42.

[16] Pohlmann D, Rossel M, Salchow DJ, et al. Outcome of a penetrating keratoplasty in a 3-month-old child with sclerocornea. GMS Ophthalmol Cases 2020;10:Doc35.

[17] Mohammad AE, Kroosh SS. Huge corneal dermoid in a well-formed eye: a case report and review of the literature. Orbit 2002;21(4):295–9.

[18] Yao Y, Zhang MZ, Jhanji V. Surgical management of limbal dermoids: 10-year review. Acta Ophthalmol 2017;95(6):e517–8.

[19] Promelle V, Lyons CJ. Management of limbal dermoids by simple excision in young children. J Pediatr Ophthalmol Strabismus 2021;58(3):196–201.

[20] Zaidman GW. Integrated intraoperative optical coherence tomography for pediatric lamellar corneal transplant surgery. Dev Ophthalmol 2021;61:1–7.

[21] Pant OP, Hao JL, Zhou DD, et al. Lamellar keratoplasty using femtosecond laser intrastromal lenticule for limbal dermoid: case report and literature review. J Int Med Res 2018;46(11): 4753–9.

[22] García-Rabasco A, De-Unamuno B, Martínez F, et al. Microphthalmia with linear skin defects syndrome. Pediatr Dermatol 2013;30(6):e230–1.

[23] Herwig MC, Loeffler KU, Gembruch U, et al. Anterior segment developmental anomalies in a 33-week-old fetus with MIDAS syndrome. Pediatr Dev Pathol 2014;17(6):491–5.

[24] Elbaz U, Strungaru H, Mireskandari K, et al. Long-term visual outcomes and clinical course of patients with peters anomaly. Cornea 2021;40(7):822–30.

[25] Bhandari R, Ferri S, Whittaker B, et al. Peters anomaly: review of the literature. Cornea 2011;30(8):939–44.

[26] Shah PR, Chauhan B, Chu CT, et al. Ocular phenotype of peters-plus syndrome. Cornea 2022;41(2):219–23.

[27] Botelho PJ, Congdon NG, Handa JT, et al. Keratoprosthesis in high-risk pediatric corneal transplantation: first 2 cases. Arch Ophthalmol 2006;124(9):1356–7.

[28] Aquavella JV, Gearinger MD, Akpek EK, et al. Pediatric keratoprosthesis. Ophthalmology 2007;114(5):989–94.

[29] Gupta DK, Mohan H, Sen DK. Congenital anterior staphyloma. J All India Ophthalmol Soc 1969;17(2):64–6.

[30] Thiagalingam S, Jakobiec FA, Chen T, et al. Corneal anomalies in newborn primary congenital glaucoma. J Pediatr Ophthalmol Strabismus 2009;46(4):241–4.

[31] Mocan MC, Mehta AA, Aref AA. Update in genetics and surgical management of primary congenital glaucoma. Turk J Ophthalmol 2019;49(6):347–55.

[32] Eldib A, Janczewski S, Nischal KK. Integrated intraoperative optical coherence tomography in pediatric glaucoma surgery. Dev Ophthalmol 2021;61:40–5.

[33] Alward WL. Axenfeld-Rieger syndrome in the age of molecular genetics. Am J Ophthalmol 2000;130(1):107–15.

[34] Hingorani M, Hanson I, van Heyningen V. Aniridia. Eur J Hum Genet 2012;20(10): 1011–7.

[35] Berlin HS, Ritch R. The treatment of glaucoma secondary aniridia. Mt Sinai J Med 1981;48(2):111–5.

[36] Grønskov K, Olsen JH, Sand A, et al. Population-based risk estimates of Wilms tumor in sporadic aniridia. A comprehensive mutation screening procedure of PAX6 identifies 80% of mutations in aniridia. Hum Genet 2001;109(1):11–8.

[37] Holland EJ, Djalilian AR, Schwartz GS. Management of aniridic keratopathy with keratolimbal allograft: a limbal stem cell transplantation technique. Ophthalmology 2003;110(1): 125–30.

[38] Reinhard T, Engelhardt S, Sundmacher R. Black diaphragm aniridia intraocular lens for congenital aniridia: long-term follow-up. J Cataract Refract Surg 2000;26(3):375–81.

[39] Dangel ME, Bremer DL, Rogers GL. Treatment of corneal opacification in mucolipidosis IV with conjunctival transplantation. Am J Ophthalmol 1985;99(2):137–41.

[40] Del Longo A, Piozzi E, Schweizer F. Ocular features in mucopolysaccharidosis: diagnosis and treatment. Ital J Pediatr 2018;44(Suppl 2):125.

[41] Williams IM, Pineda R, Neerukonda VK, et al. Mucopolysaccharidosis type I-associated corneal disease: a clinicopathologic study. Am J Ophthalmol 2021;231:39–47.

[42] Jain IS, Singh YP, Grupta SL, et al. Ocular hazards during birth. J Pediatr Ophthalmol Strabismus 1980;17(1):14–6.

[43] Merin S, Beyth Y. Uniocular congenital blindness as a complication of midtrimester amniocentesis. Am J Ophthalmol 1980;89(2):299–301.

[44] McAnena L, O'Keefe M, Kirwan C, et al. Forceps delivery-related ophthalmic injuries: a case series. J Pediatr Ophthalmol Strabismus 2015;52(6):355–9.

[45] Szaflik JP, Ołdak M, Kwiecień S, et al. Optical coherence tomography and in vivo confocal microscopy features of obstetric injury of the cornea. Cornea 2008;27(9):1070–3.

[46] Agarwal R, Singh NK, Sinha R, et al. Obstetrical forceps-induced Descemet membrane tears. Indian J Ophthalmol 2021;69(12):3432–41.

[47] Honig MA, Barraquer J, Perry HD, et al. Forceps and vacuum injuries to the cornea: histopathologic features of twelve cases and review of the literature. Cornea 1996;15(5): 463–72.

[48] Kancherla S, Shue A, Pathan MF, et al. Management of descemet membrane detachment after forceps birth injury. Cornea 2017;36(3):375–6.

[49] Scorcia V, Pietropaolo R, Carnevali A, et al. Results of descemet stripping automated endothelial keratoplasty for the treatment of late corneal decompensation secondary to obstetrical forceps trauma. Cornea 2016;35(3):305–7.

[50] Ganesh S, Arora P, Arora K. Descemet membrane breaks following forceps delivery. Indian Pediatr 2013;50(2):257.

[51] Chaurasia S, Ramappa M, Ashar J, et al. Neonatal infectious keratitis. Cornea 2014;33(7): 673–6.

[52] Redd TK, Kersten RC, Ashraf D, et al. Neonatal corneal ulcer secondary to congenital entropion. Am J Ophthalmol Case Rep 2022;25:101371.

[53] Vollmer L, Sowka J. Case report: corneal ulceration from bilateral ectropion due to congenital ichthyosis. Optom Vis Sci 2019;96(9):706–9.

[54] Scelfo C, Mantagos IS. Neurotrophic keratopathy in pediatric patients. Semin Ophthalmol 2021;36(4):289–95.

[55] Ohana M, Lipsker D, Chaigne D, et al. Unilateral ulceration of the cornea secondary to congenital trigeminal nerve agenesis. Eur J Ophthalmol 2015;25(4):e35–7.

[56] Charhi O, Saoudi Hassani S, Bendali I, et al. Chronic corneal ulcer in an infant secondary to congenital corneal anesthesia due to a neurovascular conflict. J Fr Ophtalmol 2019;42(4): e177–9.

[57] Bonini S, Rama P, Olzi D, et al. Neurotrophic keratitis. Eye 2003;17(8):989–95.

[58] Schuerch K, Baeriswyl A, Frueh BE, et al. Efficacy of amniotic membrane transplantation for the treatment of corneal ulcers. Cornea 2020;39(4):479–83.

[59] Terzis JK, Dryer MM, Bodner BI. Corneal neurotization: a novel solution to neurotrophic keratopathy. Plast Reconstr Surg 2009;123(1):112–20.

[60] Mataftsi A, Islam L, Kelberman D, et al. Chromosome abnormalities and the genetics of congenital corneal opacification. Mol Vis 2011;17:1624–40.

[61] Nischal KK, Naor J, Jay V, et al. Clinicopathological correlation of congenital corneal opacification using ultrasound biomicroscopy. Br J Ophthalmol 2002;86(1):62–9.

[62] Christie KA, Courtney DG, DeDionisio LA, et al. Towards personalised allele-specific CRISPR gene editing to treat autosomal dominant disorders. Sci Rep 2017;7(1):16174.

[63] Siebelmann S, Hermann M, Dietlein T, et al. Intraoperative optical coherence tomography in children with anterior segment anomalies. Ophthalmology 2015;122(12):2582–4.

[64] Titiyal JS, Kaur M, Falera R. Intraoperative optical coherence tomography in anterior segment surgeries. Indian J Ophthalmol 2017;65(2):116–21.

[65] Numa K, Imai K, Ueno M, et al. Five-year follow-up of first 11 patients undergoing injection of cultured corneal endothelial cells for corneal endothelial failure. Ophthalmology 2021;128(4):504–14.

[66] Schlötzer-Schrehardt U, Zenkel M, Strunz M, et al. Potential functional restoration of corneal endothelial cells in fuchs endothelial corneal dystrophy by ROCK inhibitor (Ripasudil). Am J Ophthalmol 2021;224:185–99.

[67] Maida JM, Mathers K, Alley CL. Pediatric ophthalmology in the developing world. Curr Opin Ophthalmol 2008;19(5):403–8.

[68] Gain P, Jullienne R, He Z, et al. Global survey of corneal transplantation and eye banking. JAMA Ophthalmol 2016;134(2):167–73.

[69] Córdoba A, Mejía LF, Mannis MJ, et al. Current global bioethical dilemmas in corneal transplantation. Cornea 2020;39(4):529–33.

[70] Nallasamy S, Colby K. Keratoprosthesis: procedure of choice for corneal opacities in children? Semin Ophthalmol 2010;25(5–6):244–8.

Advances in Ophthalmology and Optometry 8 (2023) 329–341

ADVANCES IN OPHTHALMOLOGY AND OPTOMETRY

Inborn Errors of Metabolism and Their Corneal Manifestations

Samantha Marek, MD*, Taylor Linaburg, MD, Brian J. Nguyen, MD

Scheie Eye Institute, University of Pennsylvania, 51 North 39th Street, Philadelphia, PA 19106, USA

Keywords
- Inborn errors of metabolism • Cornea • Metabolism

Key points
- Inborn errors of metabolism (IEM) can affect any metabolic pathway and may or may not lead to pathologic changes in the body.
- IEM are individually rare, but cumulatively can affect a significant portion of the population.
- IEM can affect any part of the eye, and many have specific corneal findings with variable impact on visual acuity.

INTRODUCTION

Inborn errors of metabolism (IEM) are a heterogeneous group of diseases characterized by disruption of metabolic pathways of carbohydrates, proteins, and fatty acids that lead to accumulation of byproducts that can be toxic to the body [1,2]. Although individually rare, the cumulative incidence has been shown to be upward of 1/2500 births [1]. Patients may present at any age with various systemic manifestations, depending on the type and severity of the enzyme deficiency. Ocular involvement of these conditions may manifest in any part of the eye, which may or may not be visually significant depending on the disorder. Here, we review those IEMs specifically with corneal involvement.

*Corresponding author. E-mail address: Samantha.Marek@pennmedicine.upenn.edu

https://doi.org/10.1016/j.yaoo.2023.02.015
2452-1760/23/

DISORDERS OF AMINO ACID, PROTEIN, AND MINERAL METABOLISM

Tyrosinemia

Tyrosinemia is a group of disorders that develops from inappropriate metabolism of tyrosine. Specifically, tyrosinemia type II is a deficiency in tyrosine aminotransferase leading to accumulation of tyrosine that causes cognitive impairment, painful hyperkeratotic lesions of palms and soles, and recurrent pseudodendritic keratitis or recurrent erosions [3,4]. Patients present with tearing, photophobia, and conjunctival injection. Chronic keratitis may lead to irreversible corneal scarring. Dietary restriction of tyrosine and phenylalanine can improve ocular and dermatologic symptoms as well as cognition.

Alkaptonuria

Alkaptonuria is an autosomal recessive deficiency in homogentisate 1,2-dioxygenase that leads to accumulation of homogentisic acid (HGA), tyrosine, and phenylalanine [4]. HGA accumulates in many parts of the body including kidneys, ear and joint cartilage, tendons, and sclera (Fig. 1A, B). One of the earliest signs of this disease is black urine that results from oxidization of HGA in urine when it hits air. The deposition of HGA in the eye leads to pigmentation of sclera, conjunctiva, limbus, and trabecular meshwork. Ocular pigment deposition can cause astigmatism as well as pigmentary glaucoma. Treatment is limited, but may consist of dietary restriction of tyrosine and phenylalanine in addition to enzyme replacement therapy.

Cystinosis

Cystinosis is a rare autosomal recessive disorder caused by mutations in the CTNS gene, which reduces transmembrane export of cystine in cell lysosomes, leading to accumulation and crystallization of cystine in tissue [5]. Systemic

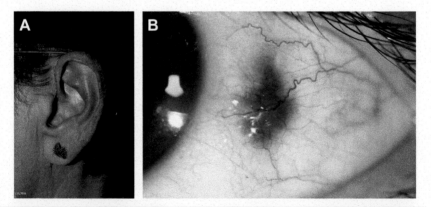

Fig. 1. (A) A photograph of a patient with alkaptonuria showing ochronosis of the ear. (B) A photograph of a patient with alkaptonuria showing ochronosis of the sclera. (*Courtesy of* Stephen E. Orlin, MD, Philadelphia, PA.)

findings include renal failure, hypothyroidism, diabetes mellitus, pulmonary dysfunction, male hypogonadism, and growth retardation [6]. Early ocular findings include visually significant anterior corneal stromal crystalline depositions that can lead to photophobia, epiphora, and secondary blepharospasm within the first year of life (Fig. 2) [5–7]. Later in life, patients may develop recurrent corneal erosions and crystal deposits in all areas of the eye including the conjunctiva, iris, ciliary body, choroid, fundus, and optic nerve [5,6]. Treatment consists of oral cysteamine, which binds cystine and allows it to exit the lysosome via the lysine transport enzyme [8]. Topical cystamine 0.44% eye drops may be used for corneal crystal formation as the oral formulation inadequately penetrates the cornea [5,8].

Wilson disease

Wilson disease is an autosomal recessive mutation of ATP7B, which leads to accumulation of copper in multiple organ systems, including liver, brain, and eyes [9]. Ocular involvement includes Kayser-Fleisher rings, a copper deposition in the Descemet membrane in the periphery of the cornea (Fig. 3), and sunflower cataracts [3,9]. Management of Wilson disease includes use of zinc to prevent copper absorption in the intestines as well as chelating agents such as penicillamine and trientine to remove excess copper from the body.

Gout

Gout is a disorder characterized by hyperuricemia leading to monosodium urate crystal deposition primarily in joints and tendons [10]. It classically is known for causing acute severe arthritis and joint nodules called tophi. Rarely, crystals can deposit in the eye and cause conjunctival or scleral inflammation, stromal nodules or tophi, corneal epithelial and stromal deposits, or band keratopathy. Management for acute inflammation includes use of indomethacin or colchicine. Long-term management may include allopurinol to reduce uric acid levels.

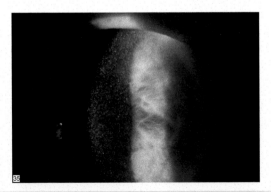

Fig. 2. A slit lamp photograph of a patient with cystinosis showing cystine crystal deposition in the cornea. (*Courtesy of* Stephen E. Orlin, MD, Philadelphia, PA.)

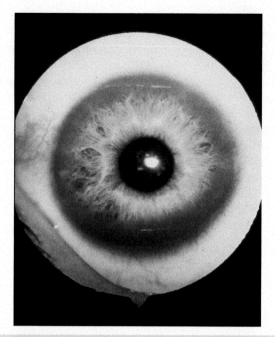

Fig. 3. Slit lamp photograph of a patient with Wilson disease demonstrating a prominent Kayser-Fleisher ring. (*Courtesy of* Stephen E. Orlin, MD, Philadelphia, PA.)

LYSOSOMAL STORAGE DISEASES
Mucopolysaccharidoses
Mucopolysaccharidosis Type I (MPS I) is an autosomal recessive condition caused by a deficiency of lysosomal hydrolase a-L-iduronidase, leading to accumulation of glycosaminoglycans including dermatan sulfate and heparan sulfate [11]. The disease spectrum includes the following disorders:

Hurler Syndrome (MPS IH) is a severe form of the disorder, presenting with systemic findings including a spinal "gibbus" deformity, persistent nasal discharge, middle ear effusions, frequent upper respiratory infections often leading to development of obstructive sleep apnea, coarse facial features, enlarged tongue, cognitive impairment, joint stiffness and contractures, and cardiac disease [11]. Well-described ocular findings include severe, visually-significant corneal clouding, and opacification (Fig. 4) as well as pigmentary retinopathy and optic nerve head swelling and atrophy [12–14].

Scheie syndrome (MPS IS) is considered the least severe form of the disease often diagnosed in adolescence, with systemic findings including hepatomegaly, joint contractures, and cardiac valve abnormalities [11]. Corneal findings include mild to moderate, often visually insignificant corneal clouding and opacification that rarely requires corneal transplantation until adulthood [15]. Other ocular findings have been described and include angle-closure glaucoma and pigmentary retinopathy [12,16].

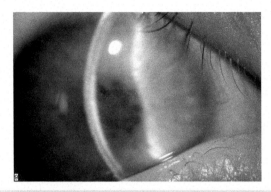

Fig. 4. A slit lamp photograph of a patient diagnosed with MPS I H demonstrating severe, visually-significant corneal clouding and opacification. (*Courtesy of* Stephen E. Orlin, MD, Philadelphia, PA.)

Hurler/Scheie syndrome (MPS IH/S) is considered a moderate form of the disease often diagnosed in childhood at approximately 6 to 7 years of age [11]. Systemic manifestations are variable, but can include joint stiffness and contractures, umbilical hernias, abnormal facies, hepatosplenomegaly, and cervical myelopathy. Ocular findings consist of moderate and diffuse corneal clouding and opacification, which sometimes can become visually significant [17]. Other ocular findings include chronic angle-closure glaucoma, open-angle glaucoma, and retinopathy [18].

Morquio Syndrome (MPS IV) historically was grouped into two autosomal recessive disorders that lead to the accumulation of glycosaminoglycans in the body; MVS IV A is caused by a deficiency of the enzyme *N*-acetyl-galactosamine-6-sulfatase, leading to accumulation of the glycosaminoglycans keratan sulfate and chondroitin sulfate MVS IV B is caused by a deficiency of the enzyme B-galactosidase leading to accumulation of the glycosaminoglycans keratan sulfate [11]. MPS IV B is now considered a variant of GM1-gangliosidosis. Systemic findings of MPS IV A include severe skeletal changes and growth retardation, cervical myelopathy, deafness, middle ear disease, restrictive respiratory disease, cardiac valve lesions, and hernias [11]. Corneal changes include development of mild corneal stromal opacities in 10% of patients, usually after 10 years of age [14]. Other ocular changes include pigmentary retinopathy and pseudoexophthalmos secondary to shallow orbits [19].

Maroteaux-Lamy Syndrome (MPS VI) is caused by an autosomal recessive deficiency of the enzyme *N*-acetylgalactosamine-4-sulfatase, leading to accumulation and deposition of the glycosaminoglycan dermatan sulfate [11]. Systemic findings include, but are not limited to, short stature with variable skeletal deformities, coarse facial features, hepatosplenomegaly, and hernias. Ocular findings consist of significant and progressive moderate corneal opacification associated with corneal edema, though the cornea may be clinically clear early in the disease process [20]. Other ocular findings include acute and chronic angle-closure and open-angle glaucoma, and optic nerve swelling and atrophy [13,14].

Sly syndrome (MPS VII) is caused by an autosomal recessive deficiency of b-glucuronidase leading to accumulation and deposition of glycosaminoglycans (GAGs) including dermatan, heparan and chondroitin sulfate [11]. Most patients with this disease have non-immune hydrops fetalis and often do not survive past birth. In those who do survive, they suffer from systemic manifestations including, but not limited to, middle ear disease and deafness, caries and dental abscesses, upper airway obstruction, obstructive sleep apnea, cardiopathy with valve lesions, hepatosplenomegaly, hernias, hydrocephalus, learning difficulties, and dysostosis multiplex. Ocular findings include mild–moderate corneal opacities as well as optic nerve head swelling and atrophy [13,21].

Treatment of the mucopolysaccharidoses

Systemic treatment of these disorders is largely supportive but may include enzyme replacement therapy and allogeneic bone marrow transplant; some regression of corneal clouding was seen in approximately one-third of patients following successful allogenic bone marrow transplant [11]. Gene transfer therapy is under investigation. Regarding the ocular manifestations, penetrating keratoplasty (PK) or deep anterior lamellar keratoplasty (DALK) can be considered for severe and visually-significant corneal opacities, though prognosis is guarded given possible re-accumulation of abnormal storage material in the graft. Visual potential also may be limited by retinal or optic nerve abnormalities.

Other forms of MPS disease occur that have either mild and visually insignificant corneal clouding or no corneal clouding, which we do not describe here. They include Hunter syndrome (MPS II), Sanfillipo syndrome (MPS III A, B, C, D), and hyaluronidase deficiency (MPS IX), and multiple sulfatase deficiency [11].

SPHINGOLIPIDOSES

Fabry disease

Fabry disease is an X-linked recessive defect of alpha-galactosidase A leading to ceramide trihexoside accumulation in lysosomes [22]. The primary organs affected are the renal and cardiovascular systems and may cause chronic kidney disease and hypertrophic cardiomyopathy, respectively. Other manifestations include angiokeratomas and aroparesthesia, or painful peripheral neuropathy. On slit lamp examination, whorl-like verticillata is often observed on the cornea, though it is not visually significant (Fig. 5). Other ocular manifestations include tortuous conjunctival and retinal vasculature, wedge or spoking posterior subcapsular cataracts, periorbital edema, macular edema, and optic atrophy, which may be visually significant. Management includes recombinant alpha-galactosidase A infusions and chaperone therapy, which binds to defective enzymes and shifts them to fold into functional conformations.

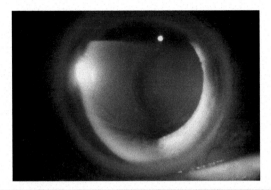

Fig. 5. Slit lamp photograph demonstrating corneal verticillata in a patient with Fabry disease. (*Courtesy of* Stephen E. Orlin, MD, Philadelphia, PA.)

Gaucher disease

Gaucher disease is an autosomal recessive disorder caused by a mutation in the gene GBA1 with subsequent deficiency of the lysosomal protein glucocerebrosidase, leading to accumulation of enzyme's metabolites, primarily glucosylceramide, and glucosylspingosine [23,24]. Three forms of the disease occur. Type I is the most common and considered non-neuronopathic; Types II, III, and IIIc manifest earlier and have neurological sequelae secondary to markedly reduced enzyme activity. In terms of ocular involvement, all subtypes have been found to be associated with functional or structural ocular abnormalities, though it is rarely sight-threatening. Regarding corneal involvement, patients can develop mild corneal clouding and calcification. Patients also can develop pingueculas of the conjunctiva. Genotype–phenotype correlations are inconsistent in Gaucher disease with the exception of a specific mutation D409H, which is associated with the unique Type-IIIc neuronopathic phenotype, however, it is not associated with Gaucher cell presence, so the accumulated material found in the cornea may represent aggregated glucosylceramide in keratocytes that has been trafficked between ocular tissues. Some but not all manifestations are amenable to treatment, which is overall limited, but can include enzyme replacement and substrate reduction therapy.

Niemann-Pick disease

Niemann-Pick disease is an autosomal recessive disorder caused by mutation in the SMPD1 gene with subsequent deficiency of sphingomyelinase leading to accumulation of sphingomyelin and cholesterol in the brain, abdominal viscera, and other tissues throughout the body [25]. Two types exist. Type A, the more severe form with earlier onset, which manifests as irritability, failure to thrive, hepatosplenomegaly, hypotonia, and pulmonary infections, and Type B, the less severe form with later onset, which manifests as hepatosplenomegaly, pulmonary infections, and hyperlipidemia. In terms of ocular findings, patients can present with subtly progressive corneal stromal haze, brownish discoloration of the anterior surface of the lens, and white spots on the posterior lens capsule, which are thought to be secondary to sphingolipid storage in the corneal stroma, corneal endothelium, and lens epithelium, respectively [26]. Patients also may have retinal opacification with a macular cherry-red spot, as well as nystagmus. Treatment of this disorder often is supportive, but enzyme replacement trials are underway. Currently, patients often have a poor life expectancy and poor visual prognosis [25].

GM1 gangliosidosis

GM1 gangliosidosis is an autosomal recessive defect of beta-galactosidase leading to accumulation of GM1 gangliosides in lysosomes [27,28]. This accumulation leads to a broad systemic presentation including developmental delay, hypotonia, cardiomyopathy, hepatosplenomegaly, and skeletal abnormalities. The GM1 gangliosides also deposit into the corneal epithelium and manifest as a mild corneal haze. Additionally, ophthalmic examination may reveal esotropia, nystagmus, cherry-red spot, retinal hemorrhage, and optic atrophy. There is currently no treatment, and management is palliative.

GM2 gangliosidosis

This group includes Tay Sachs disease and Sandhoff disease, which have ocular involvement, but they do not have significant corneal involvement, and as such will not be outlined here.

DISORDERS OF LIPID METABOLISM

Hyperlipoproteinemias

Type I–hyperchylomicronemia

Hyperchylomicronemia is an autosomal recessive disorder caused by a defect of lipoprotein lipase resulting in the reduction of chylomicron and triglyceride clearance from plasma [29]. The accumulation of the chylomicrons and triglycerides in the serum cause acute pancreatitis and hepatosplenomegaly and deposit in the skin as xanthomas. Given elevated levels of lipids, the cornea may develop arcus [30]. Lipid deposition can further cause lipemia retinalis and adult-onset Coats' disease. Management is achieved through dietary modification.

Type II–hyperbetalipoproteinemia

Hyperbetalipoproteinemia is a relatively common polygenic process most typically involving a mutation in the low-density lipoprotein (LDL) receptor [31]. Affected persons have increased serum LDL and very low-density lipoprotein (VLDL), which may cause varying degrees of early atherosclerotic disease and xanthelasma deposition. Early corneal arcus may be seen, which is not visually significant [30]. Milder heterozygous forms may be treated medically with lipid-lowering mediations, whereas severe homozygous forms are treated with adjunctive therapies including inhibitors of microsomal triglyceride transfer protein, apolipoprotein B, and angiopoietin-like protein 3.

Type III–familial dysbetalipoproteinemia
Dysbetalipoproteinemia is an autosomal recessive disorder of apolipoprotein E leading to increased serum VLDL, chylomicrons, and triglycerides [32]. This alteration in serum lipids leads to early atherosclerotic disease and cutaneous xanthoma formation. In the eye, these lipids may manifest as early corneal arcus and lipemia retinalis [30]. Management is accomplished through a combination of lifestyle modifications and lipid-lowering therapy.

Type IV–hyperbetalipoproteinemia
Hyperbetalipoproteinemia is a polygenic disorder leading to accumulation of VLDL and pre-beta lipoproteins [33]. This systemic elevation may induce acute pancreatitis, cholelithiasis, early atherosclerotic disease, hyperuricemia, and xanthomatous depositions. Ocular manifestation includes not visually-significant corneal arcus [30]. Like many other lipid disorders, management includes both lifestyle modifications and lipid-lowering therapy.

Type V–hyperprebetalipoproteinemia and hyperchylomicronemia
Type V hyperlipoproteinemia is a polygenic disorder leading to increases in VLDL and chylomicrons that may cause acute pancreatitis, hepatosplenomegaly, and xanthomas [34]. The cornea may develop asymptomatic early arcus and lipemia retinalis which may affect vision [30]. Management includes lifestyle modifications and lipid-lowering therapy.

Schnyder corneal dystrophy
Schnyder corneal dystrophy usually is categorized as a corneal dystrophy. It represents an autosomal recessive defect in the UBIAD1 gene localized to the cornea [35]. Unesterified and esterified cholesterol and phospholipids are deposited into the epithelium, Bowman's membrane, and anterior stroma. This progressive opacification begins in the first decade as central corneal crystal deposition followed by eventual arcus and mid-peripheral haze (Fig. 6). Other findings include reduced corneal sensation and systemic hypercholesterolemia

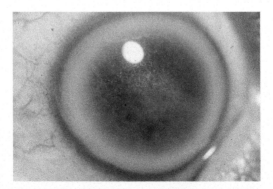

Fig. 6. A slit lamp photograph depicting arcus and mid-peripheral haze in a patient with Schnyder corneal dystrophy. (*Courtesy of* Stephen E. Orlin, MD, Philadelphia, PA.)

and genu valgum. PK, DALK, or phototherapeutic keratectomy may be performed, but recurrence may occur.

Hypolipoproteinemias

Hypolipoproteinemias are a heterogenous group of disorders comprised of five disorders including lecithin-cholesterol acyltransferase (LCAT) deficiency, fish eye disease, Tangier disease, familial hypobetalipoproteinemia, and Bassen-Kornzweig syndrome. Only the first three result in corneal disease.

Lecithin-cholesterol acyltransferase (LCAT) deficiency

Lecithin-cholesterol acyltransferase (LCAT) deficiency is an autosomal recessive disorder of the LCAT enzyme leading to a defect in the formation of unesterified cholesterol from cholesterol, leading to deposition in peripheral tissues [36]. Systemic manifestations include atherosclerosis, kidney disease, and anemia. Corneal examination may reveal arcus, nebular stromal haze, and crocodile shagreen, though none of these are visually significant. Additionally, fundus findings may include angioid streaks, vascular dilation, and peripapillary hemorrhage. No treatment exists, and management is supportive.

Fish eye disease

Fish eye disease is an allelic variant of LCAT disease with normal LCAT levels, but with functional loss leading to increased VLDL and triglycerides [37]. Minimal systemic findings occur, and the most prominent manifestation is an early progressive diffuse corneal clouding of all layers, sparing the epithelium. Though visual acuity typically is preserved, contrast sensitivity may be reduced.

Tangier disease

Tangier disease is an autosomal recessive mutation of the ABCA1 gene resulting in very low high-density lipoproteins leading to accumulation of cholesterol and phospholipids within cells [38]. This may lead to characteristic orange tonsils, hepatosplenomegaly, lymphadenopathy, and peripheral neuropathy. The cornea may develop late central stromal clouding with posterior stromal opacities, though this is not visually significant. Other ocular findings include retinal pigment epithelium mottling, exposure keratopathy, and lagophthalmos. No treatment currently exists, and management is mainly supportive.

MISCELLANEOUS

Zellweger spectrum

The Zellweger spectrum is an autosomal recessive spectrum of syndromes of varying severity united by a defect in the PXE gene. This affects peroxisomal biogenesis and biochemical functions, affecting multiple downstream pathways including lipid metabolism [39]. The least severe form is infantile Refsum disease followed by neonatal adrenoleukodystrophy and finally the most severe Zellweger syndrome. Systemic manifestations vary in severity and include developmental delay, hypotonia, seizures, sensorineural deafness, hepatic dysfunction, adrenocortical dysfunction, and renal defects. Multiple corneal manifestations include diffuse corneal edema, iridocorneal adhesion, attenuation of the Descemet membrane, band keratopathy, and enlarged corneal nerves. Beyond the cornea, patients may have pigmentary retinopathy, optic atrophy, cataract, nystagmus, microphthalmia, hypoplastic supraorbital ridges, epicanthal folds, and hypertelorism. Prognosis is very poor, and most patients pass within 1 year of birth. Management is supportive.

SUMMARY

Here we have reviewed IEM that specifically affect the cornea. The dysfunction of metabolic pathways and subsequent substrate accumulation can affect any system of the body, depending on the disorder. The spectrum of disease of IEM is even vaster than what is outlined here, but many do not have ocular, and more specifically, corneal involvement. It is important to be familiar with these various diseases because as a collective group, they are not uncommon in the population.

CLINICS CARE POINTS

- When seeing a patient with an inborn error of metabolism, eye examination may reveal various corneal pathologies.
- When seeing a new corneal finding in a patient, consider the inborn error of metabolism on the differential diagnosis.

DISCLOSURE

The authors have nothing to disclose.

References

[1] Jeanmonod R, Asuka E, Jeanmonod D. Inborn errors of metabolism. Treasure Island (FL): StatPearls Publishing; 2022 [Updated 2022 Jul 18]. In: StatPearls [Internet].

[2] Ferreira CR, van Karnebeek CDM. Inborn errors of metabolism. Handb Clin Neurol 2019;162:449–81.

[3] Davison J. Eye involvement in inherited metabolic disorders. Therapeutic Advances in Ophthalmology 2020;12:1–20.

[4] Moshirfar M, Kuang GT, Ronquillo Y. Ocular manifestations of Alkaptonuria. Treasure Island (FL): StatPearls Publishing; 2022 [Updated 2022 Aug 22]. In: StatPearls [Internet].

[5] Naik MP, Sethi HS, Dabas S. Ocular cystinosis: rarity redefined. Indian J Ophthalmol 2019;67(7):1158–9.

[6] Baker DR, Thavikulwat AT, Magone MT. The sparkle in her eye: crystal deposits in cornea, conjunctiva, meibombian glands, and iris in uncontrolled cystinosis. Am J Ophthalmol Case Rep 2021;23:101169.

[7] Tsilou E, Zhou M, Gahl W, et al. Ophthalmic manifestations and histopathology of infantile nephropathic cystinosis: report of a case and review of the literature. Surv Ophthalmol 2007;52(1):97–105.

[8] Tsilou ET, Rubin BI, Reed G, et al. Nephropathic cystinosis: posterior segment manifestations and effects of cysteamine therapy. Ophthalmology 2006;113(6):1002–9.

[9] National institute of diabetes and digestive and kidney diseases. Wilson disease. 2018. Available at: https://www.niddk.nih.gov/health-information/liver-disease/wilson-disease/all-content. Accessed November 13, 2022.

[10] Ao J, Goldblatt F, Casson RJ. Review of the ophthalmic manifestations of gout and uric acid crystal deposition. Clin Experiment Ophthalmol 2017;45:73–80.

[11] Ashworth JL, Biswas S, Wraith E, et al. Mucopolysaccharidoses and the eye. Surv Ophthalmol 2006;51(1):1–17.

[12] Caruso RC, Kaiser-Kupfer MI, Muenzer J, et al. Electroretinographic findings in the mucopolysaccharidoses. Ophthalmology 1986;93(12):1612–6.

[13] Collins ML, Traboulsi EI, Maumenee IH. Optic nerve head swelling and optic atrophy in the systemic mucopolysaccharidoses. Ophthalmology 1990;97(11):1445–9.

[14] Kenyon KR, Quigley HA, Hussels IE, et al. The systemic mucopolysaccharidoses. Ultrastructural and histochemical studies of conjunctiva and skin. Am J Ophthalmol 1972;73(6): 811–33.

[15] Quantock AJ, Meek KM, Fullwood NJ, et al. Scheie's syndrome: the architecture of corneal collagen and distribution of corneal proteoglycans. Can J Ophthalmol 1993;28(6): 266–72.

[16] Quigley HA, Maumenee AE, Stark WJ. Acute glaucoma in systemic mucopolysaccharidosis I-S. Am J Ophthalmol 1975;80(1):70–2.

[17] François J. Metabolic disorders and corneal changes. Dev Ophthalmol 1981;4:1–69.

[18] Jensen OA, Pedersen C, Schwartz M, et al. Hurler/Scheie phenotype. Report of an inbred sibship with tapeto-retinal degeneration and electron-microscopie examination of the conjunctiva. Ophthalmologica 1978;176(4):194–204.

[19] Käsmann-Kellner B, Weindler J, Pfau B, et al. Ocular changes in mucopolysaccharidosis IV A (Morquio A syndrome) and long-term results of perforating keratoplasty. Ophthalmologica 1999;213(3):200–5.

[20] Alroy J, Haskins M, Birk DE. Altered corneal stromal matrix organization is associated with mucopolysaccharidosis I, III and VI. Exp Eye Res 1999;68(5):523–30.

[21] Cantor LB, Disseler JA, Wilson FM 2nd. Glaucoma in the maroteaux-lamy syndrome. Am J Ophthalmol 1989;108(4):426–30.

[22] Zarate YA, Hopkin RJ. Fabry's disease. Lancet 2008;372(9647):1427–35.

[23] Eghbali A, Hassan S, Seehra G, et al. Ophthalmological findings in Gaucher disease. Mol Genet Metab 2019;127(1):23–7.

[24] Winter AW, Salimi A, Ospina LH, et al. Ophthalmic manifestations of Gaucher disease: the most common lysosomal storage disorder. Br J Ophthalmol 2019;103(3):315–26.

[25] Schuchman EH. The pathogenesis and treatment of acid sphingomyelinase-deficient Niemann-Pick disease. J Inherit Metab Dis 2007;30(5):654–63.

[26] Walton DS, Robb RM, Crocker AC. Ocular manifestations of group A niemann-pick disease. Am J Ophthalmol 1978;85(2):174–80.

[27] Emery JM, Green WR, Wyllie RG, et al. GM1-gangliosidosis: ocular and pathological manifestations. Arch Ophthalmol 1971;85(2):177–87.

[28] Brunetti-Pierri N, Scaglia F. GM1 gangliosidosis: review of clinical, molecular, and therapeutic aspects. Mol Genet Metab 2008;94(4):391–6.

[29] Stalenhoef AF, Casparie AF, Demacker PN, et al. Combined deficiency of apolipoprotein C-II and lipoprotein lipase in familial hyperchylomicronemia. Metabolism 1981;30(9): 919–26.

[30] Vinger PF, Sachs BA. Ocular manifestations of hyperlipoproteinemia. Am J Ophthalmol 1970;70(4):563–73.

[31] Hegele RA, Borén J, Ginsberg HN, et al. Rare dyslipidaemias, from phenotype to genotype to management: a European Atherosclerosis Society task force consensus statement. Lancet Diabetes Endocrinol 2020;8(1):50–67.

[32] Brewer HB Jr, Zech LA, Gregg RE, et al. Type III hyperlipoproteinemia: diagnosis, molecular defects, pathology, and treatment. Ann Intern Med 1983;98(5_Part_1):623–40.

[33] Schreibman PH, Wilson DE, Arky RA. Familial type IV hyperlipoproteinemia. N Engl J Med 1969;281(18):981–5.
[34] Rengarajan R, McCullough PA, Chowdhury A, et al. Identifying suspected familial chylomicronemia syndrome. SAVE Proc 2018;31(3):284–8.
[35] Weiss JS. Schnyder corneal dystrophy. Curr Opin Ophthalmol 2009;20(4):292–8.
[36] Kuivenhoven JA, Pritchard H, Hill J, et al. The molecular pathology of lecithin: cholesterol acyltransferase (LCAT) deficiency syndromes. J Lipid Res 1997;38(2):191–205.
[37] Carlson LA, Phillipson B. Fish eye disease: a new familial condition with massive corneal opacities and dyslipoproteinemia. Lancet 1979;2:921.
[38] Oram JF. Tangier disease and ABCA1. Biochim Biophys Acta 2000;1529(1–3):321–30.
[39] Braverman NE, Raymond GV, Rizzo WB, et al. Peroxisome biogenesis disorders in the Zellweger spectrum: an overview of current diagnosis, clinical manifestations, and treatment guidelines. Mol Genet Metab 2016;117(3):313–21.

Oculoplastics

Advances in Ophthalmology and Optometry 8 (2023) 343–356

ADVANCES IN OPHTHALMOLOGY AND OPTOMETRY

Blepharospasm
Review of Current Concepts in Diagnosis and Treatment

Tiffany C. Ho, MD[a,*], John B. Holds, MD[b,c,d]

[a]Oculoplastic Associates of Texas, 8230 Walnut Hill Lane, Suite #508, Dallas, TX 75231, USA; [b]Ophthalmic Plastic and Cosmetic Surgery Inc., 12990 Manchester Road, Suite #102, St. Louis, MO 63131, USA; [c]Department of Ophthalmology, Saint Louis University, 1008 South Spring Avenue, St. Louis, MO 63110, USA; [d]Department of Otolaryngology–Head and Neck Surgery, Saint Louis University, 1008 South Spring Ave, St. Louis, MO 63110, USA

Keywords
• Benign essential blepharospasm • Botulinum toxin • Myectomy • Dystonia

Key points
• Benign essential blepharospasm is a distressing and debilitating focal dystonia characterized by involuntary spasms of the bilateral orbicularis oculi, involuntary closure of the eyelids, and enhanced spontaneous blinking.
• Periorbital botulinum A toxin injections are the mainstay of treatment.
• Myectomy can be an effective adjunct in patients who are refractory to botulinum toxin, refuse serial injections, or require concurrent surgery to correct ptosis, brow ptosis, dermatochalasis, or lateral canthal tendon laxity.
• Oral medications have a role in some patients but have not proven to be terribly effective in most.

INTRODUCTION

Involuntary facial movement disorders, or dyskinesias, have been recognized for centuries. This broad category includes disorders of increased or decreased movement including tics, tremors, and dystonias. Dystonia describes movement disorders characterized by sustained twisting, pulling, or squeezing movements, and can be generalized or focal. In the sixteenth century, Flemish Renaissance painter Pieter Brueghel the Elder painted a subject with the appearance of spasms of the eyelids and jaw opening dystonia in a work named "Yawning Man" or *De*

Corresponding author. E-mail address: drho@oatexas.com

https://doi.org/10.1016/j.yaoo.2023.02.003
2452-1760/23/© 2023 Elsevier Inc. All rights reserved.

Gaper (Fig. 1). [1] As this painting may be the first potential source recognizing the symptoms associated with blepharospasm-oromandibular dystonia, Marsden used the eponym "Brueghel's syndrome" to describe the syndrome [2]. Although the painting likely represents a yawning man in a nightshirt to illustrate the cardinal sin of sloth, the appearance is consistent with facial dystonia. Earlier, Henry Meige, a French neurologist, in 1910 described 10 patients with facial convulsions of the eyelid muscles as well as lower face, jaw, and tongue [3].

Although benign essential blepharospasm (BEB) is now recognized as one of the most common forms of adult-onset dystonia, the condition was historically misdiagnosed as a manifestation of a psychiatric disorder until formally recognized as a focal dystonia in the 1970s. Primary blepharospasm or BEB is a clinical diagnosis with involuntary bilateral spasm of the orbicularis oculi, procerus, and corrugator muscles (Fig. 2). This article highlights the clinical features and current management options for BEB. Furthermore, this article discusses several medical and surgical treatment options.

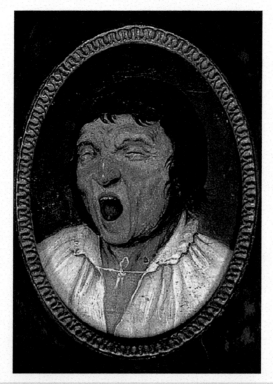

Fig. 1. Painting of the "Yawning Man" or "De Gaper." Pieter Brueghel the Elder, around 1560. Musées Royaux des Beaux – Arts Bruxelles. Purported to show a case of oromandibular dystonia with blepharospasm, this is almost certainly a depiction of a yawning man illustrating the cardinal sin of sloth. (*From* Carelli F. Brueghel: his art and his syndrome. London J Prim Care (Abingdon). 2017;9(3):43-44. Published 2017 Apr 23.)

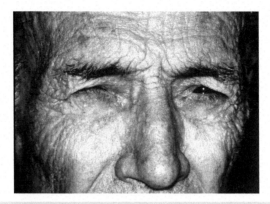

Fig. 2. Patient with BEB before any treatment.

Clinical features

The estimated worldwide prevalence of BEB ranges from 1.4 to 13.3 cases per 100,000 people with rates varying by geographic region [4,5]. It more commonly occurs in women with onset during the fifth to sixth decade of life [6]. Patients present with a spectrum of symptoms ranging from increased blink rate to sustained eyelid closure that can lead to functional blindness. Approximately 20% of patients have symptoms isolated to the eyelids but the majority may develop variable muscle spasms progressing to other muscular groups in the head and neck [7]. Symptoms can progress over months to years with periods of fluctuations in spasms. Patients have a variable evolution of symptoms. Most patients reach a plateau within 5 years, but remission is rare.

Conditions aggravating blepharospasm include bright lights, stress, fatigue, driving, and reading [8]. Patients with dystonia often adopt proprioceptive tricks to minimize spasms and to alleviate their symptoms (Fig. 3) [9–11]. These tricks include tapping or pressing on specific areas of the face, whistling, humming, singing, mouth opening, yawning, and nose pinching [9,12].

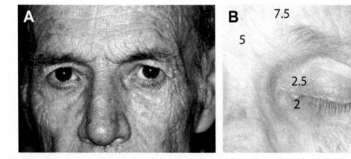

Fig. 3. (A) Patient shown in Fig. 2, 2 weeks after 40 units of periorbital botulinum toxin. (B) Typical injection sites in treatment of BEB.

Blepharospasms often can have a high psychological impact on patients. Unfortunately, diagnosis delay is common with blepharospasm. Previous studies have shown that patients saw an average of four physicians before the correct diagnosis was made [8]. Patients often felt people thought they were malingering and also were told by physicians that they were malingering. Although the link between blepharospasm and psychiatric conditions is debated, patients often have pronounced anxiety, depression, and reduced quality of life [13]. Spasms can also become severe enough to limit activities of daily living with patients reporting an inability to drive, read, watch television, or work [8].

Various syndromes are associated with blepharospasm. Patients can develop spasms of the mid or lower face referred to as Meige's syndrome. Brueghel's syndrome (idiopathic oromandibular dystonia) involves severe lower facial, mandibular, and cervical muscle involvement [12]. A subset of patients may display extracranial and generalized dystonia. Occasionally, the patient may have concurrent apraxia of eyelid opening—a nonparalytic inability to open the eyes in the absence of active eyelid contractions [14]. Primary blepharospasm must be distinguished from secondary causes of blepharospasm including medications, eye disease, or structural lesions such as Parkinson's or midbrain stroke. Reflex blepharospasm is another secondary blepharospasm caused by ocular surface irritation, inflammation, or dry eye. BEB patients commonly are aggravated by ocular surface disease such as dry eye and treating that ocular surface disease will typically provide some degree of relief from the BEB symptoms.

Pathophysiology of blepharospasm

To date, the pathophysiology of blepharospasm remains unclear. Positron emission tomography and functional magnetic resonance imaging (fMRI) investigations have demonstrated activation of the basal ganglia, cerebellum, thalamus, and midbrain during blepharospasm. These areas are thought to be important for the regulation of blinking [15,16]. In addition, patients demonstrate dysfunctional trigeminal blink reflex. Animal models have shown dopamine depletion within the substantia nigra that leads to an increase in the inhibitory output of the basal ganglia and increased reflex blind excitability [17]. Dopamine depletion, γ-aminobutyric acid (GABA) hypofunctioning, and acetylcholine excess also have been implicated in the basal ganglia signaling pathway [18]. Future research elucidating the pathogenesis of blepharospasm could help develop strategies to prevent and reverse the disease.

Treatment of blepharospasm

Upon diagnosis of blepharospasm, we provide patients with information about the Benign Essential Blepharospasm Research Foundation (BEBRF). Mattie Lou Koster founded BEBRF in 1981 and dedicated herself to educating physicians and patients about blepharospasm. What started as a grassroots organization has transitioned into a national organization providing funding for blepharospasm research and supporting thousands of patients through patient advocacy groups throughout the United States and the world [19,20]. The

BEBRF collaborates closely with the Dystonia Medical Research Foundation to promote awareness and education as well as advance research. In patients receiving a new diagnosis of blepharospasm, we advocate referral to the BEBRF for additional familial and psychological support as well as educational resources.

Currently, no cure exists for blepharospasm, and treatments are aimed at diminishing symptoms. Conservative management techniques include aggressive lubricant drops to alleviate dry eye symptoms. When evaluating blepharospasm patients, it is important to rule out reflex blepharospasm, which usually is caused by ocular surface disease. Management of underlying ocular surface disease can be effective for managing secondary blepharospasm. The blepharospasm patients also report debilitating photophobia. FL-41 lenses have a rose-colored tint that blocks wavelengths of light in the blue-green spectrum and have been shown to be superior to gray-tinted and rose-tinted lenses with identical optical density. The FL-41 tint improves blink frequency, light sensitivity, and decreases functional limitations in blepharospasm patients [21]. Thus, FL-41 lenses are a non-invasive and inexpensive adjunctive treatment of some blepharospasm patients with significant photophobia.

Botulinum toxin management

Since its introduction, botulinum toxin treatment has been established as the first-line treatment of choice for blepharospasm. It is produced by *Clostridium botulinum*. There are seven botulinum neurotoxin subtypes (labeled A–G). Serotypes A and B have clinical applications while studies are exploring applications for subtypes C–G [22]. Botulinum A has proven to be the most clinically efficacious subtype and is synthesized as single-chain polypeptides. To activate the molecule, endogenous proteolytic enzymes cleave the single-chain molecules into heavy chain and light chain. Botulinum A toxin binds to cholinergic nerve terminals of the neuromuscular junction and blocks acetylcholine release by cleaving plasma membrane synaptosome-associated protein (SNAP-25), a cell membrane cytoplasmic protein required for neurotransmitter release [23]. The affected terminals are inhibited from stimulating muscle contractions temporarily [22]. After exposure to botulinum toxin, muscle strength recovers as nerve axonal sprouts establish new connections within the neuromuscular junction. Muscle activity gradually returns, so repeated botulinum injections are required to maintain the clinical effect [24]. The toxin requires 24 to 72 hours to take effect, although some individuals may require as many as 10 days for full effect to occur. The peak effect of botulinum toxin occurs at approximately 10 days and lasts 3 to 4 months [25].

In 1981, Scott reported that botulinum toxin type A injections into hyperactive extraocular muscles in monkeys corrected strabismus [26]. The United States Food and Drug Administration (FDA) approved botulinum A toxin in 1989 for blepharospasm and adult strabismus [27]. Currently, there are five commercially available botulinum A toxins in the United States: onabotulinumtoxinA (Botox), abobotulinumtoxinA (Dysport), incobotulinumtoxinA (Xeomin), prabotulinum-toxinA (Juveau), and daxxibotulinumtoxinA (Daxxify). One botulinum toxin B is available in the United States, rimabotulinumtoxinB (MyoBloc) which is approved for cervical dystonia. Although generally less clinically effective than the botulinum A toxins, botulinum B may be useful in some refractory blepharospasm cases [28].

As mentioned above, the five preparations of botulinum A toxin have the same active molecule but differ in their purification processes and presence of complexing proteins. OnabotulinumtoxinA does not contain complexing proteins. The dose equivalency of onabotulinumtoxinA, prabotulinumtoxinA, and incobotulinumtoxinA is 1:1 whereas abobotulinumtoxinA is three times less potent than the other two botulinum toxins, and daxxibotulinumtoxinA requires twice the unit dose of onabotulinumtoxinA, but appears to last twice as long in cosmetic patients due to the presence of a proprietary 30 amino acid peptide that binds it at the injection site [15,29]. Anderson and colleagues found that onabotulinumtoxinA injections are effective in up to 86% of patients [8]. Comparative trials have found no significant difference in the efficacy, safety profile, and duration of effect between onabotulinumtoxinA and incobotulinumtoxinA [30–32]. In a small study of 50 patients, Chundury and colleagues evaluated patients' preference after switching from onabotulinumtoxinA to incobotulinumtoxinA and noted that patients preferring incobotulinumtoxinA had a significantly shorter treatment interval. In addition, those patients who preferred incobotulinumtoxinA thought it was more effective, whereas those who preferred onabotulinumtoxinA thought it had a longer duration [33].

Botulinum toxin injections into the orbicularis oculi, procerus, and corrugator muscles have been found to be the most effective treatment of blepharospasm (see Fig. 3). Careful observation during physical examination is paramount to identify the muscles of the face involved in spasm. As blepharospasm can be a progressive condition, additional muscle groups may become involved as the disease process evolves. The amount of toxin injected into each muscle (and muscles) should be individualized per patient. Several studies have shown that pretarsal injections are more effective than preseptal or orbital injections [34,35]. Pretarsal injections have been found to have longer duration of response and higher response rates [19]. In regard to injection pattern and dosage, significant variation exists between different providers. The FDA-approved patient labeling (Medication guide) sheet enclosed with each bottle of onabotulinumtoxinA is largely restrained by original clinical studies and FDA oversight. This recommends an initial injection pattern that includes a maximum of six injection sites per side with a maximum toxin dose of 15 units per side. However, a survey of practice patterns of oculoplastic surgeons found the mean initial dose of onabotulinumtoxinA was 22.5 units per side with greater than seven injection sites per side [36].

One concern with the repeated use of botulinum toxin is the development of blocking or neutralizing antibodies and subsequent nonresponse to treatment. Current formulations of botulinum toxin contain less neurotoxin complex protein and are significantly less antigenic [22]. A meta-analysis reviewing the incidence of neutralizing antibody formation across all clinical indications for botulinum toxin injections found a higher prevalence in clinically nonresponsive patients. However, the development of neutralizing antibodies did not always predict responsiveness to botulinum toxin therapy [37]. Most patients developing antibodies are treated with very high doses of toxin to larger muscle groups for torticollis or limb spasticity. Although the correlation between these antibodies and clinical response is not fully understood, keeping the treatment dose as low as possible and extending treatment intervals may be important in maintaining a beneficial botulinum toxin response.

Adverse effects with botulinum toxin injections occur in up to 20% of treated patients but are generally mild and reversible as the drug effect wanes [15,23,38]. The most common side effects are ptosis followed by diplopia, lagophthalmos, corneal exposure, and epiphora [38,39].

Oral pharmacology

Although patients with generalized dystonia often are treated with oral medications, the efficacy and duration are variable in blepharospasm patients. Commonly used medications include anticholinergics, dopaminergic, GABAergic agents, and muscle relaxants. Although botulinum toxin has FDA approval, the use of these oral therapies is "off-label" and often are added as an adjunct to botulinum toxin.

Dopamine deficiency has been implicated in blepharospasm [18]. Methylphenidate (Ritalin) is a central nervous system stimulant traditionally used to treat attention-deficit/hyperactivity disorder that inhibits the reuptake of dopamine and norepinephrine. Studies have measured decreased orbicularis oculi muscle contraction on surface electromyography after the administration of oral methylphenidate. Patients also demonstrate decreased disability and improved functional benefit with oral methylphenidate [16]. A case series described patients with blepharospasm and apraxia of eyelid opening who were refractory to botulinum toxin and eyelid myectomy and improved with methylphenidate therapy [40]. In both studies, the typical dosage of methylphenidate was 10 to 20 mg daily as needed [16,18,40]. Prescribers should note that methylphenidate is a schedule II substance under the Controlled Substance Act, which indicates high potential for abuse, and the age group of BEB patients generally mandates coordinating with the patient's primary care physician before prescribing methylphenidate.

GABA antagonists play a central role in dopamine release and have been shown to decrease blink amplitude and hypersensitivity [17,18]. GABA-ergic agents such as benzodiazepines increase the frequency of chloride ion channel opening to amplify GABA's inhibitory effects. Benzodiazepines are approved to treat anxiety, seizures, and spastic disorders. The most commonly prescribed medications for blepharospasm include lorazepam (Ativan), clonazepam (Klonopin), and diazepam (Valium) [8,18,41]. Benzodiazepines can cause compromising psychological and physical effects. Their use can be limited by adverse effects including sedation, memory disruption, dizziness, and ataxia.

Finally, acetylcholine contributes to the signaling pathway in the substantia nigra, and anticholinergics have been found to suppress acetylcholine activity and blink rates [18]. Variable clinical responses with anticholinergics have been observed in blepharospasm and commonly used medications include trihexyphenidyl and orphenadrine (Norflex) [5,18]. The authors have always preferred orphenadrine in this class due to a low side-effect profile and moderate efficacy.

Given the absence of large, controlled studies, lack of evidence-based prescribing strategies exist. There is also no clear order for the introduction of medications. In our clinical practice, commonly prescribed oral medications (used as needed 1–2 times per day) include 0.5 to 1.0 mg clonazepam, 100 mg orphenadrine, and 0.5 to 1.0 mg lorazepam as needed.

Surgical management

At the beginning of the twentieth century, the treatment of blepharospasm was aimed at destroying the facial nerve including alcohol injections into the facial nerve, neurotomy, neurectomy, and selective avulsion of facial nerve branches to the orbicularis muscle [7,8]. The facial nerve's overlapping nerve branches and ability to regenerate limited this treatment's effectiveness. The recurrence rates were high at approximately 35% to 40% at 15 months and 50% to 55% after 2 years [42,43]. Patients also suffered significant sequelae from facial nerve paralysis such as brow ptosis, ectropion, and exposure keratitis. "Successful" procedures often resulted in patients with a bilateral facial droop [44]. As a result, physicians transitioned away from peripheral facial neurectomy procedures in favor of surgical myectomy.

In 1965, Henderson provided an early description of myectomy with limited muscle stripping providing short duration of effect [45]. In the 1970s, Anderson developed radical myectomy surgery in which extensive protractor excision is performed to physically remove the majority of the spasming muscle. The entire orbicularis oculi muscle in the upper eyelid and brow region, corrugator, and procerus muscles are excised through brow and eyelid incisions [46]. Aponeurotic ptosis repair and lateral canthopexy for eyelid tightening are generally performed as part of the myectomy procedure. Although Anderson and colleagues found that 88% of their patients had improvement in blepharospasm, patients frequently experienced postoperative complications including extensive lymphedema for greater than 6 months, forehead anesthesia, and lagophthalmos [8,19].

Given its surgical morbidity, radical myectomy has fallen out of favor. Most current myectomy procedures are performed as a more limited myectomy in which a less extensive excision of the orbicularis muscle is performed through an eyelid crease incision alone (Fig. 4) [8,19,44,47]. Patients have fewer complications with more cosmetically acceptable results (Fig. 5), although it is assumed that botulinum injection will continue postoperatively. Today, surgical myectomy serves as an adjunctive procedure for patients who are resistant or refractory to botulinum toxin injection. Indications for limited myectomy

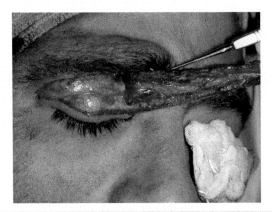

Fig. 4. Intraoperative view of limited myectomy through an upper eyelid crease incision in the upper eyelid with the removal of pretarsal and preseptal orbicularis muscle.

include patients with limited or short (<10 week) duration of botulinum toxin effect, declining efficacy, or intolerant of serial injections. Myectomy allows concurrent surgical treatment of ptosis, dermatochalasis, brow ptosis, or canthal tendon laxity. In blepharospasm patients, the years of eyelid squeezing and spasms contribute to the earlier development of eyelid malposition than the general population [44].

After limited myectomy, patients can expect continued postoperative botulinum toxin therapy. Kent and colleagues demonstrated that botulinum toxin treatment intervals increased from 10.1 to 15.7 weeks with a reduced total botulinum toxin dosage after myectomy [48].

Chemomyectomy

To provide a more permanent treatment of blepharospasm, chemomyectomy with doxorubicin injections has been reported. Doxorubincin is an antineoplastic agent used against numerous cancers that have myotoxic properties.

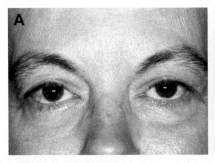
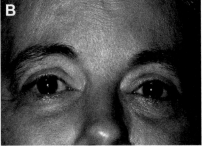

Fig. 5. (A) Preoperative view of BEB patient with spasm and blepharoptosis before myectomy surgery. (B) Same patient months postoperatively following limited myectomy and ptosis repair.

Direct injection into the orbicularis oculi muscles results in permanent muscle loss. Chemomyectomy allows for permanent muscle destruction through chemotherapeutic injection rather than surgery. Repeated injections of 1 to 1.5 mg of doxorubicin with a maximum cumulative dose of 7 mg of doxorubicin were required for improvement. Patients received a median of three injections [49]. In their clinical trial, Wirtschafer and colleagues included 27 patients (18 with blepharospasm and 9 with hemifacial spasm). In the blepharospasm group, 10 of the 18 patients (55%) completed treatment with 90% of patients having symptom relief for greater than 1 year [50]. The main drawbacks of doxorubicin are the local complications. Doxorubicin inject induces a severe inflammatory response in which patients may develop skin ulcerations and severe swelling lasting 1 to 8 weeks following injections (Fig. 6) [49]. Some patients ceased treatment as a result of this adverse effect.

Recent work has shown the possible utility of other chemodestructive agents. Doxil is a liposome-encapsulated form of doxorubicin, which has the same chemomyectomy effect as doxorubicin. This formulation provides additional skin protection [51]. IRB expiration and the lack of a commercial model led to the abandonment of these chemomyectomy trials. Ricin-mAb35 is an immunotoxin conjugated to nicotinic acetylcholine receptors that target adult skeletal muscles that have shown to paralyze extraocular muscles histologically in animal models [51,52].

Treatment horizons

To date, established treatments for blepharospasm are only symptomatic in nature with no viable medication or treatment that slows or reverses disease progression. Given that the etiology of blepharospasm is still unknown and no optimal central drug targets exist, physical therapy methods including electrical stimulation have been applied to dystonia.

Deep brain stimulation (DBS) is an invasive neuromodulation technique in which stimulating electrodes implanted in the brain use internal pulse generators

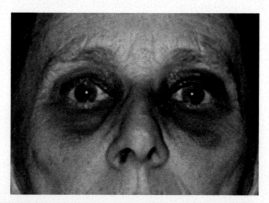

Fig. 6. Doxorubicin-treated patient showing intense erythema after injection. (*Courtesy of Andrew Harrison, MD, Minneapolis, MN.*)

to target specific areas of the brain [53]. Whereas large, randomized controlled studies have documented the efficacy of DBS for generalized and cervical dystonia, only case reports have described the use of DBS in blepharospasm [14,54,55]. Case reports describe DBS targeting the globus pallidus interna and the subthalamic nucleus as targets for refractory blepharospasm treatment [56–58]. Although early success is documented in these reports, exacerbation of blepharospasm is also reported [59]. DBS complications, although rare, can be severe and include brain hemorrhage, infection, stimulation-induced side effects (sensory, motor, visual, mood, cognitive), and hardware malfunction [14]. Longer-term and larger studies are needed to demonstrate DBS's efficacy and safety.

Repetitive transcranial magnetic stimulation (rTMS) has gained traction as a non-invasive therapeutic tool for blepharospasm. This technique uses pulsed magnetic fields to stimulate the cerebral cortex and can decrease blink rate and spasms [60]. rTMS has been studied as a novel adjunct to botulinum toxin and may improve associated anxiety and depression [61,62].

Finally, controversies regarding botulinum toxin still exist. Areas that need exploration include a comparison of the efficacy and duration among different dosing, preparation, and injection techniques. Optimal dilution parameters, treatment patterns, and treatment intervals for different toxin types are yet to be established.

SUMMARY

Although no cure exists for blepharospasm, several medical and surgical advances have been made in the past several decades to alleviate the significant functional disability in patients affected by this disease. Botulinum toxin injections remain the cornerstone of blepharospasm therapy with several adjuncts including surgery, oral medications, and brain stimulation. Although effective, botulinum toxin therapy remains transient with generally mild side effects. In the future, research regarding longer-acting medications, refinements in surgical therapy, and possibly genetic engineering may provide more lasting relief for blepharospasm patients.

CLINICS CARE POINTS

- When diagnosing blepharospasm, evaluate and adequately treat concurrent dry eye or ocular surface disease.
- Botulinum toxin is the first-line treatment of blepharospasm. There does not appear to be a significant difference in the efficacy, adverse effects, or patient preference between incobotulinumtoxinA (Xeomin) and onabotulinumtoxinA (Botox).
- Reconstitution of Xeomin and Botox is similar. If a patient is switching between the two formulations, dosage amounts are equivalent.

- When injecting botulinum toxins, pretarsal injections have a longer duration and higher response rates than preseptal or orbital injections. Injections given too deeply below the periosteum can increase the risk of ptosis.

- Although surgical myectomy is a good alternative for treatment-resistant blepharospasm, patients likely still require botulinum toxin injections although at a lower dose.

DISCLOSURE

J.B. Holds is a shareholder of Revance Therapeutics. Dr T.C. Ho has no financial conflict of interest to disclose.

References

[1] Carelli F. Brueghel: his art and his syndrome. London J Prim Care 2017;9(3):43–4.
[2] Marsden CD. Blepharospasm-oromandibular dystonia syndrome (Brueghel's syndrome). A variant of adult-onset torsion dystonia? Neurol Neurosurg Psychiatry 1976;39(12): 1204–9.
[3] Meige H. Les convulsion de la face une form clinique de convulsion faciale, bilateral et mediane. Rev Neurol 1907;10:437–43.
[4] Steeves T, Day L, Jonathan D. The prevalence of primary dystonia: a systematic review and meta-analysis. Mov Disord 2012;27:1789–96.
[5] Bradley EA, Hodge DO, Bartley GB. Benign essential blepharospasm among residents of Olmsted county, Minesota, 1976 to 1995: An epidemiologic study. Ophthal Plast Reconstr Surg 2003;19(3):177–81.
[6] Peckham EL, Lopez G, Shamim EA, et al. Clinical features of patients with blepharospasm: A report of 240 patients. Eur J Neurol 2011;18(3):382–6.
[7] Leyngold I, Berbos Z, Georgescu D, et al. Essential Blepharospasm and Hemifacial Spasm. In: Black E, editor. Smith and Nesi's ophthalmic plastic and reconstructive surgery. 2012. 2012. p. 345–54.
[8] Anderson RL, Patel BC, Holds JB, et al. Blepharospasm:Past, Present, and Future. Ophthalmic Plast Reconstr Surg 1998;14(5):305–17.
[9] Kilduff CLS, Casswell EJ, Salam T, et al. Use of alleviating maneuvers for periocular facial dystonias. JAMA Ophthalmol 2016;134(11):1247–52.
[10] Loyola D, Camargos S, Maia D, et al. Sensory tricks in focal dystonia and hemifacial spasm. Eur J Neurol 2013;20(4):704–7.
[11] Martino D, Liuzzi D, Macerollo AAM, et al. The phenomenology of the geste antagoniste in primary blepharospasm and cervical dystonia. Mov Disord 2010;25(4):407–12.
[12] Jordan DR, Patrinely JR, Anderson RLTS. Essential blepharospasm and related dystonias. Surv Ophthalmol 1989;34(2):123–32.
[13] Hall TA, McGwin G, Searcey K, et al. Health-related quality of life and psychosocial characteristics of patients with benign essential blepharospasm. Arch Ophthalmol 2006;124(1):116–9.
[14] Hwang CJ, Eftekhari K. Benign Essential Blepharospasm : What We Know and What We Don't. Int Ophthalmol Clin 2018;58(1):11–24.
[15] Ozzello DJ, Giacometti JN. Botulinum toxins for treating essential blepharospasm and hemifacial spasm. Int Ophthalmol Clin 2018;58(1):49–61.
[16] Price KM, Ramey NA, Richard MJ, et al. Can methylphenidate objectively provide relief in patients with uncontrolled blepharospasm? A pilot study using surface electromyography. Ophthal Plast Reconstr Surg 2010;26(5):353–6.
[17] Basso MA, Powers ASEC. An explanation for reflex blink hyperexcitability in Parkinson's disease. I. Superior colliculus. J Neurosci 1996;16(22):7308–17.

[18] Hirabayashi KE, Reza Vagefi M. Oral pharmacotherapy for benign essential blepharospasm. Int Ophthalmol Clin 2018;58(1):33–47.

[19] Yen MT. Developments in the treatment of benign essential blepharospasm. Curr Opin Ophthalmol 2018;29(5):440–4.

[20] Moore GH, Anderson RL. Blepharospasm Research Foundation 2018;58(1):25–31.

[21] Blackburn MK, Lamb RD, Digre KB, et al. FL-41 Tint Improves Blink Frequency, Light Sensitivity, and Functional Limitations in Patients with Benign Essential Blepharospasm. Ophthalmology 2009;116(5):997–1001.

[22] Jankovic J. Botulinum toxin in clinical practice. J Neurol Neurosurg Psychiatry 2004;75(7): 951–7.

[23] Duarte GS, Rodrigues FB, Marques RE, et al. Botulinum toxin type A therapy for blepharospasm. Cochrane Database Syst Rev 2020;11(11).

[24] Rogozhin AA, Pang KK, Bukharaeva E, et al. Recovery of mouse neuromuscular junctions from single and repeated injections of botulinum neurotoxin A. J Physiol 2008;586(13): 3163–82.

[25] Nigram P, Nigram A. Botulinum toxin. Indian J Dermatol 2010;55(1):8–14.

[26] AB S. Botulinum toxin injection of eye muscles to correct strabismus. Trans Am Ophthalmol Soc 1981;79:734–9.

[27] Hamil EB, Yen MT. The history of blepharospasm in medicine. Int Ophthalmol Clin 2018;58: 3–10.

[28] Dutton JJ, White JJ, Richard MJ. Myobloc® for the treatment of benign essential blepharospasm in patients refractory to Botox. Ophthal Plast Reconstr Surg 2006;22(3):173–7.

[29] Solish N, Carruthers J, Kaufman J, et al. Overview of DaxibotulinumtoxinA for Injection: A Novel Formulation of Botulinum Toxin Type A. Drugs 2021;81(18):2091–101.

[30] Wabbels B, Reichel G, Fulford-Smith A, et al. Double-blind, randomised, parallel group pilot study comparing two botulinum toxin type A products for the treatment of blepharospasm. J Neural Transm 2011;118(2):233–9.

[31] Jankovic J. Clinical efficacy and tolerability of Xeomin in the treatment of blepharospasm. Eur J Neurol 2009;16(Suppl 2):14–8.

[32] Saad JGA. A direct comparison of onabotulinumtoxina (Botox) and IncobotulinumtoxinA (Xeomin) in the treatment of benign essential blepharospasm: a split-face technique. J Neuro Ophthalmol 2014;34(3):233–6.

[33] Chundury RV, Couch SM, Holds JB. Comparison of preferences between onabotulinumtox in A (Botox) and incobotulinumtox in A (Xeomin) in the treatment of benign essential blepharospasm. Ophthal Plast Reconstr Surg 2013;29(3):205–7.

[34] Esposito M, Fasano A, Crisci C, et al. The combined treatment with orbital and pretarsal botulinum toxin injections in the management of poorly responsive blepharospasm. Neurol Sci 2014;35(3):397–400.

[35] Cakmur R, Ozturk V, Uzunel F, et al. Comparison of preseptal and pretarsal injections of botulinum toxin in the treatment of blepharospasm and hemifacial spasm. J Neurol 2002;249(1):64–8.

[36] Broadbent TJ, Wesley RE, Mawn LA. A Survey of Current Blepharospasm Treatment Patterns among Oculoplastic Surgeons. Ophthal Plast Reconstr Surg 2016;32(1):24–7.

[37] Fabbri M, Leodori G, Fernandes RM, et al. Neutralizing Antibody and Botulinum Toxin Therapy: A Systematic Review and Meta-analysis. Neurotox Res 2016;29(1):105–17.

[38] Czyz CN, Burns JA, Petrie TP, et al. Long-term botulinum toxin treatment of benign essential blepharospasm, hemifacial spasm, and Meige syndrome. Am J Ophthalmol 2013;156(1): 173–7.

[39] Mejia NI, Vuong KDJJ. Long-term botulinum toxin efficacy, safety, and immunogenicity. Mov Disord 2005;20(5):592–7.

[40] Eftekhari K, Choe CH, Vagefi MR, et al. Oral methylphenidate for the treatment of refractory facial dystonias. Ophthal Plast Reconstr Surg 2015;31(3):e65–6.

[41] Merikangas J, Reynolds C 3rd. Blepharospasm: Successful Treatment with clonazepam. Ann Neurol 1979;5(4):401–2.

[42] Callahan A. Intractable blepharospasm. Am J Ophthalmol 1965;60:788–91.

[43] Reynolds D, Smith JL, Walsh TJ. Differential section of the facial nerve for blepharospasm. Trans Am Acad Ophthalmol Otolaryngol 1967;71:656–64.

[44] Pariseau B, Worley MW, Anderson RL. Myectomy for blepharospasm 2013. Curr Opin Ophthalmol 2013;24(5):488–93.

[45] Henderson JW. Essential blepharospasm. Trans Am Ophthalmol Soc 1956;54:453–520.

[46] Gillum WNAR. Blepharospasm Surgery: An Anatomical Approach. Arch Ophthalmol 1981;99(6):1056–62.

[47] Yen MT. Surgical myectomy for essential blepharospasm and hemifacial spasm. Int Ophthalmol Clin 2018;58(1):63–70.

[48] Kent TL, Petris CK, Holds JB. Effect of upper eyelid myectomy on subsequent chemodenervation in the management of benign essential blepharospasm. Ophthal Plast Reconstr Surg 2015;31(3):222–6.

[49] Wirtschafter JD. Chemomyectomy of the orbicularis oculi muscles for the treatment of localized hemifacial spasm. J Neuro Ophthalmol 1994;14(4):199–204.

[50] Wirtschafter JD, McLoon LK. Long-term efficacy of local doxorubicin chemomyectomy in patients with blepharospasm and hemifacial spasm. Ophthalmology 1998;105(2):342–6.

[51] Harrison AR. Chemodenervation for facial dystonias and wrinkles. Curr Opin Ophthalmol 2003;14(5):241–5.

[52] Harrison AR, Skladzien S, Christiansen SPML. Myotoxic effects of the skeletal muscle-specific immunotoxin, ricin-mAb35, on orbicularis oculi muscle after eyelid injections in rabbits. Ophthalmic Plast Reconstr Surg 2004;20(4):312–6.

[53] McKinnon C, Gros P, Lee DJ, et al. Deep brain stimulation: potential for neuroprotection. Ann Clin Transl Neurol 2018;6(1):174–85.

[54] Vidailhet M, Vercueil L, Houeto JL, et al. Bilateral deep-brain stimulation of the globus pallidus in primary generalized dystonia. N Engl J Med 2005;352(5):459–67.

[55] Krauss J. Deep brain stimulation for dystonia in adults. Overview and developments. Stereotact Funct Neurosurg 2002;78:168–82.

[56] Luthra NS, Mitchell KT, Volz MM, et al. Intractable Blepharospasm Treated with Bilateral Pallidal Deep Brain Stimulation. Tremor Other Hyperkinet Mov (N Y) 2017;7:472.

[57] Wang X, Mao Z, Cui Z, et al. Predictive factors for long-term clinical outcomes of deep brain stimulation in the treatment of primary Meige syndrome. J Neurosurg 2019;132(5):1267–375.

[58] Yamada K, Shinojima N, Hamasaki TKJ. Pallidal stimulation for medically intractable blepharospasm. BMJ Case Rep 2016;2015214241; https://doi.org/10.1136/bcr-2015-214241.

[59] Vagefi MR, Lin CC, McCann JDAR. Exacerbation of blepharospasm associated with craniocervical dystonia after placement of bilateral globus pallidus internus deep brain stimulator. Mov Disord 2008;23(3):454–6.

[60] Kranz G, Shamim EA, Lin PT, et al. Transcranial magnetic brain stimulation modulates blepharospasm: a randomized controlled study. Neurology 2010;75(16):1465–71.

[61] Wagle Shukla A, Hu W, Legacy J, et al. Combined effects of rTMS and botulinum toxin therapy in benign essential blepharospasm. Brain Stimul 2018;11(3):645–7.

[62] Yin B, Peng B, Luo Y, et al. Efficacy of Repetitive Transcranial Magnetic Stimulation Combined with Botulinum Toxin Type A for Benign Essential Blepharospasm Patients Accompanied by Anxiety and Depression. Neuropsychiatr Dis Treat 2021;2707–11.

Advances in Ophthalmology and Optometry 8 (2023) 357–373

ELSEVIER
MOSBY

ADVANCES IN OPHTHALMOLOGY AND OPTOMETRY

Nasolacrimal Duct Obstruction

Gabriela Mabel Espinoza, MD[a,*],
Ulrich Lachmund, MD[b]

[a]Department of Ophthalmology, Saint Louis University, 1225 South Grand Boulevard, Saint Louis, MO 63104, USA; [b]Department of Neuroradiology, University of Zurich, Rämistrasse 100, CH- 8091, Zürich, Switzerland

Keywords
• Nasolacrimal duct obstruction • Dacryocystography • Lacrimal duct dilatation
• Dacryocystoplasty • Dacryocystorhinostomy

Key points

- Nasolacrimal duct obstruction can lead to dacryocystitis and periorbital cellulitis.
- Evaluation of epiphora can be done effectively and efficiently in the office with targeted history and physical exam and simple lacrimal testing.
- Imaging can be helpful in diagnosing obstruction and tailoring treatment for best outcomes.
- Identifying and treating secondary causes of nasolacrimal duct obstruction can help prevent recurrence.
- The latest technologies and advances in lacrimal surgery are making treatment easier and less complicated in a surgical field that already has a high success rate.

INTRODUCTION

Epiphora is a common complaint that is seen in both children and adults that can present to any eye care provider. Congenital nasolacrimal duct obstruction (CNLDO) is found in 1 in 9 live births, with a reported range of 5–20% occurrence in newborns [1]. Acquired nasolacrimal duct obstruction has been noted to occur in 20.24 per 100,000, with 90 percent of these having primary acquired nasolacrimal duct obstruction (PANDO) [2]. No gender predilection exists in CNLDO, however, a higher likelihood of NLDO occurs in patients over the age of 40 with a predilection for women

*Corresponding author. E-mail address: gabriela.espinoza@health.slu.edu

https://doi.org/10.1016/j.yaoo.2023.02.016
2452-1760/23/© 2023 Elsevier Inc. All rights reserved.

Symptoms of nasolacrimal duct obstruction in children can resolve spontaneously in up to 90%, however, a significant impact may occur to families prior to resolution. CNLDO can cause intermittent mucoid discharge, which easily can be mistaken by childcare providers for pink eye and cause parents to have to pull their child out of daycare and bring them to their pediatrician or primary care physician for treatment. In a retrospective study, 46% of infants with CNLDO were prescribed antibiotics, which can be a sign of increased severity [3]. Massage of the tear duct with or without antibiotic treatment was found to have a higher rate of nonsurgical resolution of CNLDO than observation alone. When these children are referred to an eye care provider, they will likely require surgical intervention and parents often are tired of conservative management. Tearing often will cause irritation of the thin eyelid skin and lead to excess rhytids, increased appearance of dark circles, hyperpigmentation, or erythema, and even breakdown of the skin.

Epiphora in adults may originate from many different ophthalmic conditions, though this article is going to focus on nasolacrimal duct obstruction which accounts for approximately 68% of all tear drainage system obstructions [2]. Many patients will have the same eyelid symptoms and signs as noted in children but will additionally complain of difficulties reading, driving, and being self-conscious due to the appearance that they are constantly crying. During the COVID pandemic, patients with NLDO were more aware of how often they had to wipe their eyes and risk contamination.

The most problematic result of NLDO is the infection of the lacrimal sac. Chronic dacryocystitis may cause persistent mucopurulent drainage with eyelid irritation and mattering of the eyelashes along with blurry vision as noted above. Acute dacryocystitis can lead to pain and swelling of the eyelid with potential extension as a preseptal or orbital cellulitis. Fistulas can form when the infection bursts through the thin skin of the tear trough to drain the abscess that forms in the lacrimal sac. These may resolve with oral antibiotics or require intravenous antibiotics and subsequent surgical correction of the NLDO. A survey of ophthalmologists in southwest England found that 70% of respondents evaluated patients with epiphora frequently or sometimes [4]. Ultimately, diagnosis and treatment of NLDO is important for clinicians to familiarize themselves with to improve patient satisfaction and reduce the impact of disease.

Anatomy of lacrimal obstruction

The outflow of tears through the nasolacrimal duct system can be blocked in several areas. Normal tear drainage occurs when tears travel from the ocular surface into the upper and lower eyelid puncta and through the upper and lower eyelid canalicular system into the lacrimal sac. Each blink creates a pump action as the orbicularis muscles contract medially to dilate the lacrimal sac to create a suctioning effect on the tears as the upper and lower eyelid meet to occlude the puncta. In 90% of people, the tears will travel through a common canaliculus into the lacrimal sac which then drains down the nasolacrimal duct into the inferior meatus of the nose. The nasolacrimal duct is surrounded by bone as it connects the lacrimal sac to the inferior meatus. Reflux of tears from the lacrimal sac is prevented by the "valve" of Rosenmuller, which is the angulation of the common canaliculus as it enters the lacrimal sac, and backflow from the nose is prevented by the valve of Hasner, which is present at the opening of the nasolacrimal duct into the inferior meatus [5]. Thus, the lacrimal system contains the eyelids and the lacrimal duct system (Fig. 1).

Functional obstruction occurs when the anatomical pathway is patent based on irrigation through the puncta, but tears still do not drain properly. This may be related to eyelid issues interfering with the pump such as weakness of the

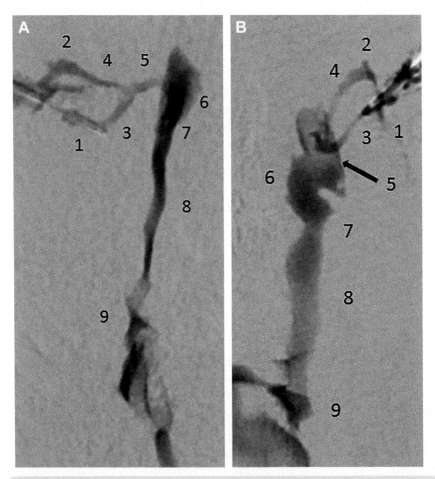

Fig. 1. Digital-Subtraction-Dacryocystography (DS-DCG) images of a normal lacrimal system labeled 1-inferior punctum, 2-superior punctum, 3-inferior canaliculus, 4-superior canaliculus, 5-common canaliculus (*arrow*), 6-lacrimal sac, 7-beginning of lacrimal duct, 8-lacrimal duct, 9-valve of Hasner. (**A**) antero-posterior view; (**B**) lateral view.

orbicularis oculi muscle (eg, facial palsy, botulinum toxin injections) or malposition of the eyelids (eg, entropion, ectropion, eyelid laxity). Some patients may be labeled with functional obstruction but have partial nasolacrimal duct obstruction due to stenosis or mechanical obstruction (eg, retained silicone tube material or punctal plug, dacryoliths, primary tumors in the lacrimal system).

The anatomy surrounding the lacrimal sac is important to understand when performing surgical correction of NLDO. The review by Rajak and Psaltis provides an excellent description of the lacrimal fossa and a three-dimensional understanding of this space [6]. The lacrimal fossa is formed by the lacrimal bone posteriorly, which is very thin, and the thicker frontal process of the maxilla. The middle meatus lies on the nasal side of the lacrimal fossa, with the axilla of the middle turbinate acting as a reliable internal landmark to this region. The agger nasi air cell is the anterior most ethmoid air cell, which occasionally will extend anteriorly between the lacrimal fossa and the middle meatus.

DIAGNOSIS

When a patient presents with epiphora to your office, a thorough history can be helpful in confirming the presence of a nonobstructive vs. an obstructive diagnosis. Minor, intermittent epiphora with reproducible triggers often is caused by nonobstructive diagnoses listed in Table 1. Persistent, daily watering and epiphora are more common in complete obstruction but symptoms can overlap with stenosis (Table 2) [7]. Physical examination of the eyelids with slit lamp evaluation of the corneal surface will aid in narrowing down the diagnosis, but the gold standard for diagnosis of nasolacrimal duct obstruction is the irrigation of the lacrimal drainage system via a lacrimal cannula through the punctum, otherwise known as syringing.

The Munk scale is very helpful as a classification of the teary eye. Asymmetric tearing can be easily recognized and documented after treatment to report the success rate of the operation or intervention. A zero on the Munk scale shows no epiphora, with grades I–IV showing progressive epiphora leading up to constant epiphora at grade V. This grading often corresponds with the degree of stenosis or obstruction [8].

Syringing

In children and adults who will not tolerate in-office syringe testing, a fluorescein dye disappearance test may be useful. I prefer to use a drop of proparacaine on a fluorescein dye strip and dip the strip into the inferior fornix of each eye. This tends to be less irritating than the drop of 2% fluorescein and helps control the amount of liquid added to the eye. Younger children can be difficult to assess due to cooperation and tendency to cry when undergoing any testing and often are best assessed through history and external exam only. A cobalt blue light then is used after five minutes to compare the amount of retained fluorescein. Asymmetric clearing, pooling, and gross epiphora after five minutes indicate poor outflow of tears. Examination also includes gentle pressure applied over the lacrimal crest to compress the lacrimal sac. If reflux

Table 1
Most common nonobstructive causes of epiphora

Nonobstructive diagnosis	Key findings	Basic management
Dry eye	Symptoms of burning, itching, foreign body sensation, worsened by wind; corneal staining; low tear lake (<0.25 mm)	Lubrication with artificial tears, gel drops, or ointment; Treat inflammatory component with targeted medicated topical therapy
Reflex epiphora	Surface irritation or trauma, environmental triggers	Lubrication; Limit exposure to airborne irritants (eg, perfume, hair spray, body spray, smoke, allergens), removal of foreign bodies (eg, eyelash, makeup, contact lens)
Eyelid malpositioning • Ectropion • Entropion • Laxity (floppy eyelid, facial palsy) • Retraction	• Exposure of the tarsal conjunctiva or visible puncta • Rotation of the eyelashes toward the globe • Poor snapback test, lagophthalmos, facial droop • Scleral show	Lubrication; Treat inflammatory component if related to infection or blepharitis; Surgical intervention is often required, though eyelid taping can be a temporizing measure
Gustatory epiphora	Precipitated by eating; History of facial palsy with aberrant regeneration	Transconjunctival botulinum toxin injection; Rarely perform surgical intervention

Table 2
Most common obstructive causes of epiphora (stenosis or occlusion)

Obstructive diagnosis	Key findings	Basic management
Congenital Nasolacrimal Duct Obstruction	Persistent tearing, mattering of the eyelashes, and intermittent mucoid discharge in an infant	Observation if asymptomatic; Massage of the lacrimal sac; Topical antibiotic as needed; Surgery if persists despite conservative management
Punctal stenosis	Narrowing of the puncta to less than 0.3 mm in diameter, increased tear lake (>0.6 mm)	Observation if asymptomatic; Dilation; Punctoplasty; Silicone tube placement
Canalicular obstruction Figs. 2 and 3	Increased tear lake, epiphora, difficulty passing a lacrimal dilator; History often reveals a secondary cause such as concurrent ocular disease, topical or systemic medication, allergy, or trauma, infection with actinomyces (canaliculitis) or dry eyes	Treat the underlying cause or remove the offending agent; Canalicular dilation and silicone tube placement if caught early, conjunctivodacryocystorhinostomy when severe.
Primary Acquired Nasolacrimal Duct Obstruction Figs. 4 and 5	History of chronic intermittent watering and tearing, more often in middle-aged women. In younger people, dacryoliths are more common.	Observation if asymptomatic; Massage of the lacrimal sac if distended; Surgery as indicated
Secondary Acquired Nasolacrimal Duct Obstruction Fig. 6 • Inflammatory	Systemic disease (eg, sarcoidosis, granulomatosis with polyangiitis); Chemical induced (eg, alkali or acidic burn, chronic allergy, glaucoma eye drops, chemotherapy such as docetaxel); Radiation or physical burn; Sinusitis or allergies	Treatment of secondary cause; Observation if asymptomatic; Massage of the lacrimal sac if distended; Surgery as indicated.

- Infectious Dacryocystitis can be caused by bacteria, viruses, fungi, or parasites. Most common pathogens: Staphylococcus, Streptococcus, and Actinomyces species (Canaliculitis); Sinusitis
- Traumatic Lacerations or fractures of the midface region
- Neoplastic Primary tumors of the nasolacrimal mucosa (eg, papillomas, lymphomas, squamous cell carcinoma, melanoma); Adjacent primary tumors (eyelid skin carcinomas, nasal mucosal carcinomas, lymphomas) Metastatic tumors (rare breast carcinoma, malignant melanoma, prostate carcinoma)
- Mechanical Dacryoliths (see Fig. 4); Sinus mucocele; Migrated punctal or intracanalicular plugs

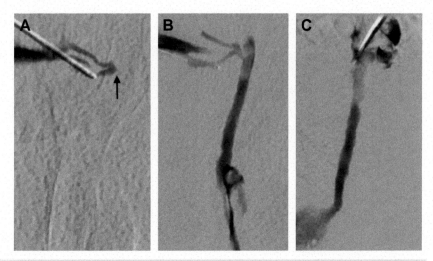

Fig. 2. Proximal occlusion of the common canaliculus. Clinical exam revealed a soft stop on irrigation and heavy reflux, Munk scale IV. **(A)** DS-DCG. The *arrow* points to the presaccal occlusion in the anterior third of the common canaliculus; **(B)** DS-DCG antero-posterior view two months after dacryoplasty with normal lacrimal system; **(C)** DS-DCG lateral view two months after dacryoplasty with the normal lacrimal system.

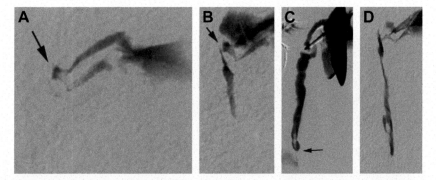

Fig. 3. High grade proximal stenosis of the common canaliculus and postsaccal distal high grade stenosis. Clinical exam revealed a soft stop on irrigation and heavy reflux, Munk scale IV. **(A)** DS-DCG antero-posterior view. The *arrow* pointing on the high-grade stenosis may be misdiagnosed as a presaccal occlusion; **(B)** DS-DCG antero-posterior view. The *arrow* pointing on the high-grade stenosis. The distal lacrimal system can only be seen after continued injection of contrast medium; **(C)** DS-DCG lateral view. The *arrow* pointing on the postsaccal high grade stenosis at the level of the valve of Hasner; **(D)** DS-DCG antero-posterior view two months after dacryoplasty shows the normal lacrimal system.

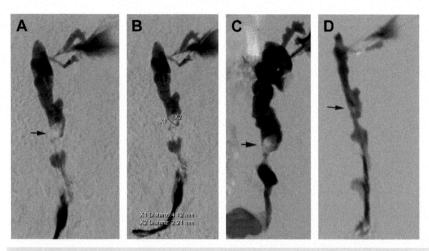

Fig. 4. Dacryolith postsaccal in the lower third of nasolacrimal duct. Clinical exam shows heavy reflux, Munk scale IV. (**A**) DS-DCG antero-posterior view. Arrow points to a filling defect in the lower third of the nasolacrimal duct which is typical for a dacryolith. (**B**) DS-DCG antero-posterior view. Measurement of dacryolith 4.12 × 2.21 mm; (**C**) DS-DCG lateral view. Filling defect of the lower third of the nasolacrimal duct with proximal lacrimal system dilation due to dacryolith (*arrow*); (**D**) DS-DCG anter-posterior view. Normal lacrimal system three months after dacryoplasty. *Arrow* points to normal filling in the area of the prior dacryolith.

of fluorescein, mucoid material, or sometimes gelatinous tears occurs, then significant nasolacrimal duct obstruction can be presumed, and a syringe test can be avoided to help prevent discomfort and possible injury or aggravation of already inflamed tissue.

Syringing is an in-office procedure which can provide significant information regarding the amount of obstruction and the location of the obstruction. Apply

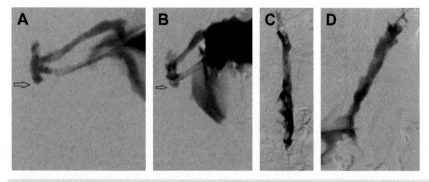

Fig. 5. (**A**) DS-DCG antero-posterior view. The lacrimal sac appears small due to post-saccal proximal occlusion (*arrow*); (**B**) DS-DCG lateral view. Post-saccal proximal occlusion (*arrow*); (**C**) DS-DCG antero-posterior view. Normal lacrimal system three months after dacryoplasty. (**D**) DS-DCG lateral view. Normal lacrimal system three months after dacryoplasty.

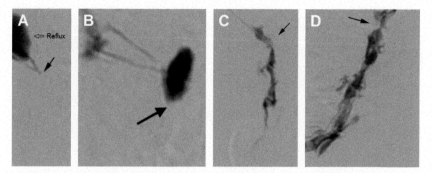

Fig. 6. Patient after failed endonasal dacryocystorhinostomy (DCR) done at an external hospital. Pre-saccal proximal occlusion of the common canaliculus with soft stop on irrigation and heavy reflux, Munk scale IV, occlusion of the anastomosis after DCR and post-saccal proximal occlusion of the nasolacrimal duct. (**A**) DS-DCG antero-posterior view. A proximal (anterior third) occlusion of the common canaliculus (*arrow*). (**B**) DS-DCG antero-posterior view. After re-opening of the common canaliculus the occlusion of the anastomosis after DCR and a proximal post-saccal occlusion can be seen (*arrow*). (**C**) DS-DCG antero-posterior view. Normal pre-saccal system and wide re-opened DCR anastomosis. The anastomosis by DCR was very low on the lacrimal sac (*arrow*). (**D**) DS-DCG lateral view. Re-opened anastomosis after failed DCR (*arrow*).

a drop of proparacaine into the eye and then place a cotton tip applicator soaked in proparacaine over the puncta for approximately 10 seconds. This will not provide complete anesthesia but helps minimize the discomfort and put the patient at ease. A 23-gauge lacrimal cannula often will go through most puncta without needing dilation, but provides more inherent resistance than a 19 gauge lacrimal cannula which commonly is available in the operating room. A small punctal dilator can be used carefully to open the puncta with a gentle twisting motion along the puncta and canalicular pathway to open the puncta wide enough to fit the cannula. A 3-cc syringe filled with 2 cc of water or saline is optimal for control of the syringe during irrigation and assessing the resistance of the lacrimal drainage system (Table 3). Occasionally, patients will find relief of epiphora from the act of syringing, possibly due to the mechanical dilation of the puncta or the hydrostatic dilation of the lacrimal drainage system. Unfortunately, this relief usually is temporary.

Imaging

The use of routine imaging for nasolacrimal duct obstruction is not common given the ability to predict the pathology based on clinical presentation and exam, however, it can be very useful when available. Computed tomography (CT) or magnetic resonance imaging (MRI) is useful when suspicion of a neoplasm, trauma, or a history of sinus disease exists, which may complicate surgical intervention. Most otolaryngologists and some ophthalmologists will perform nasal endoscopy in the office to assess. A special anterograde lacrimal endoscopy (through the canalicular system) can be performed with a small

Table 3
Irrigation results and implications

Fluid passage into the nose or throat	Possible or probable anatomical obstruction
Easy (no resistance) and immediate	None or functional obstruction
Easy with reflux through the opposite punctum	Stenosis at the common canaliculus or nasolacrimal duct
Easy with reflux through the same punctum	Stenosis or occlusion of the opposite punctum or canaliculus
Delayed without reflux	Stenosis or occlusion of the opposite punctum or canaliculus, stenosis of the nasolacrimal duct
Delayed with reflux through the opposite punctum	Stenosis of the nasolacrimal duct
Delayed with reflux through the same punctum	Stenosis or occlusion of the opposite punctum or canaliculus, stenosis of the nasolacrimal duct
None with distension of the lacrimal sac	Occlusion of the nasolacrimal duct, competent valve of Rosenmuller
None with 100% reflux from the same punctum	Occlusion of the same canaliculus
None with 100% reflux from the opposite punctum	Occlusion of the common canaliculus or nasolacrimal duct
None with 100% reflux from the opposite punctum, but positive passage once the opposite punctum is occluded	Stenosis of the nasolacrimal duct
Unable to cannulate punctum	Occlusion of the punctum, unable to assess distal lacrimal drainage system if both puncta are closed

micro-endoscope of 1.1 mm diameter in the office to provide useful information about the lacrimal system, which can detect the reason and location of the obstruction. The results of lacrimal endoscopy depend on the experience of the ophthalmologist and the resolution of the endoscope. Another diagnostic tool is the Digital-Subtraction-Dacryocystography (DS-DCG). In this procedure, a normal angiographic image (with radio-opaque contrast) is subtracted from the image without contrast. The contrast is injected through the inferior and/or superior punctum. A high-resolution image of the lacrimal system can be obtained in a less invasive technique than the micro-endoscopy, and even high-grade obstructions can be diagnosed (see Figs. 1–6). Figs. 2–6 demonstrate the diagnostics and planning for further interventions of presaccal and postsaccal obstructions, dacryoliths, filling defects, and planning for treatment in failed dacryocystorhinostomies. DS-DCG also is a good tool to diagnose fistulas.

These techniques allow for the observation of abnormalities in the tear duct such as lacrimal sac masses, diverticuli, blockages, and other anatomical abnormalities [9]. Since the endoscopy or the DS-DCG can only give information about the inside of the lacrimal system, a CT-DCG or MRI-DCG can be additionally performed to gather information about the surrounding soft tissue or bony structures to detect tumors or image the bony structures especially after trauma.

Dacryoscintigraphy (DSG) is the use of a tracer dye instilled into the cul-de-sac and followed with serial gamma camera imaging through the tear drainage system over 15–30 minutes, providing the evaluation of the dynamic flow of tears. This mostly is used in research studies and has been found to have minimal use in predicting the functional success of surgery [10].

In a 2008 survey of oculoplastic surgeons, less than 5% of respondents used any imaging to evaluate nasolacrimal duct obstruction, with CT scan being the most common type used and DSG being the least utilized [11]. The use of DSG followed by DCG or DS-DCG can provide sensitive data regarding the etiology of epiphora, however, this clinical benefit is not a major advantage over in-office evaluation of a patient with a good history, external ophthalmic and nasal examination, and the straightforward lacrimal testing noted above [12].

TREATMENT
Conservative treatment
Observation is commonly used in children with CNLDO due to the potential for spontaneous resolution of epiphora in 80 to 90% by the age of 12 months. Some adult patients also will choose observation due to a history of dry eyes and having a beneficial effect of the extra tears.

Massage of the lacrimal sac is a useful adjunct to observation in both children and adults. The hydrostatic pressure applied to a distended lacrimal sac can hasten the opening of an imperforate valve of Hasner in a child. In adults who are not interested in surgery or are poor candidates for surgery, massage can help reduce epiphora by maintaining space in the lacrimal sac available and also can reduce the risk of dacryocystitis or cellulitis by reducing the bacterial load.

Medical management of secondary causes of nasolacrimal duct obstruction is beyond the scope of this article but note that many of the secondary causes will cause complete nasolacrimal duct obstruction and require surgery to restore a patent outflow path. If a secondary cause goes undiagnosed, significant risk occurs to the patient of recurrent obstruction or worse in cases of malignancy. Topical and oral antibiotic treatment can help reduce the local inflammation related to acute and chronic dacryocystitis but will not treat the underlying obstruction.

Surgical treatment of nasolacrimal duct obstruction
Probing and irrigation of the lacrimal system is the mainstay of treatment of CNLDO. This includes the use of a lacrimal probe passed from the puncta through the entire lacrimal system into the inferior meatus. Studies show that the performance of this procedure is safe and effective in the office as well as in a facility setting with success rates of 54–100%, with the lower rates present in children older than 13 months [13].

Probing with silicone tube placement often is the second step in the treatment of CNLDO when primary probing and irrigation fails, though some will use this as a primary treatment when a child has been observed up until age 13 months. The overall success rate has been found to be similar between monocanalicular silicone tubing and bicanalicular silicone tubing at a rate of 59–100% [14–16].

Balloon catheter dilation of the lacrimal drainage system (dacryocystoplasty) is an adjunct to probing which involves the placement of a catheter that introduces an inflatable balloon into the nasolacrimal duct. The balloon then is inflated to widen the nasolacrimal duct and then is removed. This procedure can be performed with or without silicone tube placement and has been found to have an equivalent success rate to silicone tube placement in CNLDO (53–95%) [17].

Nasal endoscopy may be used in combination with probing, silicone tube intubation, and balloon catheter dilation to confirm the position of the probes in the inferior meatus and identify intranasal abnormalities that may decrease the success rate. While helpful, studies have not found an increased overall success rate with nasal endoscopy [18,19].

Acquired nasolacrimal duct obstruction also may be treated with probing and silicone tube placement or balloon dacryocystoplasty, but the success rate of either procedure is much lower in this population at 47–57% [20,21].

The author Dr. Lachmund is using an advanced minimally invasive dacryoplasty (balloon dacryocystoplasty) technique. This therapy is performed as an outpatient procedure under local anesthesia, except sometimes in children who may need light sedation. Under fluoroscopic guidance and the use of a small cannula, a flexible 0.014-inch guidewire is introduced through the superior or inferior punctum across the obstruction into the inferior meatus of the nasal cavity. In Seldinger technique, the deflated balloon catheter then is advanced antegrade over the wire to the obstruction. With water-soluble contrast medium, the balloon is then dilated. Under fluoroscopic control the result of dilation is visible immediately.

Figs. 2–6 show the diagnostic exam and treatment of lacrimal pathologies as for example presaccal obstructions (stenosis and occlusion), postsaccal obstructions (dacryoliths, stenosis, and occlusion), and therapy of failed DCR [22–24].

Another combination of minimal invasive therapies described by Javate is the use of Transcanalicular Endoscopic Lacrimal Duct Recanalization (TELDR) to recanalize the nasolacrimal duct, and then use balloon dacryocystoplasty and silicone tube placement with a success rate of 95.6% with a mean follow-up of 61 weeks [25]. TELDR is the process of using a lacrimal trephine with a microendoscope to directly visualize the lacrimal drainage system and remove obstructions. Success rates of TELDR with just silicone tube placement have been reported to be 86.2% in PANDO, with a 93.1% success rate if a focal obstruction was encountered [26]. The results of Dr. Lachmund are similar to that of the TELDR.

Dacryocystorhinostomy (DCR) is a lacrimal bypass surgery that creates a path from the lacrimal sac through the lacrimal sac fossa directly into the middle meatus. The external approach is done by creating an incision along the tear trough or the medial canthus, which provides direct visualization of the lacrimal sac fossa. The endoscopic approach is done with nasal visualization of the middle meatus and probing through the canalicular system to identify the lacrimal sac. One benefit of the endoscopic approach is that it can avoid an external scar that may also cause lagophthalmos [27]. Literature from both ophthalmic and otolaryngology surgeons show varied but statistically similar success rates of the different approaches, which are both overall in the 85–100% range in children and adults [28–31]. Transcanalicular laser-assisted DCR has been studied over the years and historically has a lower rate of success over time as noted by Kaynak and colleagues in 2014 with 85.4% initial success that decreased to 63.3% in the first year [32]. Mutlu and colleagues completed a randomized control study published in 2022 showing improved parity in outcomes of transcanalicular laser-assisted DCR to external DCR of 90% compared to 96.7% at a mean follow-up of 12.3 months [33]. It is notable that historically otolaryngologists tend to show higher success rates with endoscopic DCR, and that ophthalmologists show higher success rates with external DCR, revealing that bias occurs based on surgeon comfort and facility with the various instrumentation, and over time the outcomes improve with newer techniques. Several adjuncts to DCR exist, which have been used including antimetabolite chemical therapy to avoid scarring (5-fluorouracil and mitomycin C), though they more often are used in revision surgeries. No standard exists for the timing of silicone tube removal, although studies suggest that removal could be done within 4 weeks to avoid the formation of biofilm, which may reduce the success rate due to inflammation [34,35].

FUTURE THERAPIES

Technology continues to improve with high-resolution endoscopes and laser-based assisting devices that can improve the down time from surgery and reduce side effects such as nasal bleeding and scarring. Silicone tube material includes bicanalicular and monocanalicular silicone tubes, and recent innovations have added pushed intubation devices and self-retaining silicone tubes to the standard pulled silicone tubes. We use the term silicone tube purposefully to avoid the term "stent," which implies that a lumen for the passage of tears exists. As these instruments and devices become available and training is widespread, lacrimal surgeries will continue to be enhanced and less invasive. Of note, true lacrimal stent placements have been attempted to open nasolacrimal duct pathology in patients where a DCR cannot be performed or dacryoplasty has failed [23]. Unfortunately, the stents can become blocked or slip, but removal and replacement are simply performed when needed. Stent placement is only reserved for selected patients.

SUMMARY

Nasolacrimal duct obstruction is an issue that will commonly present to eye care providers. In patients who suffer from dacryocystitis and especially preseptal and orbital cellulitis, diagnosis and intervention are key to minimizing severe distress. Thorough history-taking can distinguish between the primary and secondary causes of nasolacrimal duct obstruction. Simple lacrimal testing during a clinical visit can effectively and efficiently evaluate the location of obstruction and direct intervention. Imaging options such as DS-DCG and DSG are uncommonly used widely due to availability but can be very helpful in conjunction with the clinical evaluation in custom tailoring surgical options as detailed by Dr. Lachmund. Treatment options have developed from external DCR to internal DCR and to more minimal invasive techniques such as dacryoplasty. Even real stent placements exist, but because of reclosure, are reserved only for few patients. Collaboration with other specialties such as industry (silicone tube design), radiology (imaging options both externally and internally), and otolaryngology (endoscopic techniques) continue to make advances in technology that strives to facilitate lacrimal surgery that makes it more efficient and less complicated.

CLINICS CARE POINTS

- When evaluating epiphora, you need to first rule out and adequately treat concurrent dry eye or ocular surface disease.
- When evaluating a child less than age 12 months, conservative management with massage of the lacrimal sac is the first line treatment due to high rates of resolution. Surgical intervention starting with probing and irrigation is indicated in an infant though if there is persistent conjunctivitis or dacryocystitis.
- Irrigation of the tear drainage can be easily done in the office to assess the presence of stenosis or obstruction in the nasolacrimal drainage system.
- Imaging with digital subtraction dacryocystography is very helpful in distinguishing the location of stenosis or obstruction and the presence of a dacryolith, which is more common in young adults with epiphora.
- Surgical intervention for nasolacrimal duct obstruction is very successful for improving tearing related to obstruction or stenosis, but it is important to recognize and treat secondary causes as epiphora may persist or recur.

CONFLICT OF INTEREST STATEMENT

The authors have no financial or other conflicts of interests to disclose.

References

[1] Sathiamoorthi S, Frank RD, Mohney BG. Incidence and clinical characteristics of congenital nasolacrimal duct obstruction. Br J Ophthalmol 2019;103(4):527–9.

[2] Woog JJ. The incidence of symptomatic acquired lacrimal outflow obstruction among residents of Olmsted County, Minnesota, 1976-2000 (an American Ophthalmological Society thesis). Trans Am Ophthalmol Soc 2007;105:649–66.

[3] Mohney BG, Sathiamoorthi S, Frank RD. Spontaneous resolution rates in congenital nasolacrimal duct obstruction managed with massage or topical antibiotics compared with observation alone. Br J Ophthalmol 2022;106(9):1196–9.

[4] Cuthbertson FM, Webber S. Assessment of functional nasolacrimal duct obstruction–a survey of ophthalmologists in the southwest. Eye 2004;18(1):20–3.

[5] Yedavalli V, Das D, Massoud TF. Eponymous "valves" of the nasolacrimal drainage apparatus. I. A historical review. Clin Anat 2019;32(1):41–5.

[6] Rajak SN, Psaltis AJ. Anatomical considerations in endoscopic lacrimal surgery. Ann Anat 2019;224:28–32.

[7] Soiberman U, Kakizaki H, Selva D, et al. Punctal stenosis: definition, diagnosis, and treatment. Clin Ophthalmol 2012;6:1011–8.

[8] Munk PL, Lin DT, Morris DC. Epiphora: treatment by means of dacryocystoplasty with balloon dilation of the nasolacrimal drainage apparatus. Radiology 1990;177(3): 687–90.

[9] Singh S, Ali MJ, Paulsen F. Dacryocystography: From theory to current practice. Ann Anat 2019;224:33–40.

[10] Kim DJ, Baek S, Chang M. Usefulness of the dacryoscintigraphy in patients with nasolacrimal duct obstruction prior to endoscopic dacryocystorhinostomy. Graefes Arch Clin Exp Ophthalmol 2019;257(7):1535–40.

[11] Nagi KS, Meyer DR. Utilization patterns for diagnostic imaging in the evaluation of epiphora due to lacrimal obstruction: a national survey. Ophthal Plast Reconstr Surg 2010;26(3):168–71.

[12] Barna S, Garai I, Kukuts K, et al. Clinical utility of SPECT/CT and CT-dacryocystography-enhanced dacryoscintigraphy in the imaging of lacrimal drainage system obstruction. Ann Nucl Med 2019;33(10):746–54.

[13] Morrison DG, Binenbaum G, Chang MY, et al. Office- or facility-based probing for congenital nasolacrimal duct obstruction: a report by the american academy of ophthalmology. Ophthalmology 2021;128(6):920–7.

[14] Pediatric Eye Disease Investigator Group. Primary treatment of nasolacrimal duct obstruction with nasolacrimal duct intubation in children younger than 4 years of age. J AAPOS 2008;12(5):445–50.

[15] Eshraghi B, Aghajani A, Kasaei A, et al. "Pushed" silicone tube intubation for treatment of complex congenital nasolacrimal duct obstruction. Eur J Ophthalmol 2014;24(5):650–4.

[16] Hamed Azzam S, Hartstein M, Dolmetsch A, et al. Assessment of Lacrijet monocanalicular intubation for congenital nasolacrimal duct obstruction. Eur J Ophthalmol 2022;32(6): 3340–5.

[17] Pediatric Eye Disease Investigator Group. Balloon catheter dilation and nasolacrimal duct intubation for treatment of nasolacrimal duct obstruction after failed probing. Arch Ophthalmol 2009;127(5):633–9.

[18] Couch SM, White WL. Endoscopically assisted balloon dacryoplasty treatment of incomplete nasolacrimal duct obstruction. Ophthalmology 2004;111(3):585–9.

[19] Gardiner JA, Forte V, Pashby RC, et al. The role of nasal endoscopy in repeat pediatric nasolacrimal duct probings. J AAPOS 2001;5:148–52.

[20] Bleyen I, van den Bosch WA, Bockholts D, et al. Silicone intubation with or without balloon dacryocystoplasty in acquired partial nasolacrimal duct obstruction. Am J Ophthalmol 2007;144(5):776–80.

[21] Bleyen I, Paridaens AD. Bicanalicular silicone intubation in acquired partial nasolacrimal duct obstruction. Bull Soc Belge Ophtalmol 2008;23–6, 309-310.

[22] Lachmund U, Ammann-Rauch D, Forrer A, et al. Balloon catheter dilatation of common canaliculus stenoses. Orbit 2005;24(3):177–83.

[23] Lachmund U, Wilhelm K, Remonda L, et al. Interventionelle radiologische Therapie der Tränenwege. Klin Neuroradiol 2005;15:50–61.

[24] Lachmund U, Wilhelm K. Diagnostic and therapeutic interventional radiology of the lacrimal system. In: Ali M, editor. Principles and practice of lacrimal surgery. Singapore: Springer; 2018; https://doi.org/10.1007/978-981-10-5442-6_34.

[25] Javate RM. Optimizing clinical outcomes for endoscopic lacrimal duct recanalization in patients with complete PANDO. Int Ophthalmol 2022; https://doi.org/10.1007/s10792-022-02414-2.

[26] Lee SM, Lew H. Transcanalicular endoscopic dacryoplasty in patients with primary acquired nasolacrimal duct obstruction. Graefes Arch Clin Exp Ophthalmol 2021;259(1): 173–80.

[27] Haefliger IO, Meienberg O, Pimentel de Figueiredo AR. Temporary medial upper eyelid lagophthalmos after external dacryocystorhinostomy. Klin Monbl Augenheilkd 2016;233(4): 406–8, English.

[28] Su PY. Comparison of endoscopic and external dacryocystorhinostomy for treatment of primary acquired nasolacrimal duct obstruction. Taiwan J Ophthalmol 2018;8(1):19–23.

[29] Karasu B, Kiray G, Eris E, et al. Comparison of success between external and endonasal dacryocystorhinostomy in primary acquired nasolacrimal duct obstruction in Turkish cohort. North Clin Istanb 2020;7(6):579–84.

[30] Wong WK, Dean S, Nair S. Comparison between endoscopic and external dacryocystorhinostomy by using the lacrimal symptom questionnaire: a pilot study. Am J Rhinol Allergy 2018;32(1):46–51.

[31] Sobel RK, Aakalu VK, Wladis EJ, et al. A comparison of endonasal dacryocystorhinostomy and external dacryocystorhinostomy: a report by the american academy of ophthalmology. Ophthalmology 2019;126(11):1580–5.

[32] Kaynak P, Ozturker C, Yazgan S, et al. Transcanalicular diode laser assisted dacryocystorhinostomy in primary acquired nasolacrimal duct obstruction: 2-year follow up. Ophthal Plast Reconstr Surg 2014;30(1):28–33.

[33] Mutlu D, Bayram N, Arici MK, et al. Comparison of outcomes of external dacryocystorhinostomy and transcanalicular laser-assisted dacryocystorhinostomy in patients with primary acquired nasolacrimal duct obstruction. Klin Monbl Augenheilkd 2022;239(6):799–803, English.

[34] Bispo PJ, Haas W, Gilmore MS. Biofilms in infections of the eye. Pathogens 2015 Mar 23;4(1):111–36.

[35] Ali MJ. Lacrimal Stents and Biofilms. In: Atlas of lacrimal drainage disorders. Singapore: Springer; 2018; https://doi.org/10.1007/978-981-10-5616-1_62.

Uveitis

Advances in Ophthalmology and Optometry 8 (2023) 375–394

ADVANCES IN OPHTHALMOLOGY AND OPTOMETRY

Multimodal Imaging in Infectious Uveitis

Maura Di Nicola, MD*, Pooja Bhat, MD,
Ann-Marie Lobo-Chan, MD, MS

Department of Ophthalmology and Visual Sciences, University of Illinois at Chicago, 1009 South Wood Street, Chicago, IL 60612, USA

Keywords

- Acute retinal necrosis • Fluorescein angiography • Fundus photography
- Infectious uveitis • Multimodal imaging • Optical coherence tomography
- Syphilis • Toxoplasmosis

Key points

- A number of infectious processes can cause intraocular inflammation affecting virtually every structure of the eye.
- Clinical diagnosis of infectious uveitis can sometimes be challenging.
- The use of multimodal imaging (fundus photography, fundus autofluorescence, fluorescein/indocyanine green angiography, optical coherence tomography, optical coherence tomography angiography, and ultrasonography) can aid the ophthalmologist in distinguishing the underlying infectious cause.
- Certain imaging modalities have been helpful in elucidating the pathogenetic mechanisms of ocular infections.
- Multimodal imaging also can aid in monitoring disease progression and response to treatment.

INTRODUCTION

Diagnosis of infectious uveitis has historically been achieved through clinical examination and laboratory testing. Although some of the most common infectious causes of uveitis, including viruses, bacteria, and protozoa, present with typical ophthalmoscopic findings, other conditions may have more subtle findings, creating diagnostic dilemmas. Multimodal imaging uses a combination of

*Corresponding author. 900 Northwest 17th Street, Suite 266A, Miami, FL 33136. E-mail address: mauradinicola@gmail.com

https://doi.org/10.1016/j.yaoo.2023.02.017
2452-1760/23/© 2023 Elsevier Inc. All rights reserved.

different imaging modalities to aid the ophthalmologist in the diagnosis, management, and follow-up of both typical and atypical presentations of infectious uveitis. This article will focus on the use of fundus photography (FP), fundus autofluorescence (FAF), fluorescein angiography (FA), indocyanine green angiography (ICGA), optical coherence tomography (OCT), optical coherence tomography angiography (OCTA), and ultrasonography in the context of the most common causes of infectious uveitis.

HUMAN HERPESVIRUSES

Human herpesvirus infection can cause intraocular inflammation that affects virtually every part of the eye. Multimodal imaging is particularly helpful in the diagnosis, documentation, and management of posterior uveitis secondary to the most commonly involved herpesviruses, including herpes simplex virus 1 and 2 (HSV-1 and HSV-2), varicella zoster virus (VZV), and cytomegalovirus (CMV).

Acute retinal necrosis (ARN) is a sight-threatening emergency, most commonly secondary to VZV, HSV-1 or HSV-2 infection, with an incidence of 0.63 cases per million per year [1]. It is characterized by unifocal or multifocal peripheral foci of retinal necrosis with discrete borders, rapid, circumferential progression in the absence of treatment, evidence of occlusive vasculopathy with arteriolar involvement, and prominent inflammation in the anterior chamber and vitreous [2]. Optic neuritis or optic atrophy, scleritis, and pain can be variably present [2]. Progressive outer retinal necrosis (PORN) is a highly destructive and rapidly progressive variant of ARN, which occurs in immunocompromised patients with very low CD4+ counts and is caused by VZV [3]. In PORN, patches of necrotizing retinitis initially involve the outer retina and present at the posterior pole. As the disease progresses, the patches of retinitis rapidly coalesce and spread to the peripheral retina, with full thickness retinal necrosis. Anterior chamber and vitreous inflammation are absent or minimal given the immunocompromised state [3,4]. CMV retinitis also typically occurs in immunocompromised patients, especially in individuals with a CD4+ count less than 50 cells/μL [5]. Clinical features include necrotizing hemorrhagic peripheral retinitis with a perivascular distribution and centrifugal progression, vasculitis, and only mild anterior chamber inflammation and minimal vitritis [4,5]. The most feared complication of viral retinitis is retinal detachment, which usually occurs secondary to retinal breaks at the border of retinal necrosis [4,5].

Fundus photography and fundus autofluorescence

Wide-field FP is extremely helpful in the context of viral retinitis to determine the extent of the disease, monitor its progression, and document response to therapy. Ultra-wide-field imaging (UWFI) can capture 200° of the retina in a single image, as opposed to conventional fundus cameras, which have a field capacity of 30° or 50°. In the context of ARN, UWFI especially is useful for detecting peripheral retinal lesions through opaque media (Fig. 1A) [6,7].

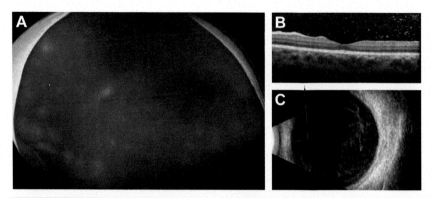

Fig. 1. Wide-field fundus photography in a case of acute retinal necrosis shows hazy media and multifocal patches of peripheral retinal whitening (A). OCT demonstrates the presence of hyperreflective foci in the vitreous, secondary to inflammation (B). Ultrasonography confirms the presence of dense vitritis (C).

UWFI helps to document and monitor the shape, extent, and location of the necrotic lesions [6]. UWFI also can be used to detect and document necrotic retinal breaks, which can lead to retinal detachment [7]. The use of digital FP and UWFI has been investigated in the screening for CMV retinitis (Fig. 2A) and might be particularly helpful in human immunodeficiency virus (HIV) patients who lack access to ophthalmological care [8].

FAF is a noninvasive imaging modality used to map fluorophores distribution to detect the health of the retinal pigment epithelium (RPE). It has been used to help delineate the extent of retinal necrosis in ARN, with areas of retinitis appearing hypoautofluorescent with well-defined hyperautofluorescent borders [9]. In PORN, it has been used to document various stages of the disease [10]. Early in the course of the disease, discrete areas of outer retinal opacification appear hypoautofluorescent, whereas stippled areas of hypoautofluorescence and hyperautofluorescence are seen as the retinitis resolves [10]. FAF is particularly helpful in detecting areas of active CMV retinitis and possible recurrence, with hyperautofluorescence typically seen at the border of active, advancing retinitis (Fig. 2B) [11,12].

Fluorescein angiography and indocyanine green angiography

FA and indocyanine green angiography (ICGA) are imaging modalities that assess the retinal and choroidal vasculature after the intravenous injection of a dye. Several angiographic patterns have been described in the context of viral retinitis. ARN can present with obliterative necrotizing vasculitis, areas of retinal nonperfusion, and variable amounts of vascular inflammation and leakage [13,14]. If optic nerve inflammation is present, FA demonstrates late leakage and staining [15]. Active areas of confluent retinitis in PORN demonstrate leakage on FA [16]. Active CMV lesions demonstrate early and late

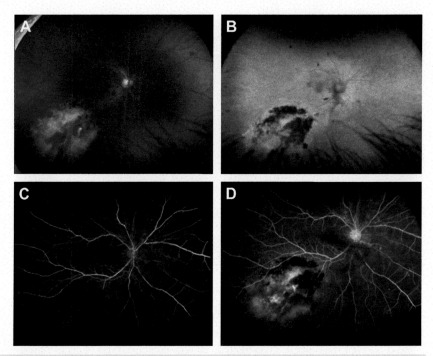

Fig. 2. Wide-field fundus photography demonstrating cytomegalovirus retinitis in the infero-temporal midperiphery (A). Autofluorescence shows corresponding hypoautofluoresence with a surrounding hyperautofluorescent rim (B). Fluorescein angiography demonstrates early hypofluorescence (C) with some late leakage (D).

hypofluorescence on FA (Fig. 2C,D) [17]. Frosted-branch angiitis associated with CMV retinitis demonstrates early perivascular hypofluorescence, corresponding to the yellow material seen clinically and on FP, and late vascular staining [13,18].

Optical coherence tomography and optical coherence tomography angiography

OCT is a noninvasive imaging technique that renders an in vivo cross-sectional view of the retina. In the acute phase of ARN, high reflectivity of the inner retina has been described in areas of retinitis [19,20]. With the progression of the disease, full thickness involvement with disorganization and loss of normal retinal architecture is observed [20]. Significant hyperreflectivity of the vitreous cavity also can be present, secondary to inflammation (Fig. 1B) [21]. Associated findings documented on OCT include subretinal fluid and cystoid macular edema [19]. Significant retinal thinning and hyperreflectivity is observed after resolution of the acute lesions. OCT can help in detecting retinal breaks and subsequent detachment, which usually occur at the margin of retinal necrosis [20,21]. The choroid underlying the area of retinal necrosis may present only minimal alteration of the choriocapillaris, or can seem slightly thickened on enhanced-depth imaging-OCT [21,22]. OCT findings in the early phases of PORN include edema and hyporeflectivity of the outer retina, likely due to shadowing from the hyperreflective, thickened inner retinal layers [23,24]. Because the disease progresses, full-thickness involvement of the retina, total loss of retinal layers, and subsequent retinal thinning occur, similarly to ARN [23,24]. CMV retinitis demonstrates a similar OCT pattern, with initial disorganization and subsequent atrophy of the affected retina [21,25,26].

OCTA has emerged as a noninvasive technique to visualize the microvasculature of the retina and choroid without the need for intravenous dye injection. Introduction of OCTA has allowed characterization of macular microvascular abnormalities in eyes with viral retinitis without macular involvement on clinical examination or OCT. Vascular density at the level of both the superficial and deep capillary plexus was decreased in a case of ARN, with an improvement of vascular density after treatment [27]. Similar findings were observed in eyes with CMV retinitis, with persistent decreased macular vascular density after 12 months [28]. Given the limited number of cases reported in the literature, the clinical significance of these OCTA findings has yet to be determined.

Ultrasonography
B-scan ultrasonography in the context of ARN highlights vitreous inflammation (Fig. 1C). It can also be particularly useful to detect retinal detachment in cases with dense vitreous opacity.

SYPHILIS
Syphilis is an infectious disease caused by *Treponema pallidum*, with an estimated incidence of 10 to 12 million new cases per year worldwide and a resurgence in recent years [29,30]. The association between HIV and syphilis coinfection is well known, with syphilis increasing the risk of contracting HIV infection, and HIV modifying the course of syphilitic disease and increasing progression to neurosyphilis [30]. The disease can affect different organ systems and potentially every structure in the eye, leading to conjunctivitis, interstitial keratitis, scleritis, chorioretinitis, neuroretinitis, and/or retinal vasculitis [31]. Ocular involvement most commonly occurs in the secondary and tertiary stages but it can occur at any point during the course of the disease [32].

Fundus photography and fundus autofluorescence
Posterior uveitis is the most common manifestation of ocular syphilis [33]. Both FP and FAF are helpful in documenting and monitoring its numerous findings. Acute syphilitic posterior placoid chorioretinitis (ASPPC) presents as a yellowish, placoid area at the level of the outer retina involving the posterior pole (Fig. 3A, E) [34]. In syphilitic retinitis, areas of active retinochoroiditis appear as white, often wedge-shaped patches with variable degrees of vitritis on FP [33]. The presence of "ground glass" retinitis with creamy, round, yellow superficial retinal precipitates helps differentiate syphilis from other causes of necrotizing retinitis [35]. FP is helpful in monitoring response to treatment

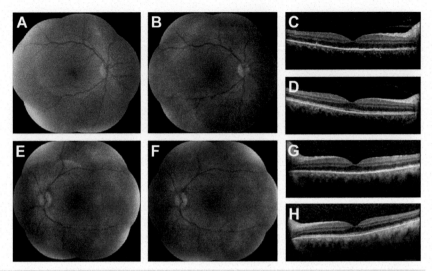

Fig. 3. Montage fundus photography demonstrating yellowish, placoid areas involving the posterior pole, secondary to syphilis (*A, E*). OCT shows the disruption of the ellipsoid zone and granular irregularities at the level of the RPE (*C, G*). The placoid areas are completely resolved after antibiotic therapy (*B, F*), with reconstitution of the outer retinal layers (*D, H*).

because these findings resolve after appropriate antibiotic therapy with penicillin G (Fig. 3B, F) [35]. Similarly, cicatricial changes can be seen and documented after treatment and resolution of the acute phase, with possible RPE mottling, hyperplasia, and retinal fibrosis. Optic nerve hyperemia, edema with blurring of the margins, and atrophy with pallor all can be seen throughout the course of the disease and documented on FP [31,36].

In ASPPC, FAF helps to clearly delineate the affected placoid area, which can be subtle on clinical examination or FP, as it appears as a hyperautofluorescent geographic area with punctate areas of both increased and decreased autofluorescence within it [34,37].

Fluorescein angiography and indocyanine green angiography

FA is helpful in determining the extent of inflammation of the posterior segment. Subtle vasculitis may not be appreciated clinically but vascular leakage and staining can be seen on FA [38]. Inflammatory vascular occlusion and subsequent retinal ischemia also can be appreciated on FA. Patches of retinitis seem hypofluorescent, with leakage at the margins and possible overlying hypofluorescent spots corresponding to the preretinal precipitates seen with this phenotype [33]. The level of optic nerve inflammation can also be documented on FA, with late leakage and staining [38].

On FA, ASPPC demonstrates a typical pattern with early hypofluorescence and progressive late hyperfluorescence corresponding to the placoid yellowish area seen clinically and on FP [34,37,39]. The same placoid area demonstrates variable hypofluorescence in both the early and intermediate/late phases of ICGA, likely due to possible choriocapillaris hypoperfusion or blockage from the overlying infected RPE [37,39]. This determines a characteristic FA-ICGA dissociation of the placoid areas in the late phase [37].

Optical coherence tomography and optical coherence tomography angiography

OCT findings of ASPPC include disruption and loss of the ellipsoid zone with subsequent granular irregularities at the level of the RPE (Fig. 3C, G), and punctate hyperreflectivity of the choroid [39]. Retinal abnormalities completely resolve after appropriate antibiotic treatment in the vast majority of patients (Fig. 3D, H) [39]. OCT also is helpful in distinguishing multifocal retinitis from superficial preretinal deposits seen with confluent retinochoroiditis [40]. The latter seem as hyperreflective circular deposits on the retinal surface, whereas in multifocal retinitis, OCT demonstrates the intraretinal location of the hyperreflective infiltrates [33,40].

Most recently, several findings on OCTA have been described in the context of ASPPC, including flow voids at the level of the chori ocapillaris, which normalize after treatment, suggesting a possible pathogenic role of choriocapillaris inflammation in the disease process [41,42].

TOXOPLASMOSIS

Toxoplasmosis is the most common cause of infectious posterior uveitis in the United States, where the prevalence of ocular toxoplasmosis ranges from 0.6% to 2% [43]. Serologic evidence of toxoplasmosis is found in 15% to 30% of the population in the United States and up to 70% of individuals in other countries [43]. Clinically, toxoplasmosis presents as a necrotizing retinochoroiditis, accompanied by vitritis and anterior chamber inflammation [44].

Fundus photography and fundus autofluorescence

Active toxoplasmosis retinochoroiditis usually presents as a white inflammatory focus orginating from the border of a pigmented scar (Fig. 4A). Acute or new lesions appear as white areas with overlying vitreous inflammation, giving the classic "headlight in a fog" appearance that can be documented on FP [45]. Atypical presentations include neuroretinitis, papillitis and multifocal, punctate lesions termed punctate outer retinal toxoplasmosis in some immunocompetent patients [45]. Although anterior chamber and vitreous inflammation can obscure visualization of active lesions and previous scars, FP still provides a useful way to monitor treatment response. Serial photographs should demonstrate a decrease in vitritis, sharpening of the lesion borders, and increased pigmentation of the lesions (Fig. 4E) [46]. Additionally, FP is capable of documenting findings that may be difficult to identify clinically like segmental retinal arteritis, previously called Kyrieleis arteritis [47].

Blue-light FAF has a unique pattern when active lesions regress to resultant scars [45]. Active lesions have subtle hyperautofluorescence or isoautofluorescence and become more hyperautofluorescent with a hypoautofluorescent

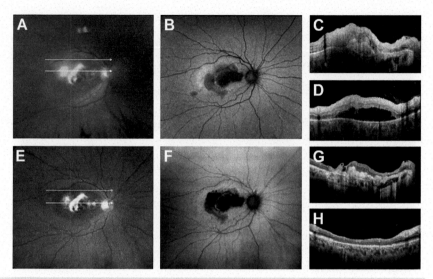

Fig. 4. Fundus photography showing an ill-defined focus of active toxoplasmosis superotemporal to a pigmented scar with some vitreous haze (A). The active area seems hyperautofluorescent (B). OCT demonstrates a full-thickness lesion (C, corresponding to *white arrow* on A), with an adjacent exudative detachment (D, corresponding to *green arrow* on A). After treatment, the area appears well-defined and pigmented, with resolution of vitreous haze (E), and complete hypoautofluorescence (F). OCT shows retinochoroidal atrophy (G, corresponding to *white arrow* on E), and resolution of subretinal fluid (H, corresponding to green *arrow* on E).

rim over time (Fig. 4B). Eventually, the hypoautofluorescent rim progresses centripetally until a complete absence of autofluorescence occurs in clinically healed lesions (Fig. 4F) [45].

Fluorescein angiography and indocyanine green angiography

Active toxoplasmosis lesions demonstrate early hypofluorescence centrally with leakage at the margin of the lesion that progresses toward the center on FA [48]. Additional angiographic features include optic nerve and blood vessel leakage, retinochoroidal vascular anastomosis, and leakage from choroidal neovascular membranes [45]. FA has also been used to assess segmental retinal arteritis, which demonstrates early hypofluorescence and intermediate hyperfluorescence. This is notable in comparison to vascular sheathing or frosted branch angiitis, which involve both arteries and veins with full-thickness vessel inflammation and subsequent extensive leakage [47].

ICGA in toxoplasmosis primarily is helpful in documenting inflammatory infiltration of the choroid. This causes blockage of choroidal perfusion and subsequent focal hypofluorescence that seems more extensive than the overlying retinal lesion [45,48]. Diffuse hypofluorescent choroidal dots may be seen during active inflammation, and these areas resolve with resolution of inflammation with or without treatment.

Optical coherence tomography and optical coherence tomography angiography

Typical OCT findings of toxoplasmosis include full-thickness, hyperreflective retinal lesions, denser in the inner retinal layers, with posterior shadowing and some blurring of the retinal layers (Fig. 4C) [46]. In cases of active toxoplasmosis with vitritis, OCT shows hyperreflective fine dots over the retinal surface [46]. Chorioretinal lesions may be accompanied by a serous retinal detachment, which can be detected on OCT (Fig. 4D) [46]. The choroid may demonstrate focal hyporeflectivity, thickening, and obscuration of details [22,46]. OCT in patients with inactive lesions may demonstrate residual vitritis; scar formation is documented by retinal atrophy, hypertrophy, or a combination of the two (Fig. 4G, H). The RPE often is thickened and hyperreflective, and the choroid seems thin with indistinguishable vascular structures [46]. When patients present with punctate outer retinal toxoplasmosis, OCT reveals RPE-choriocapillaris changes with retinal infiltrates in the deep retinal layers [45]. OCT also can be used to localize segmental retinal arteritis, which demonstrates hyperreflectivity of the vessel wall with a narrow but otherwise normoreflective lumen [49].

In the context of acute retinochoroiditis, retinal infiltration demonstrates vascular attenuation on OCTA, with focal hypoperfusion of the underlying choriocapillaris [45]. The vascular damage to the choriocapillaris progressively decreases during the healing phase, resulting in focal areas of vascular dropout [45,50]. OCTA through retinal arterioles with segmental arteritis demonstrate a narrowed intraluminal flow signal, which may persist even after successful treatment [47,49].

TUBERCULOSIS

Around one-third of the world's population has been infected by *Mycobacterium tuberculosis*, with the highest incidence rates of active tuberculosis in Africa, Southeast Asia, and India [51]. The overall case rate of active tuberculosis in the United States is around 3 per 100,000 persons, with foreign-born individuals representing the majority of cases [51]. Among patients with active tuberculosis, the reported prevalence of intraocular involvement varies widely from 1% (in patients with the pulmonary form) to more than 20% (in patients with extrapulmonary involvement) [52]. When causing intraocular inflammation, tuberculosis may present as anterior, intermediate, posterior, or panuveitis and usually is granulomatous in nature [52]. Given the myriad of presentations of intraocular tuberculosis, multimodal imaging may be particularly helpful in differentiating intraocular tuberculosis from simulating conditions, including sarcoidosis, Vogt-Koyanagi-Harada disease, sympathetic ophthalmia, and other causes of granulomatous uveitis.

Fundus photography and fundus autofluorescence

FP is useful to document the variety of posterior segment presentations that can be seen clinically in ocular tuberculosis including retinal vasculitis, multifocal choroiditis, choroidal tubercles (multiple ill-defined deep lesions), tuberculomas (large usually unilateral elevated masses), and serpiginous-like choroiditis (Fig. 5A) [53].

FAF often has been used in posterior uveitis as a noninvasive way to characterize disease activity. In limited reports, FAF of tuberculomas demonstrates hyperautofluorescence with central hypoautofluorescence, with ultimate isoautofluorescence as the disease resolves [54]. Autofluorescence of tubercular serpiginous-like choroiditis is better defined because inactive lesions appear hypoautofluorescent; however, lesions that have reactivated at the margin will demonstrate hyperautofluorescent borders (Fig. 5B) [55].

Fluorescein angiography and indocyanine green angiography

FA is useful to assess the retina, choroid, and optic nerve involvement, as well as differentiating active from inactive disease and monitoring response to treatment. Active tubercles demonstrate early hypofluorescence and late hyperfluorescence [53], whereas inactive lesions show transmission hyperfluorescence [56]. This pattern is similar for active tuberculomas and focal choroiditis. Tubercular serpiginous-like choroiditis also shows initial hypofluorescence with diffuse staining of the active edge. In contrast, inactive lesions have peripheral hyperfluorescence with central hypofluorescence (Fig. 5C, D). The retinal vessels, predominantly veins, may demonstrate leakage during active vasculitis, and the optic nerve may demonstrate leakage.

Given that tuberculosis uveitis often affects the choroid, ICGA is a particularly useful imaging modality. Partial thickness choroidal tuberculomas are primarily hypofluorescent early and isofluorescent late. Full thickness choroidal lesions remain hypofluorescent throughout the duration of the test, and the vast majority of tuberculomas are full thickness [53]. ICGA shows similar early and late hypofluorescent findings in tubercular serpiginous-like choroiditis, and when healed, ICGA shows a well-delineated atrophic choroid [56].

Optical coherence tomography and optical coherence tomography angiography

On OCT, tuberculomas appear as round or oval hyporeflective and homogenous lesions that may have full thickness choroidal involvement, often with associated subretinal fluid [53]. In active tubercular serpiginous-like choroiditis, OCT can show a "double-layer" sign, where disruption of the external limiting membrane and ellipsoid zone results in a gap between Bruch membrane and hyperreflective RPE [57]. The underlying choroid may demonstrate thickening and infiltration with mixed reflectivity [58]. These areas correspond with hyperautofluorescent areas on FAF. As the disease resolves, the double layer sign regresses and is replaced by irregular, hyperreflective elevations of the outer retina, corresponding with hypoautofluorescence (Fig. 5E) [57]. The localized region of choroiditis results in choroidal fibrosis and thinning with the resolution of disease in comparison to the remaining choroid, which returns to normal thickness [58].

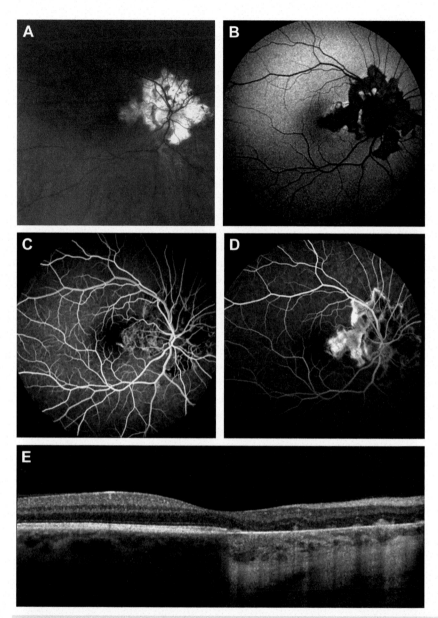

Fig. 5. Fundus photography demonstrating serpiginous-like tubercular chorioretinitis (*A*). The lesion appears hypoautofluorescent, with minimal hyperautofluorescence along the temporal border (*B*). Fluorescein angiography shows early hypo/isofluorescence (*C*) with late hyperfluorescence (*D*). OCT demonstrates atrophy of the outer retinal layers and hyperreflective elevations with partial sparing of the fovea (*E*).

OCTA of choroidal granulomas shows flow void lesions, some of which may not be detectable on ICGA [59]. Similarly, in cases of tubercular serpiginous-like choroiditis, OCTA reveals localized loss of choriocapillaris blood flow that is not apparent on conventional angiography [60]. OCTA is even more helpful in those cases that have an associated choroidal neovascular membrane not clearly defined on ICGA [61].

BARTONELLOSIS

Cat-scratch disease is a zoonosis mainly caused by *Bartonella henselae*, which typically presents with regional lymphadenopathy, fever, and malaise with other constitutional symptoms; ocular bartonellosis occurs in 5% to 10% of patients with cat-scratch disease [62,63]. The disease most commonly occurs in patients aged younger than 20 years and is transmitted from the scratch or bite of an infected cat, which causes a nonpruritic papule or pustule that resolves without scarring [63]. Common ocular manifestations include Parinaud oculoglandular syndrome (unilateral granulomatous conjunctivitis associated with regional lymphadenopathy), neuroretinitis, focal or multifocal retinochoroiditis, vascular occlusions, macular edema, exudative retinal detachment, vitritis, and choroidal and optic nerve granulomas [63,64].

Fundus photography and fundus autofluorescence

The most typical sign of ocular bartonellosis, although not pathognomonic, is neuroretinitis, which is characterized by optic nerve edema and peripapillary exudation, followed by macular star formation [65]. FP is helpful in documenting the evolution of this condition. The acute stages are characterized by a swollen optic nerve with surrounding exudative detachment often involving the macula. Later in the course of the disease and with appropriate treatment, optic nerve edema resolves, variably causing residual optic nerve pallor and atrophy; radial or stellate lipid precipitates appear in the macula [66,67]. Isolated or multiple foci of retinochoroiditis are easily seen and documented on FP and appear as discrete areas of retinal whitening [65]. UWFI can help in detecting peripheral granulomas, which have been rarely reported in ocular bartonellosis [64,65].

FAF is helpful in clearly delineating the extent of macular star exudates, which are located in the outer plexiform layer, and therefore appear hypoautofluorescent secondary to blockage of the underlying RPE [68].

Fluorescein angiography and indocyanine green angiography

In the early stages of neuroretinitis, FA demonstrates diffuse or sectoral leakage of the inflamed optic nerve and pooling of the associated macular detachment. Hyperfluorescence of the optic nerve also can be secondary to the presence of angiomatous lesions or staining due to residual fibrosis after resolution of optic nerve edema [65]. Vascular occlusion has been described in ocular bartonellosis [64,65]. Discrete areas of retinitis can demonstrate early blockage and late staining on FA [65]. Choroidal ischemia characterized by hypofluorescence along watershed zones has been reported [69].

ICGA is not routinely used in the diagnosis and management of ocular bartonellosis but it can demonstrate areas of hyperfluorescence, corresponding to regions of choroiditis [65].

Optical coherence tomography and optical coherence tomography angiography

In patients with neuroretinitis, OCT shows variable amounts of intraretinal and subretinal fluid with retinal thickening and loss of foveal contour [70]. The primary inflammatory process is thought to originate in the disc microvasculature, with subsequent exudation of fluid through the outer plexiform layer. Because the fluid gets reabsorbed, the residual lipid exudates appear as hyperreflective foci in the outer plexiform layer on OCT and resolve in 2 to 4 weeks on average [65,70]. OCT through areas of discrete retinitis demonstrates highly reflective inner retinal lesions with masking of the underlying outer retina and choroid. Resolved areas of retinitis demonstrate decreased reflectivity and persistent disorganization of the inner retinal layers [71]. Intrinsic vascularity of focal retinitis has been demonstrated at the level of the deep capillary plexus on OCTA [71].

TOXOCARIASIS

Toxocariasis is a helminthic infection most commonly caused by *Toxocara canis*, which mainly affects children [72]. Patients with systemic disease rarely demonstrate concomitant ocular involvement. Ocular toxocariasis accounts for only 1% of all uveitis cases in the United States. Clinically, ocular involvement is predominantly unilateral and findings have been classified into 4 types including peripheral granuloma, posterior pole granuloma, chronic endophthalmitis, and mixed type [73]. Multimodal imaging can be particularly helpful in differentiating ocular toxocariasis from simulating conditions including retinoblastoma, Coats disease, and other causes of uveitis or endophthalmitis.

Fundus photography and fundus autofluorescence

FP documents the findings seen on clinical examination and can be used to monitor signs of progression, especially in patients without significant inflammation. FP in the peripheral granuloma form demonstrates a white inflammatory mass in the retinal periphery, often associated with a traction induced retinal fold that connects the lesion with the optic nerve. UWFI may be required in some patients with the peripheral granuloma type, depending on how anterior the lesion is [74,75]. The posterior pole granuloma form presents with a retinal or subretinal mass in the posterior pole that may have wrinkling of the internal limiting membrane and tractional bands to the surrounding retina [73]. Given that toxocariasis often affects the pediatric population, clinical examination can be difficult, highlighting the value of ancillary imaging such as UWFI. In addition to the characteristic presentations, some patients may display scattered small, yellow/white lesions presumed to be microgranulomas [76].

Fluorescein angiography and indocyanine green angiography

FA in the context of toxocariasis may reveal hyperfluorescent lesions, along with leakage of small-sized and medium-sized veins, suggesting increased vascular permeability [76,77]. The optic disc may be hyperfluorescent [77]. Rarely, choroidal neovascularization may develop secondary to ocular toxocariasis [78]. ICGA is not frequently used in the diagnosis or management of this condition because toxocariasis does not present with choroidal involvement.

Optical coherence tomography and optical coherence tomography angiography

OCT analysis of ocular toxocariasis may reveal multiple presentations including hyperreflective lesions in various locations, including subretinal, outer retinal, on the retinal surface, or in the vitreous cavity [76,77,79]. Lesions tend to have well-demarcated borders [77,79], and the retina overlying the lesion or in the macula may demonstrate preretinal membranes and traction along the vitreoretinal interface [80]. The utility of OCTA in patients with toxocariasis remains unknown because the findings have yet to be well described.

Ultrasonography

B-scan ultrasonography highlights vitreous membranes and bands [76] and can document the presence of an exudative retinal detachment [81]. When tractional detachments result from an underlying granuloma, ultrasound may document cases that are more challenging to see clinically due to vitreous inflammation. Granulomas may appear as a medium-reflectivity mass, and calcification may be seen in eyes with significant ocular disruption or phthisis [73].

EMERGING VIRUSES

Infection with several emerging viruses has been associated with varying degrees of intraocular inflammation and diverse ocular manifestations. Multimodal imaging can be helpful in the differential diagnosis and monitoring of these rarer conditions.

West Nile virus (WNV) is transmitted by infected mosquitos and can be found in several parts of the world, including North America, Europe, Africa, Asia, and Australia. Infected individuals often present with a mild, self-limited febrile illness [82]. However, posterior uveitis often is associated with meningoencephalitis, hence patients with visual symptoms may present with more severe constitutional symptoms [83]. FP is used to document and monitor posterior segment manifestations, including chorioretinitis, which is often bilateral and presents with typical curvilinear clustering of yellow-white creamy lesions following the retinal nerve fiber layer course [84]. FA is helpful in distinguishing active from inactive chorioretinal lesions, with active lesions demonstrating early hypofluorescence with late staining, and inactive lesions demonstrating central hypofluorescence with peripheral ring-like hyperfluorescence [85–87]. Similarly, chorioretinal lesions appear hypofluorescent on ICGA and may be more numerous than those appreciated clinically [86,88]. On

OCT, several abnormalities in the outer retina and RPE have been reported, including granular hyperreflective specks located in the inner and outer nuclear layers in active lesions, and atrophy in inactive lesions [87,89]. Most recently, OCTA has demonstrated vascular attenuation in the superficial and deep capillary plexus in the context of WNV-associated occlusive vasculitis [90].

Zika virus infection is mostly transmitted by mosquitoes but sexual, vertical, perinatal, and breast milk transmission also have been described [91]. The most recent epidemic was reported in Brazil starting in 2015. Acquired infection often is asymptomatic or oligosymptomatic, whereas congenital infection is associated with microcephaly and vision-threatening ocular lesions in up to 30% of infants [91,92]. The most common ocular manifestations include macular pigment mottling, pigmentary clumping, atrophic chorioretinal lesions often involving the macula and the posterior pole, and optic nerve hypoplasia [92]. Wide-field FP is helpful in documenting and monitoring the extent of these lesions. On FA, window defects are seen corresponding to the areas of chorioretinal atrophy. However, FA also is helpful in demonstrating abnormalities not seen clinically or on FP, including window defects at the posterior pole and peripheral avascularity of the retina [93]. Chorioretinal lesions demonstrate several abnormalities on OCT including discontinuation of the ellipsoid zone, retinal and choroidal thinning, and coloboma-like excavation of the neurosensory retina, RPE, and choroid [94].

Ebola virus disease presents as a severe hemorrhagic fever with a high-mortality rate. The most recent epidemic started in West Africa in 2013. Hypertensive uveitis has been described among other ocular sequelae of the disease, leading to progressive visual loss in up to 20% of convalescent patients [4]. Chorioretinal lesions associated with Ebola virus usually are nonpigmented, pale gray, and tend to respect the horizontal raphe, with curvilinear peripapillary lesions following the retinal nerve fiber layer projections [95]. FP is helpful in documenting the extent and distribution of chorioretinal lesions. On OCT, small retinal lesions demonstrate discontinuity of the ellipsoid and interdigitation zones with overlying hyperreflectivity of the outer nuclear layer, whereas larger lesions demonstrate retinal thinning with the loss of retinal layers [95]. Perilesional areas of dark without pressure, demonstrating a thinned hyporeflective ellipsoid zone and an absent interdigitation zone on OCT, have also been described [95].

The ongoing coronavirus disease 2019 (COVID-19) pandemic caused by severe acute respiratory syndrome coronavirus 2 has gained attention from the international medical community since the first cases of atypical pneumonia were reported in China in 2019. The severity of COVID-19 clinical manifestations is variable, ranging from mild flu-like symptoms to severe respiratory syndrome that can lead to hospitalization and death. Asymptomatic cases also are common. Since the beginning of the pandemic, numerous ocular manifestations have been reported in the literature including conjunctivitis, episcleritis, uveitis, retinal vascular abnormalities and occlusions, and optic neuritis [96–98]. Multimodal imaging can be particularly helpful in documenting the retinal manifestations of COVID-19. FP demonstrates retinal hemorrhages, cotton wool spots, and dilated tortuous vessels [98,99]. When present, retinal vascular occlusions can be demonstrated on FA [96]. Microvasculopathy associated with COVID-19 has been demonstrated on OCTA, with reduced vessel density and enlarged foveal avascular zone in infected subjects compared with healthy subjects [97].

SUMMARY
Numerous infectious processes can involve the eye, with potentially catastrophic consequences for vision. The combination of several imaging modalities including FP, autofluorescence, FA, ICGA, OCT, and OCTA is extremely helpful for the ophthalmologist to correctly diagnose, monitor, and treat these conditions. Some of the imaging modalities also have helped to further understand the pathogenetic mechanisms of ocular infections. The advent of more advanced and less invasive imaging tools will help in further understanding and managing these conditions.

CLINICS CARE POINTS

- In the context of infectious uveitis, wide-field FP can be very helpful to easily visualize and monitor peripheral chorioretinal disease, especially in those patients with vitreous haze or in cases where clinical examination is particularly challenging.
- FAF is particularly helpful in delineating the extent of disease in ASPPC and identifying areas of reactivation in tubercular serpiginous-like choroiditis.
- Specific patterns on FA, such as early hypofluorescence and late staining in ASPPC, and ICGA, such as hypofluorescence corresponding to choroidal granulomas in tubercular uveitis, can help in quickly identifying the correct diagnosis.
- Optical coherence tomography demonstrates typical patterns in some disease entities such as ASPPC, ARN, and toxoplasmosis, and it can be used to monitor response to treatment.

FINANCIAL DISCLOSURE AND COMPETING INTERESTS
The authors have no financial interests in the contents of this article.

References
[1] Cochrane TF, Silvestri G, McDowell C, et al. Acute retinal necrosis in the United Kingdom: results of a prospective surveillance study. Eye 2012;26(3):370–7.
[2] Holland GN. Standard diagnostic criteria for the acute retinal necrosis syndrome. Executive Committee of the American Uveitis Society. Am J Ophthalmol 1994;117(5):663–7.
[3] Holland GN. The progressive outer retinal necrosis syndrome. Int Ophthalmol 1994;18(3): 163–5.
[4] Lee JH, Agarwal A, Mahendradas P, et al. Viral posterior uveitis. Surv Ophthalmol 2017;62(4):404–45.

[5] Munro M, Yadavalli T, Fonteh C, et al. Cytomegalovirus retinitis in HIV and non-HIV individuals. Microorganisms 2019;8(1):55.

[6] Lei B, Zhou M, Wang Z, et al. Ultra-wide-field fundus imaging of acute retinal necrosis: clinical characteristics and visual significance. Eye 2020;34(5):864–72.

[7] Tripathy K, Sharma YR, Gogia V, et al. Serial ultra wide field imaging for following up acute retinal necrosis cases. Oman J Ophthalmol 2015;8(1):71–2.

[8] Shah JM, Leo SW, Pan JC, et al. Telemedicine screening for cytomegalovirus retinitis using digital fundus photography. Telemed J e Health 2013;19(8):627–31.

[9] Ward TS, Reddy AK. Fundus autofluorescence in the diagnosis and monitoring of acute retinal necrosis. J Ophthalmic Inflamm Infect 2015;5:19.

[10] Yeh S, Wong WT, Weichel ED, et al. Fundus autofluorescence and OCT in the management of progressive outer retinal necrosis. Ophthalmic Surg Laser Imag 2010;41(3):1–4.

[11] Tadepalli S, Bajgai P, Dogra M, et al. Ultra-widefield fundus autofluorescence in cytomegalovirus retinitis. Ocul Immunol Inflamm 2020;28(3):446–52.

[12] Yeh S, Forooghian F, Faia LJ, et al. Fundus autofluorescence changes in cytomegalovirus retinitis. Retina 2010;30(1):42–50.

[13] Kaburaki T, Fukunaga H, Tanaka R, et al. Retinal vascular inflammatory and occlusive changes in infectious and non-infectious uveitis. Jpn J Ophthalmol 2020;64(2):150–9.

[14] Reddy AK. Peripheral vascular occlusion in acute retinal necrosis. JAMA Ophthalmol 2015;133(12):e152157.

[15] Takei H, Ohno-Matsui K, Hayano M, et al. Indocyanine green angiographic findings in acute retinal necrosis. Jpn J Ophthalmol 2002;46(3):330–5.

[16] Walton RC, Byrnes GA, Chan CC, et al. Fluorescein angiography in the progressive outer retinal necrosis syndrome. Retina 1996;16(5):393–8.

[17] Ueda N, Kamo M, Sai T, et al. Indocyanine green angiographic findings in a cytomegalovirus retinitis patient. Osaka City Med J 2005;51(1):27–31.

[18] Churgin D, Relhan N, Davis JL, et al. Perivascular hypofluorescence in frosted branch angiitis. Ophthalmic Surg Lasers Imaging Retina 2015;46(3):396–7.

[19] Suzuki J, Goto H, Minoda H, et al. Analysis of retinal findings of acute retinal necrosis using optical coherence tomography. Ocul Immunol Inflamm 2006;14(3):165–70.

[20] Ohtake-Matsumoto A, Keino H, Koto T, et al. Spectral domain and swept source optical coherence tomography findings in acute retinal necrosis. Graefes Arch Clin Exp Ophthalmol 2015;253(11):2049–51.

[21] Kurup SP, Khan S, Gill MK. Spectral domain optical coherence tomography in the evaluation and management of infectious retinitis. Retina 2014;34(11):2233–41.

[22] Invernizzi A, Agarwal AK, Ravera V, et al. Comparing optical coherence tomography findings in different aetiologies of infectious necrotising retinitis. Br J Ophthalmol 2018;102(4):433–7.

[23] Blair MP, Goldstein DA, Shapiro MJ. Optical coherence tomography of progressive outer retinal necrosis. Retina 2007;27(9):1313–4.

[24] Almony A, Dhalla MS, Feiner L, et al. Macular optical coherence tomography findings in progressive outer retinal necrosis. Can J Ophthalmol 2007;42(6):881.

[25] Invernizzi A, Agarwal A, Ravera V, et al. Optical coherence tomography findings in cytomegalovirus retinitis: a longitudinal study. Retina 2018;38(1):108–17.

[26] Gupta MP, Patel S, Orlin A, et al. Spectral domain optical coherence tomography findings in macula-involving cytomegalovirus retinitis. Retina 2018;38(5):1000–10.

[27] Costa de Andrade G, Marchesi Mello LG, Martines GC, et al. Optical coherence tomography angiography findings in acute retinal necrosis. Retin Cases Brief Rep 2021;15(3):256–60.

[28] Wongchaisuwat N, Khongpipatchaisiri S, Boonsopon S, et al. Extralesional microvascular and structural macular abnormalities in cytomegalovirus retinitis. Sci Rep 2020;10(1):21432.

[29] Hook EW 3rd, Peeling RW. Syphilis control–a continuing challenge. N Engl J Med 2004;351(2):122–4.

[30] Tsuboi M, Nishijima T, Yashiro S, et al. Prognosis of ocular syphilis in patients infected with HIV in the antiretroviral therapy era. Sex Transm Infect 2016;92(8):605–10.

[31] Dutta Majumder P, Chen EJ, Shah J, et al. Ocular Syphilis: an update. Ocul Immunol Inflamm 2019;27(1):117–25.

[32] Kiss S, Damico FM, Young LH. Ocular manifestations and treatment of syphilis. Semin Ophthalmol 2005;20(3):161–7.

[33] Pichi F, Neri P. Multimodal imaging patterns of posterior syphilitic uveitis: a review of the literature, laboratory evaluation and treatment. Int Ophthalmol 2020;40(5):1319–29.

[34] Eandi CM, Neri P, Adelman RA, et al. Acute syphilitic posterior placoid chorioretinitis: report of a case series and comprehensive review of the literature. Retina 2012;32(9):1915–41.

[35] Fu EX, Geraets RL, Dodds EM, et al. Superficial retinal precipitates in patients with syphilitic retinitis. Retina 2010;30(7):1135–43.

[36] Browning DJ. Posterior segment manifestations of active ocular syphilis, their response to a neurosyphilis regimen of penicillin therapy, and the influence of human immunodeficiency virus status on response. Ophthalmology 2000;107(11):2015–23.

[37] Marchese A, Agarwal AK, Erba S, et al. Placoid lesions of the retina: progress in multimodal imaging and clinical perspective. Br J Ophthalmol 2022;106(1):14–25.

[38] Balaskas K, Sergentanis TN, Giulieri S, et al. Fluorescein and indocyanine-green angiography in ocular syphilis: an exploratory study. Graefes Arch Clin Exp Ophthalmol 2012;250(5):721–30.

[39] Pichi F, Ciardella AP, Cunningham ET Jr, et al. Spectral domain optical coherence tomography findings in patients with acute syphilitic posterior placoid chorioretinopathy. Retina 2014;34(2):373–84.

[40] Curi AL, Sarraf D, Cunningham ET Jr, et al. Multimodal imaging of syphilitic multifocal retinitis. Retin Casess Brief Rep 2015;9(4):277–80.

[41] Mikowski M, Evans T, Wu L. Reversible choriocapillaris flow voids in acute syphilitic posterior placoid chorioretinitis. Ocul Immunol Inflamm 2021;30(7–8):1964–9.

[42] Tsui E, Gal-Or O, Ghadiali Q, et al. Multimodal imaging adds new insights into acute syphilitic posterior placoid chorioretinitis. Retinal Cases Brief Rep 2018;12(Suppl 1):S3–8.

[43] Jones JL, Kruszon-Moran D, Wilson M, et al. Toxoplasma gondii infection in the United States: seroprevalence and risk factors. Am J Epidemiol 2001;154(4):357–65.

[44] Commodaro AG, Belfort RN, Rizzo LV, et al. Ocular toxoplasmosis: an update and review of the literature. Mem Inst Oswaldo Cruz 2009;104(2):345–50.

[45] Brandão-de-Resende C, Balasundaram MB, Narain S, et al. Multimodal imaging in ocular toxoplasmosis. Ocul Immunol Inflamm 2020;28(8):1196–204.

[46] Ebrahimiadib N, Fadakar K, Hedayatfar A, et al. Expanded spectrum of optical coherence tomography findings in patients with ocular toxoplasmosis. Ocul Immunol Inflamm 2021;30(3):533–40.

[47] Pichi F, Veronese C, Lembo A, et al. New appraisals of Kyrieleis plaques: a multimodal imaging study. Br J Ophthalmol 2017;101(3):316–21.

[48] Atmaca LS, Simsek T, Atmaca Sonmez P, et al. Fluorescein and indocyanine green angiography in ocular toxoplasmosis Graefes. Arch Clin Exp Ophthalmol 2006;244(12):1688–91.

[49] Tsui E, Leong BCS, Mehta N, et al. Evaluation of segmental retinal arteritis with optical coherence tomography angiography. Retin Cases Brief Rep 2019;15(6):688–93.

[50] de Oliveira Dias JR, Campelo C, Novais EA, et al. New findings useful for clinical practice using swept-source optical coherence tomography angiography in the follow-up of active ocular toxoplasmosis. Int J Retina Vitreous 2020;6:30.

[51] Cunningham ET Jr, Rathinam SR, Albini TA, et al. Tuberculous uveitis. Ocul Immunol Inflamm 2015;23(1):2–6.

[52] Cutrufello NJ, Karakousis PC, Fishler J, et al. Intraocular tuberculosis. Ocul Immunol Inflamm 2010;18(4):281–91.

[53] Agarwal A, Aggarwal K, Pichi F, et al. Clinical and multimodal imaging clues in differentiating between tuberculomas and sarcoid choroidal granulomas. Am J Ophthalmol 2021;226:42–55.

[54] Lekha T, Karthikeyan R. Multimodal imaging of choroidal tubercles. Ind J Ophthalmol 2018;66(7):995–6.

[55] Brar M, Sharma M, Grewal SPS, et al. Comparison of wide-field swept source optical coherence tomography angiography and fundus autofluorescence in tubercular serpiginous-like choroiditis. Ind J Ophthalmol 2020;68(1):106–211.

[56] Agarwal A, Mahajan S, Khairallah M, et al. Multimodal imaging in ocular tuberculosis. Ocul Immunol Inflamm 2017;25(1):134–45.

[57] Konana VK, Bhagya M, Babu K. Double-layer sign: a new OCT finding in active tubercular serpiginous-like choroiditis to monitor activity. Ophthalmol Retina 2020;4(3):336–42.

[58] Moharana B, Bansal R, Singh R, et al. Enhanced-depth imaging by high-resolution spectral domain optical coherence tomography in tubercular multifocal serpiginoid choroiditis. Ocul Immunol Inflamm 2019;27(5):781–7.

[59] Pichi F, Smith SD, Neri P, et al. Choroidal granulomas visualized by swept-source optical coherence tomography angiography. Retina 2021;41(3):602–9.

[60] Mandadi SKR, Agarwal A, Aggarwal K, et al. Novel findings on optical coherence tomography angiography in patients with tubercular serpiginous-like choroiditis. Retina 2017;37(9): 1647–59.

[61] Demirel S, Yalçındağ N, Yanık Ö, et al. The use of optical coherence tomography angiography in the diagnosis of inflammatory type 1 choroidal neovascularization secondary to tuberculosis: a case report. Ocul Immunol Inflamm 2020;29(7–8):1431–7.

[62] Carithers HA. Cat-scratch disease. An overview based on a study of 1,200 patients. Am J Dis Child 1985;139(11):1124–33.

[63] Biancardi AL, Curi AL. Cat-scratch disease. Ocul Immunol Inflamm 2014;22(2):148–54.

[64] Kalogeropoulos D, Asproudis I, Stefaniotou M, et al. Bartonella henselae- and quintana-associated uveitis: a case series and approach of a potentially severe disease with a broad spectrum of ocular manifestations. Int Ophthalmol 2019;39(11):2505–15.

[65] McClintic J, Srivastava SK. Imaging in the diagnosis and management of ocular cat scratch disease. Int Ophthalmol Clin 2012;52(4):155–61.

[66] Freitas-Neto CA, Oréfice F, Costa RA, et al. Multimodal imaging assisting the early diagnosis of cat-scratch neuroretinitis. Semin Ophthalmol 2016;31(5):495–8.

[67] Stanescu-Segall D, Burton B, Rahman MM, et al. Multimodality imaging of multifocal ocular bartonellosis with an optic nerve head mass. Can J Ophthalmol 2019;54(1):e3–6.

[68] Ayata A, Unal M, Erşanli D, et al. Fundus autofluorescence imaging of macular star. Acta Ophthalmol 2009;87(6):690–1.

[69] Ghadiali Q, Ghadiali LK, Yannuzzi LA. Bartonella henselae neuroretinitis associated with central retinal vein occlusion, choroidal ischemia, and ischemic optic neuropathy. Retin Cases Brief Rep 2020;14(1):23–6.

[70] Habot-Wilner Z, Zur D, Goldstein M, et al. Macular findings on optical coherence tomography in cat-scratch disease neuroretinitis. Eye 2011;25(8):1064–8.

[71] Pichi F, Srivastava SK, Levinson A, et al. A focal chorioretinal bartonella lesion analyzed by optical coherence tomography angiography. Ophthalmic Surg Lasers Imaging Retina 2016;47(6):585–8.

[72] Despommier D. Toxocariasis: clinical aspects, epidemiology, medical ecology, and molecular aspects. Clin Microbiol Rev 2003;16(2):265–72.

[73] Arevalo JF, Espinoza JV, Arevalo FA. Ocular toxocariasis. J Pediatr Ophthalmol Strabismus 2013;50(2):76–86.

[74] Li S, Sun L, Liu C, et al. Clinical features of ocular toxocariasis: a comparison between ultra-wide-field and conventional camera imaging. Eye 2021;35(10):2855–63.

[75] Hernanz I, Moll-Udina A, Llorenç BV, et al. Ocular toxocariasis: beyond typical patterns through the new imaging technologies. Ocul Immunol Inflamm 2020;29(7–8):1252–8.

[76] Guo X, Liu H, Li M, et al. Multimodality image analysis in a cohort of patients with atypical juvenile ocular toxocariasis. J Ophthalmol 2021;2021:4853531.

[77] Hashida N, Nakai K, Nishida K. Diagnostic evaluation of ocular toxocariasis using high-penetration optical coherence tomography. Case Rep Ophthalmol 2014;5(1):16–21.

[78] Yoon DY, Woo SJ. Intravitreal administration of ranibizumab and bevacizumab for choroidal neovascularization secondary to ocular toxocariasis: a case report. Ocul Immunol Inflamm 2018;26(4):639–41.

[79] do Lago A, Andrade R, Muccioli C, et al. Optical coherence tomography in presumed subretinal Toxocara granuloma: case report. Arq Bras Oftalmol 2006;69(3):403–5.

[80] Carvalho da Silva FT, Yamamoto JH, Hirata CE, et al. Optical coherence tomography of a subretinal granuloma in simultaneous visceral and ocular larva migrans. Retin Cases Brief Rep 2008;2(4):316–8.

[81] Ahn SJ, Ryoo NK, Woo SJ. Ocular toxocariasis: clinical features, diagnosis, treatment, and prevention. Asia Pac Allergy 2014;4(3):134–41.

[82] Hayes EB, Sejvar JJ, Zaki SR, et al. Virology, pathology, and clinical manifestations of West Nile virus disease. Emerg Infect Dis 2005;11(8):1174–9.

[83] Hasbun R, Garcia MN, Kellaway J, et al. West Nile virus retinopathy and associations with long term neurological and neurocognitive sequelae. PLoS One 2016;11(3):e0148898.

[84] Khairallah M, Ben Yahia S, Attia S, et al. Linear pattern of West Nile virus-associated chorioretinitis is related to retinal nerve fibres organization. Eye 2007;21(7):952–5.

[85] Khairallah M, Ben Yahia S, Ladjimi A, et al. Chorioretinal involvement in patients with West Nile virus infection. Ophthalmology 2004;111(11):2065–70.

[86] Golshani C, Venkat A, Srivastava SK. Multimodal imaging findings in acute West Nile virus chorioretinitis, Retin Cases Brief Rep 2021; https://doi.org/10.1097/ICB.0000000000001162.

[87] Learned D, Nudleman E, Robinson J, et al. Multimodal imaging of West Nile virus chorioretinitis. Retina 2014;34(11):2269–74.

[88] Khairallah M, Ben Yahia S, Attia S, et al. Indocyanine green angiographic features in multifocal chorioretinitis associated with West Nile virus infection. Retina 2006;26(3):358–9.

[89] Wang R, Wykoff CC, Brown DM. Granular hyperreflective specks by spectral domain optical coherence tomography as signs of West Nile virus infection: the stardust sign. Retin Cases Brief Rep 2016;10(4):349–53.

[90] Khairallah M, Kahloun R, Gargouri S, et al. swept-source optical coherence tomography angiography in West Nile virus chorioretinitis and associated occlusive retinal vasculitis. Ophthalmic Surg Lasers Imaging Retina 2017;48(8):672–5.

[91] Jampol LM, Goldstein DA. Zika Virus infection and the eye. JAMA ophthalmology 2016;134(5):535–6.

[92] de Paula Freitas B, de Oliveira Dias JR, Prazeres J, et al. Ocular findings in infants with microcephaly associated with presumed Zika virus congenital infection in Salvador, Brazil. JAMA ophthalmology 2016;134(5):529–35.

[93] Ventura CV, Gois AL, Freire BO, et al. Fluorescein angiography findings in children with congenital Zika syndrome. Ophthalmic Surg Lasers Imaging Retina 2019;50(11):702–8.

[94] Ventura CV, Ventura LO, Bravo-Filho V, et al. Optical coherence tomography of retinal lesions in infants with congenital Zika syndrome. JAMA ophthalmology 2016;134(12):1420–7.

[95] Steptoe PJ, Momorie F, Fornah AD, et al. Multimodal imaging and spatial analysis of Ebola retinal lesions in 14 survivors of Ebola virus disease. JAMA ophthalmology 2018;136(6):689–93.

[96] Lin TPH, Ko CN, Zheng K, et al. COVID-19: Update on its ocular involvements, and complications from its treatments and vaccinations. Asia Pac J Ophthalmol 2021;10(6):521–9.

[97] Teo KY, Invernizzi A, Staurenghi G, et al. COVID-19-related retinal micro-vasculopathy - A review of current evidence. Am J Ophthalmol 2021;235:98–110.

[98] Marinho PM, Marcos AAA, Romano AC, et al. Retinal findings in patients with COVID-19. Lancet (Lond) 2020;395(10237):1610.

[99] Invernizzi A, Torre A, Parrulli S, et al. Retinal findings in patients with COVID-19: results from the SERPICO-19 study. EClinicalMedicine 2020;27:100550.

Advances in Ophthalmology and Optometry 8 (2023) 395–410

ADVANCES IN OPHTHALMOLOGY AND OPTOMETRY

Inflammatory Choroidal Neovascular Membranes

Willy Carpio-Rosso, MD[a], David Wu, BS[b], Pooja Bhat, MD[a],*

[a]Department of Ophthalmology and Visual Sciences, University of Illinois at Chicago, Chicago, IL 60612, USA; [b]The University of Illinois at Chicago College of Medicine, Chicago, IL 60612, USA

Keywords

- Inflammatory choroidal neovascularization • Uveitis complications
- Multimodal imaging • Corticosteroids • Immunosuppression • Anti-VEGF

Key points

- Inflammatory choroidal neovascularization is a rare sight-threatening complication in uveitis that occurs in up to 4.8% of cases.
- Multifocal choroiditis, punctate inner choroidopathy, and serpiginous choroiditis are the diseases that have the highest incidence of this complication.
- Inflammation-related fundus changes make the diagnosis of choroidal neovascularization challenging, and multimodal imaging, particularly angiotomography, can be helpful in diagnosis.
- Corticosteroids, immunosuppression, and/or combination antimicrobial treatment will help reduce the neovascular complex.
- Antiangiogenics are specific molecules that target the main stimulus for choroidal vessels proliferation and are the mainstay of treatment along with inflammation control.

INTRODUCTION AND EPIDEMIOLOGY

Inflammatory choroidal neovascular membranes (CNVs) are a sight-threatening complication in uveitis that affect the retina and choroid [1–8], can develop late in the uveitic disease process, and even after inflammation has been seemingly controlled [1]. Inflammation is the third most common cause of CNV after age-related macular degeneration and myopia and occurs

*Corresponding author. UIC Department of Ophthalmology & Visual Sciences, 1905 West Taylor Street, Chicago, IL 60612. *E-mail address:* pbhat@uic.edu

https://doi.org/10.1016/j.yaoo.2023.02.004
2452-1760/23/© 2023 Elsevier Inc. All rights reserved.

in 2% to 4.8% of patients [1–4]. It is more frequent in the young population, with a median age of 38 years [5,6].

Inflammatory CNV can become difficult to identify because of abnormalities in the retina and choroid that have occurred from the primary disease process [7,8]. Bansal and colleagues reported factors leading to the delayed diagnosis of inflammatory CNV such as fundus scarring, sunset glow fundus, cataract, poorly dilating pupil, media haze due to vitritis, cystoid macular edema, and multiple chorioretinal scars [9]. In rare instances, inflammatory CNV may be a presenting sign of uveitis and requires newer imaging methodologies and multimodal imaging for diagnosis.

Published studies exist in CNV emergence and treatment, most focusing on those secondary to age-related macular degeneration. This article aims to comprehensively synthesize etiologies of CNVs secondary to ocular inflammation, its diagnostic testing, and its treatment. A PubMed search was conducted using key words CNV, uveitis, inflammatory CNV, and anti-vascular endothelial growth factor (anti-VEGF). A total of 138 articles were found of which 99 articles most relevant to this review are included and are referenced below.

ETIOLOGY: DISEASE ASSOCIATIONS AND CLINICAL FEATURES
CNV is an abnormal ingrowth of the choroidal vasculature into the subretinal pigment epithelial or the subretinal or intraretinal space. The choroidal vessels penetrate through a break in the Bruch's membrane [10,11]. Inflammatory CNV typically presents as a type 2 neovascular membrane, with abnormal growth of vessels from the choroid into the subretinal space [4,7,8,12,13]. Etiology of uveitis with resultant CNV formation may be infectious or noninfectious and is detailed below.

Noninfectious diseases
Noninfectious uveitis associated with inflammatory CNVs, their incidence if known, location, and treatment are listed in Table 1.

Among the granulomatous panuveitis, CNV has been reported in 7% to 15% of the patients in the chronic stage of Vogt–Koyanagi–Harada (VKH), and the presence of CNV is associated with poor visual outcome [14,15]. In a series of 14 patients with chronic VKH followed for a mean duration of 5 years, Agarwal and colleagues found persistent macular edema in 59% of patients and CNV in 30%. The location of CNV was predominantly foveal or extrafoveal; patients were treated with serial anti-VEGF injections. The authors noted that despite treatment, inflammatory CNV is associated with poor visual outcomes, and early diagnosis is essential to establish early treatment plan with adjustment of systemic therapies and addition of anti-VEGFs [15]. Data are sparse on the incidence of CNV in patients with sympathetic ophthalmia, limited to case series and case reports as listed in Table 1, and are perhaps reflective of the rarity of this condition as well as the need for aggressive immunosuppression in disease management. CNV was reported in 1.1% of 32 patients of pulmonary-biopsy-proven ocular sarcoidosis (OS) in the Serbian population

Table 1
Noninfectious etiologies, incidence, location, and treatment of inflammatory choroidal neovascularization

Disease	Incidence	Location	Treatment
Vogt–Koyanagi–Harada [14–19]	7%–15%	Subfoveal, peripapillary, and peripheral	Anti-VEGF
Sympathetic ophthalmia [20–25]	Rare	Subfoveal, disc, and peripheral	Laser photocoagulation, immunosuppression, and anti-VEGF
Ocular sarcoidosis [26–29]	1.10%	Subfoveal and peripheral	Laser photocoagulation, corticosteroids, and anti-VEGF
Behcet's disease [30]	Rare	Subfoveal and disc	Immunosuppression
Pars planitis [31–35]	<1%	Subfoveal, peripapillary, and peripheral	Laser photocoagulation, cryotherapy, corticosteroids, immunosuppression, and anti-VEGF
Multifocal choroiditis [3,36–40]	22%–33%	Subfoveal and peripheral	Laser photocoagulation, immunosuppression, anti-VEGF, and PDT
Punctate inner choroidopathy [5,41–44]	40%–75%	Subfoveal and extrafoveal	Corticosteroids, immunosuppression, anti-VEGF, and PDT
Acute zonal occult outer retinopathy [45–48]	Rare	Subfoveal and peripapillary	Immunosuppression, anti-VEGF, and PDT
Acute posterior multifocal placoid pigment epitheliopathy [49,50]	8.50%	Subfoveal and extrafoveal	Corticosteroids, anti-VEGF, and PDT
Birdshot chorioretinopathy [51–54]	3.2%–14%	Subfoveal, peripapillary, and peripheral	Corticosteroids, immunosuppression, and anti-VEGF
Multiple evanescent white-dot syndrome [55–59]	Rare	Subfoveal and peripapillary	Corticosteroids, anti-VEGF, and PDT
Tubulointerstitial nephritis and uveitis [60–64]	4.3%–18%	Subfoveal, peripapillary, and disc	Corticosteroids, immunosuppression, and anti-VEGF
Serpiginous choroiditis [65,66]	10%–35%	Subfoveal and extrafoveal	Corticosteroids, immunosuppression, and anti-VEGF

Abbreviations: Anti-VEGF, anti-vascular endothelial growth factor; PDT, photodynamic therapy.

by Radosavljevic and colleagues, but its location was not defined further [29]. Case reports exist on CNV in OS treated with anti-VEGFs, and likely the incidence of CNV in OS is related to development of multifocal choroiditis (MFC) in patients with OS [27,28] (Fig. 1).

Among the inflammatory choroidopathies, MFC and punctate inner choroidopathy (PIC) seem to have the highest incidence of CNV formation. Thorne and colleagues reported CNV incidence of 22% in a series of 122 eyes with MFC, with CNV formation being the leading cause of poor visual acuity (VA). More than half of the eyes had presenting VA of 20/200 or worse. CNV was the most common cause of incident vision loss, with approximately 45% of vision loss attributed to new-onset or recurrent CNV. The authors also found that the use of immunosuppressive drug therapy was associated with an 83% reduction in the risk of posterior pole complications, and a 92% reduction in the risk of 20/200 or worse VA in affected eyes [36]. CNV have been described between 40% and 75% of the reported series in patients with PIC [41,42,44]. Niederer and colleagues in a series of 318 eyes with PIC, followed for a median of 8.4 years, found that CNV was present at presentation in 152 eyes (47.8%). New CNV occurred in 58 eyes (33.5% of affected eyes and 4.3% of initially unaffected eyes). An increased risk of developing CNV was associated with the presence of a CNV in the fellow eye, and the previous oral corticosteroid treatment was associated with halving of the risk of developing CNV.

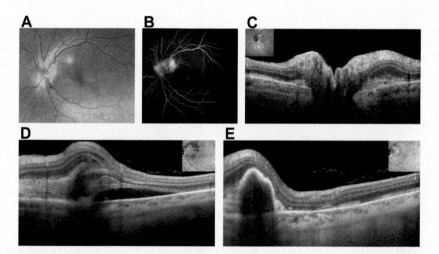

Fig. 1. Ocular sarcoidosis. A 68-year-old woman diagnosed with sarcoidosis 16 months ago, evaluated for chronic uveitis and optic disc leakage (A, B). Treatment with corticosteroids and immunosuppressants (methotrexate and adalimumab) was started with improvement and decrease of disc leakage, at which time OCT showed a juxtapapillary hyperreflective subretinal lesion, s/o of CNV with no signs of activity (C). One month ago, the patient presented with decreased visual acuity, and fundus examination showed hemorrhages and subretinal fluid by OCT (D). The patient has received two intravitreal injections of bevacizumab so far with improvement (E). s/o, suspected of.

No difference was observed in visual outcome with oral corticosteroids, but subjects treated with anti-VEGF had better visual outcomes. The authors concluded that treatment with oral corticosteroids may help to reduce the risk of CNV development. Anti-VEGF therapy for CNV was associated with better clinical outcomes [67].

Acute posterior multifocal placoid pigment epitheliopathy (APMPPE) and birdshot chorioretinopathy have higher incidences of CNV formation at 8.5% and 3.2% to 14%, respectively [49,51–54]; CNV may develop years after the initial diagnosis of the disease. Bowie and colleagues reported a case of a 55-year-old woman who developed subfoveal CNV 29 years after being diagnosed with APMPPE without resurgence of overt disease activity. The CNV resolved with local steroids and photodynamic therapy (PDT) [50]. CNV formation is rare in acute zonal occult outer retinopathy (AZOOR) and multiple evanescent white dots syndrome, limited to case series and case reports. Given the significant changes seen within the fundus from the disease itself, authors have emphasized the need for multimodal imaging to identify CNV in cases with AZOOR [45]. An interesting report by Introini and colleagues describes four patients with AZOOR who were treated successfully with anti-VEGF injections for CNV, where the VA stabilized; however, progression of the AZOOR lesions was noted subsequently, and a causal relationship between anti-VEGF therapy and disease progression was questioned [46].

CNV is a complication reported in 18% of cases of tubulointerstitial nephritis and uveitis (TINU) by Koreishi [61] and 4.3% of cases by Takemoto [63]. Takemoto and colleagues reported two cases in young children with TINU who presented with CNV, one of which responded to systemic corticosteroids alone and the other needed intravitreal anti-VEGF treatment. In both cases, residual subretinal fibrosis ensued and was related to poor final VA despite treatment [63].

Serpiginous choroiditis (SC) presents with focal choroidal inflammation followed by chorioretinal scarring and minimal vitritis. Recurrences occur at the edge of the scarred lesion, giving it the characteristic serpentine appearance. CNV originates from the border of the choroidal lesions in about 10% to 35% of the cases [65]. Saatci and colleagues reported a patient with active CNV lesion in her better seeing eye, who was treated with immunosuppressive medication and a single intravitreal injection of dexamethasone implant and ranibizumab with resolution of fluid, improvement of VA, and stabilization during 22 months of follow-up [66] (Fig. 2).

Infectious diseases

Infectious uveitis associated with inflammatory CNVs, their incidence if known, location, and treatment used are listed in Table 2.

Infections can cause chorioretinitis and breaks in Bruch's membrane and can result in CNV. The early recognition of the infection and its appropriate treatment results in limiting the extent of inflammatory damage and decrease in risk of CNV. In a large Brazilian study of 262 patients ($n = 344$ eyes) with active or inactive toxoplasmosis found that only one patient had CNV [69]. As neovascularization can

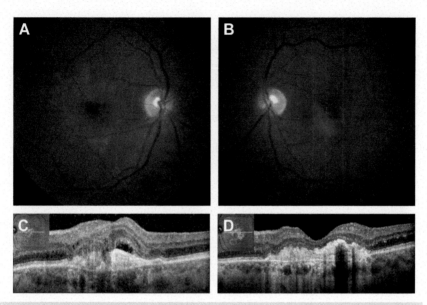

Fig. 2. Macular serpiginous. A 67-year-old male patient with a diagnosis of macular serpiginous OU (A, B), who presented recurrent CNV in the left eye despite intravitreal treatment with anti-VEGF and immunosuppressive management (methotrexate, high-dose infliximab every 4 weeks and oral prednisone) (C). At last visit, fibrotic tissue with no activity was observed in OCT (D). OU, Oculus Uterque (means both eyes).

regress with the resolution of inflammation, the number is likely an underrepresentation [70]. The management of CNV secondary to toxoplasmosis involves treatment of the underlying infection and secondary inflammation with systemic and/or local antibiotic and steroid combination therapies along with intravitreal anti-VEGF [70]. In a cohort study of 29 patients serologically confirmed to have West Nile virus (WNV) infection, 20 patients developed multifocal chorioretinitis, a pathology known to lead to CNV, but none developed CNV during the follow-up of this study [72]. WNV-associated CNV can be self-limited with successful management of the underlying infection [8,71].

CNV formation in tuberculous SC (Tb-serpiginous) can develop. A retrospective cohort study by Bansal and colleagues showed efficacy in treating 105 patients (141 eyes) afflicted by Tb-serpiginous by combined antitubercular and steroid therapy [9]. Only five eyes (3.5%) developed CNV, most within the macular region, emphasizing the importance of early treatment and prevention. Similarly, ocular histoplasmosis can result in multifocal chorioretinal scars. In the 5% of ocular histoplasmosis cases that are complicated by CNV, laser therapy and submacular surgery were previously indicated in older reports, but have since been replaced by administration of anti-VEGF [78,79]. CNV secondary to ocular syphilis (*Treponema pallidum*), ocular candidiasis (*Candida albicans*), and ocular toxocariasis (*Toxocara canis* and *Toxocara cati*) is rare, and data are limited to case reports, with successful treatment with anti-VEGFs and combination antibiotic/antifungal and anti-inflammatory agents.

Table 2
Infectious etiologies, incidence, location, and treatment of inflammatory choroidal neovascularization

Disease	Incidence	Location	Treatment
Toxoplasmosis [68–70]	Rare	Subfoveal	Antibiotics and Corticosteroids
West Nile virus [71,72]	Rare	Not defined	Supportive; self-limited
Tuberculosis serpiginous choroiditis [9,73]	Rare	Macular	Antituberculous drugs and corticosteroids
Syphilis [74–76]	Rare	Subfoveal	Antibiotics and anti-VEGF
Fungi (histoplasmosis + candidiasis) [77–80]	5% (Histoplasmosis)	Subfoveal, extrafoveal, and juxtafoveal	Anti-VEGF
Toxocara [81]	Rare	Juxtafoveal	Laser photocoagulation

Abbreviation: Anti-VEGF, anti-vascular endothelial growth factor.

Diagnosis of inflammatory choroidal neovascularization: multimodal imaging

Contrast dye images

Fluorescein angiography (FA) and indocyanine green angiography (ICG) are dye tests used to characterize the blood-retinal barriers [82] and help with the diagnosis of CNV by revealing the neovascular lesion as hyperfluorescent/hypercyanescent with late leakage. These tests also can be used as a follow-up tool after treatment of CNV with decrease of leakage in the late phases of the study [83,84]. Ultra-wide field fundus angiography has allowed the visualization of changes anterior to the equator, where peripheral leakage, ischemia, and neovascularization can often be found [30] (Fig. 3).

However, both FA and ICG can provide limited information in patients with multifocal scarring and can be sometimes inconclusive in the diagnosis of inflammatory CNV in these patients [7]. As well, both tests are invasive, time-consuming, with a potential for adverse reactions [15,85].

Optical coherence tomography

Optical coherence tomography (OCT) is a noninvasive optical imaging technology that uses light waves to create highly detailed cross-sectional images of the retina [86]. Active CNV appears on OCT as a hyperreflective area in a dome shape, fusiform or nodular formation [87]. The higher resolution of OCT imaging technology has enabled more precise diagnoses such as distinguishing between classic and occult CNV by the level of invasion into the subretinal space [88]. OCT provides a quick and noninvasive method for both diagnosing and following inflammatory CNVs that are juxtapapillary or within the macula, but is challenging to use in patients with peripheral CNV.

Optical coherence tomography angiography

OCT angiography (OCTA) is used as a noninvasive study of the retinochoroidal vasculature without the need of a dye [89,90]. It detects motion contrast in flowing blood of normal and abnormal vessels [30,84,90]. Unlike FA or ICG, this test can segment-specific layers within the retinal vasculature and choriocapillaris [44,91]

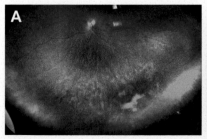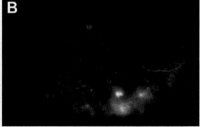

Fig. 3. Wide-field FA. Post-treatment wide-field fundus pseudocolor (A) and fluorescein angiography (B) of a 32-year-old man diagnosed with intermediate uveitis and retinal vasculitis, who presented vitreous hemorrhages in OS treated with laser photocoagulation and a single intravitreal injection of bevacizumab, who has been stable for almost 2 years.

and is able to detect CNV not seen via traditional dye testing either due to small size of the new vessels and/or the potential leakage being obscured by staining of an adjacent inflammatory scar within the retina [90] (Fig. 4).

However, OCTA has limitations such as small field of view, segmentation errors, and artifacts; some newer OCTA models address these limitations [8,44].

Management of inflammatory choroidal neovascularization

No consensus exists for the treatment of inflammatory CNV [85,92], but individual or combined treatments with local or systemic corticosteroids, immunosuppressive treatment, and anti-VEGF have been described [85].

Some of the older treatment modalities such as laser photocoagulation, PDT, and surgical removal of the CNV may not be adequate and are related to high recurrence rates and complications [11,13,93].

Specific to disease

The main goal in the management of uveitis is to suppress the intraocular inflammation in the acute phase and prevent sequelae of chronic uveitis that are associated with complications such as CNV [21,94]. Treatment typically includes high-dose systemic corticosteroid therapy with transition to steroid sparing immunomodulatory therapy.

Anti-vascular endothelial growth factor therapy

Anti-VEGF are molecules designed to bind all subtypes of VEGF to treat CNV. VEGF also can cause inflammation. Anti-VEGF therapy is used for its antiangiogenic, and anti-inflammatory properties [12,83].

Inflammatory CNV has a favorable response to anti-VEGF injections [31,42,56] due to inhibition of pro-inflammatory mediators that contribute to this response [8]. Intravitreal injections are a relatively safe procedure, with almost no systemic adverse events [11,13].

Anti-VEGF treatment protocol is not defined in inflammatory CNV [14,95]. Pro re nata treatment with a relative low number of injections demonstrates efficacy in the management of CNV, particularly in CNV of small size and focal

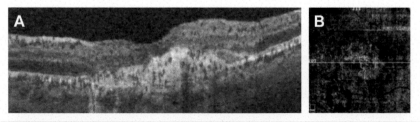

Fig. 4. OCT. A 67-year-old male patient with a diagnosis of macular serpiginous and CNV in OS. Angiotomography clearly shows neovessels in the subretinal space (A) in a fundus with changes that would make it difficult to identify CNV. En-face image shows the neovessels complex (B).

CNV; however, control of the underlying inflammatory processes is key, so combination therapy often is used [1,85].

Corticosteroid
Corticosteroid therapy has proven useful in the management of CNV as solo therapy or in conjunction with anti-VEGF [8,96]. Owing to the inflammatory nature of CNV, the administration of topical, local, or systemic corticosteroids are ideal to curb the sustained release of pro-inflammatory cytokines and angiogenic factors [97].

Corticosteroids have successfully been used in conjunction with PDT for inflammatory subfoveal CNV in OS and VKH [93,96]. Importantly, administration should be carefully monitored to avoid the significant side effects [98]. The benefits of local corticosteroids include minimal systemic exposure, sustained release over time, and improved patient compliance, examples of which include intravitreal implants of dexamethasone, fluocinolone acetonide, and triamcinolone acetonide, the latter also being of sub-tenon application [97].

Immunomodulatory therapy
Although corticosteroids are the initial mainstay of treatment in inflammatory diseases, for chronic steroid-dependent diseases, steroid sparing therapy is initiated [42,84].

Immunosuppressive therapy not only helps control inflammation but also prevents corticosteroid adverse effects. Many therapeutic agents have been used, such as antimetabolites, biologics, and alkylating agents [84,99]. Systemic immunomodulation prevents angiogenesis and limits CNV formation [8], and combination therapy with anti-VEGF has been recommended for improved results and in recalcitrant cases [13].

SUMMARY
The prompt diagnosis of ocular inflammation is important for achieving better visual outcomes and avoiding ocular complications such as CNV. Multimodal imaging allows for detection, monitoring and differentiation of inflammatory changes versus CNV.

Corticosteroids and immunomodulatory therapy are the mainstay of treatment, but close follow-up is required in patients with uveitis to monitor for development of CNV and additional treatment with mainly anti-VEGF injections but also in some instances with PDT and laser photocoagulation for CNV may be indicated.

CLINICS CARE POINTS

- Monitor uveitic patients for choroidal neovascular membrane (CNV) development, especially patients with chorioretinal scarring and breaks in Bruch's membrane.

- Disc and peripapillary changes may be associated with Bruch's membrane compromise and inflammatory CNV, and targeted imaging of the optic nerve head with optical coherence tomography (OCT) radial scan or OCT angiography may help characterize these changes further and help guide treatment.
- Wide-field angiography is particularly helpful in uveitis patients to evaluate for early detection of peripheral CNV formation.
- Combination therapy with anti-inflammatories and anti-vascular endothelial growth factor therapy is typically used for treatment of CNV.
- Continued and extended follow-up is advised in uveitis patients, as CNV formation may occur many months or years after uveitis onset and diagnosis.
- Higher incidence of CNV is seen in patients with multifocal choroiditis, punctate inner choroidopathy, and serpiginous choroidopathy, and counseling patients about the possibility of this complication and its treatment is important.

CONFLICT OF INTEREST

The authors declare that they have no conflicts of interest.

References

[1] Rouvas A, Petrou P, Douvali M, et al. Intravitreal ranibizumab for the treatment of inflammatory choroidal neovascularization. Retina 2011;31:871–9.

[2] Cornish KS, Williams GJ, Gavin MP, et al. Visual and optical coherence tomography outcomes of intravitreal bevacizumab and ranibizumab in inflammatory choroidal neovascularization secondary to punctate inner choroidopathy. Eur J Ophthalmol 2011 Jul;21(4): 440–5.

[3] Kaza H, Gala JM, Rani PK. Subfoveal retinal pigment epithelium inflammatory lesion presenting as a sign of reactivation of tubercular multifocal choroiditis. BMJ Case Rep 2021;14(5): e240280.

[4] Karti O, Can Ipek S, Ates Y, et al. Inflammatory Choroidal Neovascular Membranes in Patients With Noninfectious Uveitis: The Place of Intravitreal Anti-VEGF Therapy. Med Hypothesis Discov Innov Ophthalmol 2020;9(2):118–26.

[5] Patel KH, Birnbaum AD, Tessler HH, et al. Presentation and outcome of patients with punctate inner choroidopathy at a tertiary referral centeer. Retina 2011;31:1387–91.

[6] Baxter SL, Pistilli M, Pujari SS, et al. Risk of choroidal neovascularization among the uveitides. Am J Ophthalmol 2013;156(3):468–77.e2.

[7] Ebrahimiadib N, Maleki A, Fadakar K, et al. Vascular abnormalities in uveitis. Surv Ophthalmol 2021;66(4):653–67.

[8] Agarwal A, Invernizzi A, Singh RB, et al. An update on inflammatory choroidal neovascularization: epidemiology, multimodal imaging, and management. J Ophthalmic Inflamm Infect 2018 Dec 1;8(1):13.

[9] Bansal R, Bansal P, Gupta A, et al. Diagnostic Challenges in Inflammatory Choroidal Neovascular Membranes. Ocul Immunol Inflamm 2017 Jul 4;25(4):554–62.

[10] Safi H, Ahmadieh H, Tofighi Z. Choroidal neovascularization as the initial manifestation of multiple evanescent white dot syndrome. Eye Sci 2016;31(3):185–8.

[11] Troutbeck R, Bunting R, van Heerdon A, et al. Ranibizumab therapy for choroidal neovascularization secondary to non-age-related macular degeneration causes. Clin Exp Ophthalmol 2012 Feb;40(1):67–72.

[12] Amer R, Lois N. Punctate inner choroidopathy. Surv Ophthalmol 2011 Jan;56(1):36–53.

[13] D'Souza P, Ranjan R, Babu U, et al. Inflammatory choroidal neovascular membrane Long-Term Visual and Anatomical Outcomes After Intravitreal Anti-vascular Endothelial Growth Factor Therapy. Retina 2018;38:1307–15.

[14] Can Ipek S, Ayhan Z, Emre S, et al. Favorable clinical outcome with intravitreal aflibercept treatment in a case with bilateral choroidal neovascular membrane and quiescent Vogt-Koyanagi-Harada syndrome. GMS Opthalmol Cases 2020;10:Doc23.

[15] Agarwal M, Radosavljevic A, Patnaik G, et al. Diagnostic Value of Optical Coherence Tomography in the Early Diagnosis of Macular Complications in Chronic Vogt-Koyanagi-Harada Disease. Ocul Immunol Inflamm 2022;30(4):801–8.

[16] Wu L, Evans T, Saravia M, et al. Intravitreal bevacizumab for choroidal neovascularization secondary to Vogt-Koyanagi-Harada syndrome. Jpn J Ophthalmol 2009 Jan;53(1):57–60.

[17] Read RW, Rechodouni A, Butani N, et al. Complications and Prognostic Factors in Vogt-Koyanagi-Harada Disease. Ophthalmology 2001;131(5):599–606.

[18] Tugal-Tutkun I, Ozyazgan Y, Akova YA, et al. The spectrum of Vogt-Koyanagi-Harada disease in Turkey: VKH in Turkey. Int Ophthalmol 2007 Jun;27(2–3):117–23.

[19] Ranjan R, Agarwal M. Rebound inflammation after an intravitreal injection in Vogt-Koyanagi-Harada syndrome. Indian J Ophthalmol 2018 Jun 1;66(6):863–5.

[20] Borkowski LM, Weinberg D v, Delany CM, et al. Laser Photocoagulation for Choroidal Neovascularization Associated with Sympathetic Ophthalmia. Am J Ophthalmol 2001;132(4): 585–7.

[21] Nunes Galvarro Vianna R, Özdal P, Pessoa Souza Filho J, et al. Choroidal neovascularization associated with sympathetic ophthalmia: case report. Arq Bras Oftalmol 2005;68(3): 397–400.

[22] Chew EY, Crawford J. Sympathetic Ophthalmia and Choroidal neovascularization. Arch Ophthalmol 1988;106:1507–8.

[23] Sampangi R, Venkatesh P, Mandal S, et al. Recurrent neovascularization of the disc in sympathetic ophthalmia. Indian J Ophthalmol 2008;56:237–9.

[24] Gupta V, Gupta A, Dogra MR. Posterior sympathetic ophthalmia: A single centre long-term study of 40 patients from North India. Eye 2008;22(12):1459–64.

[25] Saatçi AO, Ayhan Z, İpek ŞC, et al. Intravitreal aflibercept as an adjunct to systemic therapy in a case of choroidal neovascular membrane associated with sympathetic ophthalmia. Turk J Ophthalmol 2018 Aug 1;48(4):209–11.

[26] Shoughy SS, Jaroudi MO, Tabbara KF. Regression of peripapillary choroidal neovascular membrane in a patient with sarcoidosis after oral steroid therapy. Saudi Journal of Ophthalmology 2014;28(2):160–2.

[27] Konidaris VE, Empeslidis T. Ranibizumab in choroidal neovascularisation associated with ocular sarcoidosis. BMJ Case Rep 2013;1:1–4.

[28] Shah SP, Hubschman JP, Bourges JL, et al. Limited long-term efficacy of intravitreous anti-VEGF pharmacotherapy in sarcoidosis complicated by peripapillary choroidal neovascular membrane. Acta Ophthalmol 2010;88(6):e243–4.

[29] Radosavljević A, Jakšić V, Pezo L, et al. Clinical Features of Ocular Sarcoidosis in Patients with Biopsy-proven Pulmonary Sarcoidosis in Serbia. Ocul Immunol Inflamm 2017 Nov 2;25(6):785–9.

[30] Aboul Naga SH, Moustafa Hassa L, el Zanaty RT, et al. Behçet uveitis: Current practice and future perspectives. Front Med 2022;9:968345.

[31] Nageeb MR. Intermediate Uveitis Complicated by Peripapillary Choroidal Neovascularization. Cureus 2022;14(11):e31040.

[32] Mehta S, Hariharan L, Ho AC, et al. Peripapillary choroidal neovascularization in pars planitis. J Ophthalmic Inflamm Infect 2013;3(1):1–5.

[33] de Amorim C, de Souza P, de Amorim C, et al. Intermediate uveitis complicated by choroidal granuloma following subretinal neovascular membrane: case reports. Arq Bras Ophthalmol 2008;71(6):890–3.

[34] Ozdal PC, Berker N, Tugal-Tutkun I. Pars planitis: Epidemiology, clinical characteristics, management and visual prognosis, 10. J Ophthalmic Vis Res. Wolters Kluwer Medknow Publications; 2015. p. 469–80.

[35] Kalina PH, Pach JM, Buettner H, et al. Neovascularization of the disc in pars planitis. Retina 1990;10(4):269–73.

[36] Thorne JE, Wittenberg S, Jabs DA, et al. Multifocal Choroiditis with Panuveitis. Incidence of Ocular Complications and of Loss of Visual Acuity. Ophthalmology 2006 Dec;113(12): 2310–6.

[37] Uparkar M, Borse N, Kaul S, et al. Photodynamic therapy following intravitreal bevacizumab in multifocal choroiditis. Int Ophthalmol 2008;28(5):375–7.

[38] Dardabounis D, Alvanos E, Gatzioufas Z, et al. Intravitreal ranibizumab in choroidal neovascularisation due to multifocal choroiditis and panuveitis syndrome. BMJ Case Rep 2013;2013:bcr2013009572.

[39] Coquelet P, Postelmans L, Snyers B, et al. Successful photodynamic therapy combined with laser photocoagulation in three eyes with classic subfoveal choroidal neovascularisation affecting two patients with multifocal choroiditis: case reports. Bull Soc Belge Ophtalmol 2002;283:69–73.

[40] Alvarez M, Hernaez J, Ciancas E, et al. Multifocal choroiditis after allogenic bone marrow transplantation. European J Ophthalmol 2001;12:135–7.

[41] Agarwal A, Handa S, Marchese A, et al. Optical Coherence Tomography Findings of Underlying Choroidal Neovascularization in Punctate Inner Choroidopathy. Front Med 2021;8:758370.

[42] Shmueli O, Amer R. Outcomes of adalimumab therapy in refractory punctate inner choroidopathy and multifocal choroiditis. Graefe's Arch Clin Exp Ophthalmol 2022 Jun 1;260(6): 2013–21.

[43] Rao VG, Rao GS, Narkhede NS. Flare up of choroiditis and choroidal neovasculazation associated with punctate inner choroidopathy during early pregnancy. Indian J Ophthalmol 2011 Mar;59(2):145–8.

[44] Kim EL, Thanos A, Yonekawa Y, et al. Optical Coherence Tomography Angiography Findings in Punctate Inner Choroidopathy. Ophthalmic Surg Lasers Imaging Retina 2017;48(10): 786–93.

[45] Levison AL, Baynes K, Lowder CY, et al. OCT Angiography Identification of Choroidal Neovascularization Secondary to Acute Zonal Occult Outer Retinopathy. Ophthalmic Surg Lasers Imaging Retina 2016;47:73–5.

[46] Introini U, Casalino G, Dhrami-Gavazi E, et al. Clinical course of acute zonal occult outer retinopathy complicated by choroidal neovascularization. Int J Retina Vitreous 2018;4(1):1–12.

[47] Fine HF, Spaide RF, Ryan EH, et al. Acute Zonal Occult Outer Retinopathy in Patients With Multiple Evanescent White Dot Syndrome. Arch Ophthalmol 2009;127(1):66–70.

[48] Cohen S.Y. and Jampol L.M., Choroidal neovascularization in peripapillary acute zonal occult outer retinopathy, Retin Cases Brief Rep, 1(4), 2007, 220–222.

[49] Papasavvas I., Mantovani A. and Herbort C.P., Acute Posterior Multifocal Placoid Pigment Epitheliopathy (APMPPE): A Comprehensive Approach and Case Series: Systemic Corticosteroid Therapy Is Necessary in a Large Proportion of Cases, Medicina (Lithuania), 58(8), 2022, 1–23.

[50] Bowie EM, Sletten KR, Kayser DL, et al. Acute posterior multifocal placoid pigment epitheliopathy and choroidal neovascularization. Retina 2005;25(3):362–4.

[51] Minos E., Barry R.J., Southworth S., et al., Birdshot chorioretinopathy: Current knowledge and new concepts in pathophysiology, diagnosis, monitoring and treatment, Orphanet J Rare Dis, 11, 2016, 1–17. BioMed Central Ltd.

[52] Vidas Pauk S., Vukojević N., Jandroković S., et al., Bilateral juxtapapillary choroidal neovascularization secondary to Birdshot chorioretinopathy—case report, Clin Case Rep, 9(8), 2021, 1–6.

[53] Oueghlani E, Westcott M, Pavésio CE. Anti-VEGF therapy for choroidal neovascularisation secondary to birdshot chorioretinopathy. Klin Monbl Augenheilkd 2010;227(4):340–1.

[54] Phasukkijwatana N, Iafe N, Sarraf D. Optical coherence tomography angiography of A29 Birdshot Chorioretinopathy complicated by retinal neovascularization. Retin Cases Brief Rep 2017;11:68–72.

[55] Papadia M, Herbort CP. Idiopathic choroidal neovascularisation as the inaugural sign of multiple evanescent white dot syndrome. Middle East Afr J Ophthalmol 2010;17(3):270.

[56] Burova M., Stepanov A., Almesmary B., et al., Choroidal neovascularization in a patient after resolution of multiple evanescent white dot syndrome: A case report, Clin Case Rep, 10(5), 2022, 1–5.

[57] Savastano M.C., Rispoli M. and Lumbroso B., Choroidal juxtapapillary neovascularization regression in multiple evanescent white dot syndrome by optical coherence tomography angiography: A case report, J Med Case Rep, 13(1), 2019, 1–5.

[58] Demirel S, Yalçindağ N, Yanik Ö, et al. Unusual presentation of multiple evanescent white dot syndrome and importance of optical coherence tomography angiography to diagnose choroidal neovascularization under inflammed choriocapillaris. Indian J Ophthalmol 2020;68:1948–50, Wolters Kluwer Medknow Publications.

[59] Um T, Lee JY. Choroidal Neovascularization after Multiple Evanescent White Dot Syndrome in a Patient with Pre-existing Pigment Epithelial Detachment. Journal of Retina 2017 May 31;2(1):38–41.

[60] Heymann H.B., Colon D. and Gill M.K., Choroidal neovascularization secondary to tubulointerstitial nephritis and uveitis syndrome (TINU) in an adult patient, J Ophthalmic Inflamm Infect, 5(1), 2015, 1–4.

[61] Koreishi AF, Zhou M, Goldstein DA. Tubulointerstitial Nephritis and Uveitis Syndrome: Characterization of Clinical Features. Ocul Immunol Inflamm 2021;29(7–8):1312–7.

[62] Nishi T, Tamura H, Miyashita Y, et al. Tubulointerstitial nephritis and uveitis syndrome with concurrent macular edema caused by granulomatous uveitis. Clin Case Rep 2020 Dec 1;8(12):2545–9.

[63] Takemoto Y, Namba K, Mizuuchi K, et al. Two cases of subfoveal choroidal neovascularization with tubulointerstitial nephritis and uveitis syndrome. Eur J Ophthalmol 2013;23(2):255–7.

[64] Paroli M.P., Cappiello D., Staccini D., et al., Juxtapapillary Choroidal Neovascularization in a Young Woman with Tubulointerstitial Nephritis and Uveitis (TINU) Syndrome with Onset in Pediatric Age, Medicina (Lithuania), 58(9), 2022, 1–8.

[65] Perente A, Kotsiliti D, Taliantzis S, et al. Serpiginous choroiditis complicated with choroidal neovascular membrane detected using optical coherence tomography angiography: A case series and literature review. Turk J Ophthalmol 2021;51(5):326–33.

[66] Saatci AO, Ayhan Z, EnginDurmaz C, et al. Simultaneous single dexamethasone implant and ranibizumab injection in a case with active serpiginous choroiditis and choroidal neovascular membrane. Case Rep Ophthalmol 2015;6(3):408–14.

[67] Niederer RL, Gilbert R, Lightman SL, et al. Risk Factors for Developing Choroidal Neovascular Membrane and Visual Loss in Punctate Inner Choroidopathy. In: Ophthalmology. Elsevier Inc.; 2018. p. 288–94.

[68] Kalogeropoulos D, Sakkas H, Mohammed B, et al. Ocular toxoplasmosis: a review of the current diagnostic and therapeutic approaches. Int Ophthalmol 2022 Jan 1;42(1):295–321.

[69] Arruda S, Vieira BR, Garcia DM, et al. Clinical manifestations and visual outcomes associated with ocular toxoplasmosis in a Brazilian population. Sci Rep 2021 Dec 1;11(1):3137.

[70] Delair E, Latkany P, Noble AG, et al. Clinical manifestations of ocular toxoplasmosis. Ocul Immunol Inflamm 2011 Apr;19(2):91–102.

[71] Bakri SJ, Kaiser PK. Ocular manifestations of West Nile Virus. Curr Opin Ophthalmol 2004;15:537–40.

[72] Khairallah M, ben Yahia S, Ladjimi A, et al. Chorioretinal involvement in patients with West Nile virus infection. Ophthalmology 2004 Nov;111(11):2065–70.

[73] Invernizzi A, Agarwal A, di Nicola M, et al. Choroidal neovascular membranes secondary to intraocular tuberculosis misdiagnosed as neovascular age-related macular degeneration. Eur J Ophthalmol 2018 Mar 1;28(2):216–24.

[74] Swierczynska M.P., Sedlak L.S., Nowak M.A., et al., Choroidal neovascularization secondary to ocular syphilis, Rom J Ophthalmol, 65(4), 2022, 406–410.

[75] Balaskas K, Spencer S, D'Souza Y. Peripapillary choroidal neovascularisation in the context of ocular syphilis is sensitive to combination antibiotic and corticosteroid treatment. Int Ophthalmol 2013 Apr;33(2):159–62.

[76] Giuffrè C, Marchese A, Cicinelli MV, et al. Multimodal imaging and treatment of syphilitic choroidal neovascularization. Retin Cases Brief Rep 2019;1–4.

[77] Jampol LM, Sung J, Walker JD, et al. Choroidal Neovascularization Secondary to Candida albicans Chorioretinitis. Ophthalmology 1996;121(6):643–9.

[78] Callanan D, Fost BF. New findings in ocular histoplasmosis. Curr Opin Ophthalmol 1995;6.

[79] Thuruthumaly C, Yee DC, Rao PK. Presumed ocular histoplasmosis. Curr Opin Ophthalmol 2014;25(6):508–12.

[80] Nachiappan K, Kadekar A, Bhagawan S, et al. Intravitreal ranibizumab in the treatment of fungal endophthalmitis scar-related choroidal neovascular membrane. Retin Cases Brief Rep 2011;5:175–8.

[81] Monshizadeh R, Ashrafzadeh MT, Rumelt S. Choroidal neovascular membrane: A Late Complication Of Inactive Toxocara Chorioretinitis. Retina 2000;20(2):219–20.

[82] Howe L, Stanford M, Graham E, et al. Indocyanine green angiography in inflammatory eye disease. Eye 1998;12:761–7.

[83] Lina Raffa, Ahmed Bawazeer. Intravitreal bevacizumab injection in a 14-year-old Vogt-Koyanagi-Harada patient with choroidal neovascular membrane. Can J Ophthalmol 2009;44(5):615–6.

[84] Paulbuddhe V, Addya S, Gurnani B, et al. Sympathetic Ophthalmia: Where Do We Currently Stand on Treatment Strategies? Clin Ophthalmol 2021 Oct;15:4201–18.

[85] Kongwattananon W, Grasic D, Lin H, Oyeniran E, Nida Sen H, Kodati S. Role of optical coherence tomography angiography in detecting and monitoring inflammatory choroidal neovascularization. Retina 2022;42:1047–56.

[86] Podoleanu AG. Optical coherence tomography. J Microsc 2012 Sep;247(3):209–19.

[87] Garcia-Layana A, Ciuffo G, Zarranz-Ventura J, Alvarez-Vidal A. Optical Coherence Tomography in Age-related Macular Degeneration. 2017.

[88] Hughes EH, Khan J, Patel N, Kashani S, Chong NV. In vivo demonstration of the anatomic differences between classic and occult choroidal neovascularization using optical coherence tomography. Am J Ophthalmol 2005;344–6.

[89] Cerquaglia A, Lupidi M, Fiore T, Iaccheri B, Perri P, Cagini C. Deep inside multifocal choroiditis: an optical coherence tomography angiography approach. Int Ophthalmol 2017;37(4):1047–1051.22.

[90] Invernizzi A, Carreno E, Pichi F, Munk MR, Agarwal A, Zierhut M, et al. Experts opinion: OCTA vs. FFA/ICG in uveitis–which will survive?: "Ten questions to find one answer. Ocular Immunol Inflamm 2022 Taylor and Francis Ltd.

[91] Yan C, Li F, Hou M, Ye X, Su L, Hu Y, et al. Vascular abnormalities in peripapillary and macular regions of behcet's uveitis patients evaluated by optical coherence tomography angiography. Front Med (Lausanne) 2021;8.

[92] Leung AK, Weisbrod DJ, Schwartz C. Intravitreal ranibizumab in the treatment of choridal neovascular membrane secondary to punctate inner choroidopathy. Canadian J Ophthalmol 2010;45(3):300.

[93] Dhingra N, Kelly S, Majid MA, Bailey CB, Dick AD. Inflammatory choroidal neovascular membrane in posterior uveitis-pathogenesis and treatment. Indian J Ophthalmol 2010;58(1):3.

[94] AlBloushi AF, Alfawaz AM, AlZaid A, Alsalamah AK, Gikandi PW, Abu El-Asrar AM. Inci-
     dence, risk factors and surgical outcomes of cataract among patients with vogt-koyanagi-
     harada disease. Ocul Immunol Inflamm 2021;29(1):128–36.
[95] Ketata A, ben Zina Z, Hajji D, Sellami D, Abdelkefi A, Kharrat W, et al. Neovaisseaux cho-
     roidiens compliquant une maladie de Vogt-Koyanagi-Harada Two cases of subretinal neo-
     vascular membrane in Vogt-Koyanagi-Harada syndrome. J Fr Ophtalmol 2006;29:302–6.
[96] Bodaghi B, Touitou V, Fardeau C, et al. Ocular sarcoidosis. Presse Med 2012;41(6 Pt 2):
     e349–54.
[97] McHarg M, Young LA, Kesav N, et al. Practice patterns regarding regional corticosteroid
     treatment in noninfectious Uveitis: a survey study. J Ophthalmic Inflamm Infect
     2022;12(1):13.
[98] Kornelsen E, Mahant S, Parkin P, et al. Corticosteroids for periorbital and orbital cellulitis.
     Cochrane Database Syst Rev 2021;2021(4).
[99] Read RW. Vogt-Koyanagi-Harada disease. Ophthalmol Clin N Am 2002;15(3):333–41.

Advances in Ophthalmology and Optometry 8 (2023) 411–426

ADVANCES IN OPHTHALMOLOGY AND OPTOMETRY

Viral Retinitis

Abhishek Sethi, BS[a], Pooja Bhat, MD[a],
Ann-Marie Lobo, MD[a], Monique Munro, MD, FRCSC[b],*

[a]Department of Ophthalmology and Visual Sciences, Illinois Eye and Ear Infirmary, University of Illinois, 1855 W. Taylor Street, Chicago, IL 60612, USA; [b]Department of Surgery, Section of Ophthalmology, University of Calgary, 100-5340 1 Street SW, Calgary, Alberta Canada

---

Keywords
- Viral retinitis • Acute retinal necrosis • Cytomegalovirus • Herpes virus • Vasculitis
- Retinitis • Vitritis • Retinal detachment

Key points
- Viral retinitis is triggered by a viral insult followed by an inflammatory response leading to retinal damage.
- Cytomegalovirus (CMV) is an opportunistic infection that can result in retinitis in immunosuppressed patients.
- Exam findings for patients with acute retinal necrosis (ARN) include retinitis, vasculitis, and anterior chamber and vitreous inflammation that rapidly progresses without antiviral therapy.
- CMV can be differentiated from ARN by eliciting a patient's history and absent or minimal vitritis and prominent retinal hemorrhages on physical exam.
- If not treated promptly, patients with viral retinitis typically have a poor visual prognosis with a high risk for ocular complications including retinal detachment.

INTRODUCTION

Viral retinitis can be classified into acute retinal necrosis (ARN) and cytomegalovirus (CMV) retinitis. ARN is an inflammatory condition characterized by rapid necrotizing retinitis due to infection, most commonly by the herpes virus family including varicella zoster virus (VZV) or herpes simplex virus (HSV) types 1 and 2 [1–3]. CMV and Epstein-Barr virus also have been associated with ARN, albeit less frequently [3,4]. ARN can affect both immunocompetent and immunosuppressed individuals at any age, but the disease is more common in immunocompetent patients [5]. CMV retinitis is a separate entity and is seen

*Corresponding author. E-mail address: moniquepmunro@gmail.com

https://doi.org/10.1016/j.yaoo.2023.02.019
2452-1760/23/© 2023 Elsevier Inc. All rights reserved.

in immunocompromised patients, most commonly in individuals with acquired immunodeficiency syndrome (AIDS), organ transplant recipients, patients on immunosuppressive drugs, and congenitally infected newborns [6]. It is recognized as the most common retinal infection in patients with AIDS and occurs late in the disease, typically when the CD4+ T-lymphocyte (CD4) count is less than 50 cells/μL [6].

The pathophysiology of ARN involves a primary, infectious trigger resulting in a severe immune-mediated response to inflammation [7]. CMV retinitis is caused by viral invasion into the vascular endothelial cells and subsequently retinal pigment epithelial cells in the retina. Both ARN and CMV retinitis can result in retinal necrosis and ensuing retinal breaks and detachments [8].

Patients with ARN may present with symptoms of uveitis including ocular pain, floaters, redness, photopsias, photophobia, and/or decreased vision [9]. Although the initial presentation is typically unilateral, bilateral ARN occurs in up to 70% of untreated patients from within a few months to several years later [10–13]. This rate is significantly lower in treated patients with one report noting a reduction in contralateral eye involvement from 70% to 13% with intravenous acyclovir [10]. Patients with CMV retinitis may present similarly with floaters and loss of peripheral vision, although not all patients are symptomatic, as the ability to mount an immune response to infection is lower in immune-suppressed patients [6].

The treatment of both ARN and CMV retinitis involves antiviral therapies. Approaches to treating viral retinitis varies with single medications or combinations with oral, intravenous, and intravitreal agents reported in the literature [11]. However, visual outcomes in ARN patients are generally poor given the extensive inflammatory response with high rates of retinal detachment. CMV retinitis can cause permanent vision loss but can be preventable with routine monitoring and prophylaxis in at-risk immunosuppressed patients [8]. The incidence of CMV retinitis has decreased in human immunodeficiency virus (HIV) patients in developed countries given the advent of antiretroviral therapy and monitoring but remains more prevalent in developing nations, where access to care is limited, and in patients who are medically immunosuppressed, such as organ transplant patients.

Given that the overall incidence of ARN and CMV retinitis is low, limited studies exist that investigate patient outcomes and treatment strategies, and large randomized controlled trials cannot be accomplished. Both diseases can cause significant ocular complications and lead to permanent vision loss despite prompt and aggressive treatment [14]. Therefore, this chapter will outline the clinical presentation of ARN and CMV retinitis with differential diagnosis and discuss medical and surgical interventions for these patients.

SIGNIFICANCE

Acute retinal necrosis Diagnosis

ARN is a rare ocular condition that affects 0.5 to 0.63 cases per one million individuals [2,15]. The disease typically affects immunocompetent individuals, which can help differentiate ARN from other similar presenting entities but can also be found in immunocompromised patients [9]. Based on guidelines from the American Uveitis Society, the diagnosis of ARN is made by clinical evidence of peripheral retinal necrosis with discrete borders, rapid progression without antiviral therapy, circumferential spread, occlusive arterial vasculopathy/periarteritis, and inflammatory reaction in the vitreous and anterior chamber manifesting as a panuveitis [16]. Patients may present with symptoms of uveitis including ocular pain, floaters, redness, photopsias, photophobia, and/ or decreased vision [9]. Other characteristics that support but are not required for diagnosis include optic atrophy and scleritis [16].

Slit lamp examination of the anterior chamber may show anterior uveitis with keratic precipitates of varying morphology (eg, stellate, granulomatous, non-granulomatous). Scleral injection secondary to inflammation of adjacent structures may occur [7]. Elevated intraocular pressure commonly is observed within 1 to 2 weeks of disease onset [17]. Fundus exam shows white and cream-colored patchy retinal lesions that become confluent, typically with rapid progression along with retinal hemorrhages/periarteritis (Figs. 1–3) [1,18]. Given these patients tend to be immunocompetent, often a robust vitritis occurs. Fluorescein angiography can be used to identify characteristic findings of ARN, including areas of occlusive arteritis, leakage of dye due to vasculitis, and hyperfluorescence of the optic nerve; however, visualization may be limited if overlying vitritis exists [7].

Polymerase chain reaction (PCR) of viral DNA from aqueous and vitreous fluid samples has revolutionized diagnosis of viral retinitis and ARN. PCR identifies viral DNA from small samples through enzymatic amplification of nucleic acid, using primers and DNA polymerase and can confirm diagnosis in suspected infectious retinitis with a positive predictive value of 99% and a negative predictive value of 68% in ARN patients [5,19]. The aqueous humor

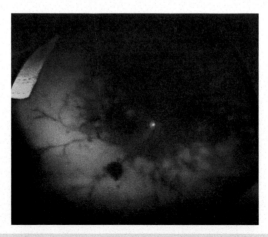

Fig. 1. An advanced ARN patient at presentation. (*Courtesy of* Pooja Bhat, MD, Chicago, IL.)

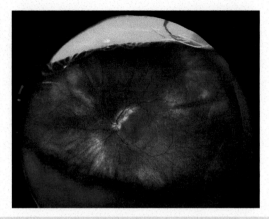

Fig. 2. The left eye with a CMV infiltrate along the superior arcade in an immunosuppressed patient. (*Courtesy of* Dr. Feisal Adatia,Clearview Eye Center, Calgary AB, Canada.)

can be more readily and cheaply acquired compared to the vitreous humor, and sampling is safe. Thus, an aqueous tap generally is recommended first line. Vitreous sampling allows for a larger quantity of intraocular fluid and may be advised in some cases [19]. Given the differential for retinal whitening can be broad, a negative PCR result may lead to an alternative diagnosis.

Prognosis

Visual outcomes in patients with ARN generally are poor and can result in irreversible blindness even if promptly diagnosed and treated. According to a

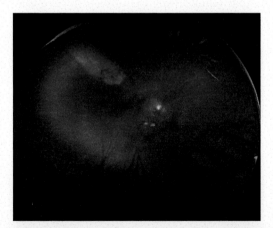

Fig. 3. The right eye of an immunosuppressed patient with CMV retinitis. This image features both a classic fulminant sectoral lesion with retinal whitening and hemorrhage as well as frosted-branch angiitis. (*Courtesy of* Monique Munro, MD, FRCSC, and Patrick Mitchell, MD, Calgary AB, CA.)

prospective study by Cochrane and colleagues, 48% of patients have a visual acuity of 20/200 or worse 6 months after diagnosis [15]. Patients who have zone 1 disease and optic nerve involvement were significantly associated with a visual acuity of 20/200 or worse [20]. The most common cause of vision loss is a rhegmatogenous retinal detachment, likely due to retinal breaks in areas within necrotic retina, with incidence reported between 20% and 73% among treated eyes [1,21]. Other causes of limited visual improvement include optic neuropathy, macular edema, macular ischemia, epiretinal membrane, and chronic vitritis [22]. Most patients initially present with unilateral symptoms, but bilateral ARN can occur in the contralateral eye within months to years. Lei and colleagues reported less severe inflammation and retinal necrosis in the eye that is later affected in 30 patients with bilateral disease [13]. However, it is associated with severe visual loss and a high rate of ocular complications [12]. Additionally, immunocompromised patients are more likely to have bilateral ocular involvement, retinal detachment, disease recurrences, and are less likely to respond to antiviral treatments [9]. Patients who undergo prompt medical treatment may have improved visual acuity and decreased risk of complications.

Treatment: antiviral medications

Antiviral therapy is the primary treatment of ARN. Intravenous acyclovir and oral valacyclovir most frequently are used [9]. Other options include oral famciclovir, valganciclovir or acyclovir, and intravenous foscarnet or ganciclovir [5,7] [Table 1]. Historically, intravenous antivirals with hospital admission were the standard of care for ARN; however, oral antivirals, including high-dose valacyclovir, have become increasingly popular with efficacious results, achieve levels within the eye effective for viral retinitis, are cost-saving, and can reduce hospital-acquired illnesses [7].

Previous papers have verified the efficacy of antiviral therapies compared to controls, and some studies have compared oral versus intravenous formulation for initial management of ARN. Palay and colleagues performed a retrospective study on patients with unilateral ARN. Compared to 30% of observed controls, 87% of patients treated with intravenous acyclovir for 7 to 10 days followed by oral acyclovir for 2 to 4 weeks were disease-free in their contralateral eye [10]. Case series by Emerson and colleagues and Taylor and colleagues reported ARN patients treated with either oral valacyclovir or famciclovir. Symptoms and visual acuity improved in 12 of 13 patients, and resolution of disease occurred within a month. Additionally, no patients developed disease reactivation or contralateral eye involvement over the study period [23,24]. Baltinas and colleagues compared visual outcomes in ARN patients treated with intravenous acyclovir versus oral valacyclovir [25]. No significant difference occurred in changes in best-corrected visual acuity, rates of severe vision loss, and rates of retinal detachment between patients treated with oral and intravenous therapy [25]. Thus, oral valacyclovir may be recommended over inpatient management. Following induction dosing with IV or oral therapy, the duration of oral therapy following this is at the discretion of the treating

Table 1
Antiviral treatments of active infectious retinitis

Systemic	Indication	Dose	Monitoring/Dose adjustment
Acyclovir	HSV, VZV	Induction: 10 mg/kg/dose divided every 8 h IV for 7 d Maintenance: 800 mg 5X daily PO	Renal impairment
Valacyclovir	HSV, VZV	1000–2000 mg TID PO	Renal impairment Elevated LFTs
Famciclovir	HSV, VZV	500 mg TID PO	Renal impairment
Ganciclovir	CMV, HSV, VZV	Induction: 500 mg IV q12 h infused over 1 h for 14–21 d Maintenance: 5 mg/kg IV daily	Blood Counts/CBC—weekly labs for thrombocytopenia, neutropenia, anemia Renal impairment Elevated LFTs
Valganciclovir	CMV	Induction: 900 mg twice daily orally for 21 d Maintenance: 450 mg twice daily po	Blood Counts/CBC weekly labs for thrombocytopenia, neutropenia, anemia Renal impairment Elevated LFTs
Foscarnet	CMV Treatment-resistant VZV, HSV ARN	Induction: 60 mg/kg q8h IV x14–21 d Maintenance: 90–120 mg/kg IV daily	Renal impairment Prolonged QT-interval Electrolyte abnormalities Seizures
Intravitreal	*Indications*	*Dose*	*Monitoring*
Ganciclovir	CMV, HSV, VZV	4 mg/0.1 mL 2 mg/0.05 mL	Post-intravitreal injection complications (endophthalmitis, retinal tear/detachment, vitreous hemorrhage, cataract)
Foscarnet	CMV, HSV, VZV Ganciclovir-resistant CMV	2.4 mg/0.1 mL 1.2 mg/0.05 mL	Post-intravitreal injection complications (endophthalmitis, retinal tear/detachment, vitreous hemorrhage, cataract)

physician and is influenced by systemic comorbidities, immunocompromised status, and concern for bilateral involvement.

Patients who are treated with antiviral medications must be regularly monitored given potential adverse effects. For example, acyclovir, famciclovir, ganciclovir, and valacyclovir require dose adjustments in geriatric and renal patients [7]. Although oral acyclovir and valacyclovir generally are well tolerated, intravenous administration of these medications can result in neurotoxicity and nephrotoxicity [26]. Additionally, immunocompromised patients are at a higher risk for nephrotoxicity and thrombocytopenia if taking valacyclovir [26]. Valganciclovir, as well as its prodrug ganciclovir, can result in bone marrow suppression and subsequent anemia, granulocytopenia, thrombocytopenia, and renal toxicity [26]. Both famciclovir and foscarnet may cause headaches and gastrointestinal symptoms; the latter has also been linked with nephrotoxicity, hypocalcemia, and neurotoxicity, and concurrent saline infusions are recommended [7,26].

Intravitreal therapy

Adjuvant intravitreal therapy has been trialed in conjunction with oral or intravenous antivirals. Wong and colleagues found that a combination of intravenous acyclovir, oral antiviral therapy, and intravitreal injection of foscarnet reduced the risk of retinal detachment (30%) compared to systemic antivirals alone (65%) [27]. Yeh and colleagues designed a similar comparative study. In this study, patients were treated with systemic antiviral therapy alone or with intravenous acyclovir or oral valacyclovir with recurrent foscarnet injections every 3 to 4 days until resolution of active disease. Patients with combination therapy also had a decreased risk for retinal detachment and were more likely to have an improvement in two lines of vision [28]. As with any intravitreal injections, a risk exists of increased intraocular pressure, endophthalmitis, vitreous hemorrhage, and retinal detachment, albeit with a low incidence. The frequency of injections has not been well established and is largely based on clinical response.

Corticosteroids

Corticosteroids have been proposed as an adjunctive treatment of ARN because of their ability to decrease the destructive inflammatory response. Some studies have suggested addition of oral corticosteroids 24 to 48 hours after antiviral therapy to reduce the risk of vitritis and retinal detachment [29]. Early use of corticosteroids should be administered cautiously, however, due to the potential to trigger viral replication and worsen the underlying retinitis [7,30]. Therefore, steroids should only be used when active infection is controlled. Intravitreal triamcinolone and dexamethasone implants have been studied in cases of persistent vitritis despite systemic antiviral therapy and in patients with cystoid macular edema [31,32].

Cytomegalovirus retinitis
Diagnosis

CMV retinitis is caused by CMV, which is usually acquired in childhood and remains latent in peripheral blood leukocytes and bone marrow until a patient becomes immunocompromised [33]. CMV retinitis is the most common opportunistic infection that affects the eyes in AIDS patients [8]. Although affected individuals are mostly HIV-positive, patients undergoing immunosuppressive treatment of hematologic malignancies, autoimmune diseases, bone marrow and solid organ transplantation, and corticosteroid administration also are at risk [34]. A CD4 count of fewer than 50 cells/μL is strongly associated with developing CMV retinitis [6]. Historically, CMV caused 90% of blindness in HIV patients, and approximately one-third of HIV patients were diagnosed with CMV retinitis [33]. With the advent of antiretroviral therapy, the incidence of CMV retinitis has decreased by 75% to 90% [35]. However, an increase occurs in the prevalence of CMV retinitis due to a decline in AIDS mortality [36].

Unlike ARN, more than half of patients with CMV retinitis are asymptomatic upon diagnosis; instead, the pathology is typically found during routine screening and examination [37]. Symptomatic patients, however, most commonly present with insidious blurred vision as well as photopsias, scotomas, and floaters [38]. A higher likelihood of visual symptoms occurs in eyes with zone 1 retinal involvement compared to peripheral retinal involvement in zones 2 and 3 [37].

CMV retinitis is a clinical diagnosis that can be confirmed with clinical history and examination. Fundus imaging will show yellow-white retinal infiltrates suggestive of necrotizing lesions or "cotton-wool spots" with variable intraretinal hemorrhages that spread inward from the periphery (images 2 and 3) [33]. The retinitis typically is distributed perivascularly and follows vessel anatomy [39]. To date, there are three variants of CMV retinitis reported in the literature [8,40].

1. Indolent variant: granular, white areas of necrotizing retinitis with little to no hemorrhage in the peripheral retina
2. Fulminant variant: full-thickness yellow-white lesions with retinal hemorrhage in a sectoral, peri-vascular distribution
3. Perivascular variant: also described as a "frosted-branch angiitis"

Several characteristic findings occur in CMV patients who are HIV-positive. These include focal or multifocal granular retinitis, mild aqueous and vitreal inflammation, and possible nonocclusive venous sheathing in the area of retinitis [41]. In contrast, in some HIV-negative patients, CMV retinitis has been associated with significant intraocular inflammation and occlusive arteritis resembling an ARN pattern. In a case series, published by Schneider and colleagues, patients also were found to have slowly progressive granular retinitis and panretinal occlusive vasculitis in areas away from the retinitis. Importantly, all patients had risk factors related to immune dysfunction, including advanced age (mean 71.0 years), diabetes mellitus, corticosteroid use, and noncytotoxic immunosuppressive medication use, but their CD4 counts at initial evaluation were within the normal range [41]. Davis and colleagues also reported that elderly patients with CMV retinitis were more likely to have occlusive vasculopathy, neovascularization, or hemorrhage compared to HIV-positive patients [42]. Aqueous or vitreous ocular fluid can be analyzed using PCR to confirm CMV infection. PCR may be useful in atypical clinical presentations and to differentiate retinitis from other causative agents [8].

Prognosis

Like ARN, CMV retinitis can cause permanent vision loss, especially if not promptly detected. In patients who are untreated, CMV can progress in 3 to 6 months to involve the entire retina, as retinitis spreads at a rate of roughly 750 microns every 3 weeks [39]. Three theories exist that account for CMV-related blindness [39].

1. Damage to the macula or optic nerve
2. Retinal detachment during acute infection or later in the disease course
3. Development of immune-recovery uveitis (IRU), an ocular inflammatory syndrome

Studies have reported complications including preretinal neovascularization, papillitis, proliferative vitreoretinopathy, and anterior segment inflammation such as iris synechiae and cataracts [35]. In addition to increasing CD4 count and decreasing HIV viral load, Kempen and colleagues found that large retinal lesions and use of intravitreal cidofovir injections were risk factors for IRU as discussed below [35].

Overall, poor prognostic factors for CMV include increased size and activity of the lesions and absence of antiretroviral therapy in HIV patients during onset of disease. Patients whose CD4 counts were less than 50 were at a significantly higher risk for contralateral ocular disease and retinal detachment compared to individuals with CD4 greater than 200 [36]. Previous studies have not shown HIV status to be a risk factor for visual prognosis and clinical course of CMV retinitis [34,43]. Patients without macular involvement and better presenting visual acuity have a better visual prognosis [36,43].

Treatment

CMV retinitis is treated with high-dose antiviral therapy. Like the treatment of ARN, patients are administered oral, intravenous, and intravitreal formulations of antiviral medications. Patients with sight-threatening lesions (ie, zone 1 involvement) are given intravitreal injections in addition to systemic therapy. The primary drugs used for CMV retinitis include valganciclovir, ganciclovir, foscarnet, and cidofovir [8]. Unlike in ARN, acyclovir is not used in treatment as CMV does not encode for a virus-specific thymidine kinase, which phosphorylates and activates the medication [8]. Induction therapy is administered for 14 to 21 days and is followed by continuous maintenance therapy; the duration of treatment is determined by clinical response, including improvement in CD4 counts in HIV patients and stability/regression of CMV lesions [8].

To date, studies have not identified a universal treatment protocol to treat CMV retinitis. Guidelines exist in the literature regarding relative efficacy of some medications. For example, Martin and colleagues determined that induction therapy with ganciclovir or its prodrug valganciclovir is equally efficacious in AIDS patients who were newly diagnosed with CMV retinitis. This study excluded patients with the advanced staged disease, specifically centrally located CMV [44]. Valganciclovir is only available in oral formulations, whereas ganciclovir is given intravenously given its poor oral bioavailability and–in addition to foscarnet–can be useful in patients unable to tolerate oral medications [8]. Additionally, AIDS patients with CMV retinitis who were treated with foscarnet had longer life expectancy compared to those given ganciclovir [45]. This must be balanced with systemic foscarnet's side effects including nephrotoxicity and electrolyte abnormalities [7,26]. Cidofovir currently is not used as first-line therapy for CMV retinitis because of side effects including nephrotoxicity and ocular inflammation [46].

Intravitreal antiviral injections commonly are combined with systemic therapy for sight-threatening lesions but also have been studied as monotherapy in some studies albeit with mixed results. Agarwal and colleagues showed that weekly intravitreal injections of ganciclovir for 6 weeks successfully resolved CMV retinitis in non-HIV immunocompromised patients [47]. Meanwhile, Jabs and colleagues found that a similar regimen in HIV-positive patients increased the rate of retinitis progression compared with systemic treatment [48].

Antiviral resistance in CMV is underestimated, especially in transplant recipients. Resistance to valganciclovir and ganciclovir may be due to mutations in UL97, involved in the initial phosphorylation of ganciclovir. Mutations in UL54 are associated with resistance to foscarnet and cidofovir after prolonged ganciclovir treatment. Awareness of this is pivotal, and new treatments are emerging against this. Letermovir targets the viral terminase complex (UL51, UL56, UL89) and recently has been approved for primary CMV infections in allogenic hematopoietic stem cell transplant recipients. Letermovir is an interesting medication in that it is used for the prevention of complications in seropositive CMV patients in allogeneic stem cell transplants [49]. Additionally, leflunomide is an anti-inflammatory agent used for inflammatory diseases and has been shown to have efficacy against ganciclovir-resistant CMV strains [50]. Leflunomide is an inhibitor of dihydroorotate dehydrogenase, thus, blocking pyrimidine synthesis and T-cell proliferation [50]. Rifkin and colleagues have reported two organ transplant recipients with CMV retinitis and UL97 mutation who were not effectively treated with valganciclovir and foscarnet but benefited from the addition of systemic leflunomide [50].

Additionally, given that the majority of CMV retinitis patients also are HIV-positive, we recommend routine ocular evaluation of immunosuppressed patients. HIV testing should be performed in patients who have CMV retinitis findings on fundus exam. If positive, antiretroviral therapy must be initiated to improve immune function.

IRU occurs in patients with CMV retinitis whose immune function recovers with the initiation of antiretroviral therapy and is defined by an increase in CD4 count by 50 or more cells/μL from the nadir. Most patients have a CD4 count > 100 cells/μL upon diagnosis of IRU [51]. IRU is recognized by vitritis and posterior segment complications, and patients have a >20-fold greater risk of cystoid macular edema and 5-fold to 6-fold higher risk for epi-retinal membrane compared to eyes without IRU. IRU can be observed in eyes with mild disease or treated with posterior sub-tenon Kenalog injections or intravitreal triamcinolone [35,52,53].

FUTURE AVENUES

Other adjunctive and prophylactic therapies

In addition to the standard treatment approaches for viral retinitis such as sys-temic antiviral medications and corticosteroids, prophylactic laser retinopexy and vitrectomy have been debated in the literature. Laser retinopexy surround-ing the areas of retinitis has been theorized to reduce the risk of retinal detach-ment, particularly in ARN; however, no clear evidence exists that recommends its use in patients with ARN [54]. Tibbetts and colleagues performed a retro-spective cohort study on 58 ARN patients, 33% of whom received a prophylac-tic retinopexy; however, rates of retinal detachment did not differ between treated and untreated patients [11]. Laser only can be used with a clear media and limited retinitis and thus precludes many patients depending on their level of inflammation. Additionally, the procedure results in increased inflammation in a disease process that has an inflammatory pathophysiology [7]. Early vitrec-tomy has also been postulated to remove inflammatory debris, reduce vitreor-etinal traction, and decrease the risk of retinal detachment [7]. One paper by Iwahashi-Shima and colleagues found no benefit to prophylactic vitrectomy; 58% of ARN patients with early vitrectomy had attached retinas compared to 75% of patients who did not undergo the procedure. Additionally, no signif-icant difference occurred between baseline and final visual acuity in patients [20]. Other studies have found improvements in visual acuity and decreased rates of retinal detachment in patients who underwent early vitrectomy but vary in the baseline characteristics of patients, use of silicone oil, and follow-up time [7].

Aspirin and warfarin have been suggested for ARN patients, as the patho-physiology of ARN includes retinal arteritis and vascular occlusions. Ando and colleagues tested platelet function in patients with bilateral ARN and de-tected platelet hyperaggregation in six out of seven patients. Visual acuity improved once 500 mg/d of aspirin was administered [55]. Meanwhile, antico-agulation has not been well studied as a treatment of patients with ARN. We suggest future research focus on using adjunct therapies along with systemic antiviral medications to analyze patient outcomes.

SUMMARY

This chapter highlights ARN and CMV retinitis, two subclasses of viral reti-nitis, and outlines the pathophysiology, epidemiology, prognosis, and treat-ment options. Rare diseases are associated with poor ocular prognosis in patients, including irreversible blindness and retinal detachment. Both pathol-ogies are challenging to diagnose clinically given the range of differential diag-noses, which include progressive outer retinal necrosis (PORN), syphilis, toxoplasmosis, Behcet's disease, fungal or bacterial endophthalmitis, idiopathic panuveitis, large cell/intraocular lymphoma, and HIV retinopathy.

Ocular syphilis can result in various degrees of uveitis including round vitreous opacities and involvement of the retinal arteries. Toxoplasmosis is associated with significant vitritis. Both pathologies can mimic the inflammation found in ARN. Findings of posterior placoid chorioretinitis can help identify posterior syphilis along with systemic skin findings of the disease. On exam, an area of visible retinitis can be seen through the vitritis in toxoplasmosis.

Like CMV retinitis, PORN can be found in immunocompromised patients, and no vitritis is seen on exam. However, minimal to no retinal hemorrhages can differentiate it from CMV. HIV retinopathy can often be confused with CMV retinitis, as both are rapidly progressive, and the former has "cotton-wool spots" akin to the yellow-white retinal infiltrates in the latter. Repeat examination in 3 to 4 weeks will show fading of the cotton-wool spots in HIV retinopathy but progression of lesions in CMV retinitis [39]. We recommend PCR testing of aqueous and vitreous fluid to confirm ARN and CMV retinitis if history and physical exam are equivocal. However, antiviral therapy should be initiated while laboratory results are pending, given the rapidly progressive nature of the diseases.

Viral retinitis needs to be treated with prompt high-dose antiviral therapy. For ARN, we recommend intravenous acyclovir or oral valacyclovir ± intravitreal foscarnet or ganciclovir + a topical steroid and cycloplegic agent as induction treatment with progression to maintenance treatment with oral valacyclovir or oral acyclovir. For CMV retinitis, we suggest oral valganciclovir or intravenous ganciclovir ± intravitreal ganciclovir or foscarnet if lesions are active and sight-threatening. Medications may be substituted, but all antiviral agents should be carefully dosed and monitored depending on patients' medical comorbidities and adverse risk profile of medications. Corticosteroids are suggested in ARN given the significant inflammatory response, but early initiation may suppress the body's immune response and exacerbate the retinitis. Some studies also have considered antiplatelet and anticoagulant agents for treatment given the vasculitis and artery involvement in ARN. Preliminary evidence exists of the benefits of aspirin, but no evidence for anticoagulants.

Previous papers have considered laser retinopexy and vitrectomy as surgical approaches for ARN. Laser retinopexy cannot be used in all patients, as the vitreous media should be clear, and many patients may have significant uveitis on examination. Rates of retinal detachment do not differ between patients who underwent laser retinopexy and controls. Studies have not found a benefit to early vitrectomy in reducing the risk of retinal detachment and improving visual acuity despite the potential to remove inflammatory debris.

Additionally, patients diagnosed with CMV retinitis are immunocompromised. Therefore, HIV testing should be performed if a patient does not have a known history of autoimmune disease or currently taking immunosuppressive drugs. Antiretroviral medications should be promptly initiated if a patient is newly diagnosed with HIV with monitoring of CD4 and viral load over time.

Patients on antiretroviral therapy are at risk for IRU, as an increased immune response can result in intraocular inflammation. IRU is defined by vitritis and posterior segment complications including cystoid macular edema and epiretinal membrane formation.

CLINICS CARE POINTS

- History: immunosuppression versus no immunosuppression
- Exam: degree of inflammation, sectoral versus circumferential retinitis
- Obtain an aqueous sample (primary sample) or vitreous sample (secondary sample) for PCR
- Orders: PCR for HSV, VZV, CMV, labs for complete blood counts, metabolic panel, kidney function, HIV, syphilis, TB, CMV titers, ± toxoplasmosis depending on clinical presentation
- Based on clinical suspicion—inject ganciclovir ± foscarnet depending on availability
- Start systemic medications based on highest probability—for example, no immunocompromise—valaciclovir or acyclovir (ARN); immunosuppression—valganciclovir (CMV)
- Adjust treatment pending PCR and clinical response
- Have suspicion of genetic resistance in unresponsive cases
- Be aware of monitoring labs required while on particular antivirals

DISCLOSURE

No financial conflicts of interest or funding sources.

References

[1] Hillenkamp J, Nölle B, Bruns C, et al. Acute Retinal Necrosis: Clinical Features, Early Vitrectomy, and Outcomes. Ophthalmology 2009;116:1971–5.e2.
[2] Muthiah MN, Michaelides M, Child CS, et al. Acute retinal necrosis: A national population-based study to assess the incidence, methods of diagnosis, treatment strategies and outcomes in the UK. Br J Ophthalmol 2007;91:1452–5.
[3] Lau CH, Missotten T, Salzmann J, et al. Acute Retinal Necrosis. Features, Management, and Outcomes. Ophthalmology 2007;114:756–63.
[4] Ganatra JB, Chandler D, Santos C, et al. Viral causes of the acute retinal necrosis syndrome. Am J Ophthalmol 2000;129:166–72.
[5] Schoenberger SD, Kim SJ, Thorne JE, et al. Diagnosis and Treatment of Acute Retinal Necrosis: A Report by the American Academy of Ophthalmology. Ophthalmology 2017;124:382–92.
[6] Au Eong KG, Beatty S, Charles SJ. Cytomegalovirus retinitis in patients with acquired immune deficiency syndrome. Postgrad Med J 1999;75:585–90.
[7] Powell B, Wang D, Llop S, et al. Management strategies of acute retinal necrosis: Current perspectives. Clin Ophthalmol 2020;14:1931–43.
[8] Munro M, Yadavalli T, Fonteh C, et al. Cytomegalovirus retinitis in HIV and non-HIV individuals. Microorganisms 2020;8:1–20.

[9] Bonfioli AA, Eller AW. Acute retinal necrosis. Semin Ophthalmol 2005;20:155–60.

[10] Palay DA, Sternberg P, Davis J, et al. Decrease in the risk of bilateral acute retinal necrosis by acyclovir therapy. Am J Ophthalmol 1991;112:250–5.

[11] Tibbetts MD, Shah CP, Young LH, et al. Treatment of Acute Retinal Necrosis. Ophthalmology 2010;117:818–24.

[12] Miserocchi E, Iuliano L, Fogliato G, et al. Bilateral Acute Retinal Necrosis: Clinical Features and Outcomes in a Multicenter Study. Ocul Immunol Inflamm 2019;27:1090–8.

[13] Lei B, Jiang R, Wang Z, et al. Bilateral acute retinal necrosis syndrorne. Retina 2018;40: 145–53.

[14] Mojarrad A, Omidtabrizi A, Ansari Astaneh M, et al. Acute retinal necrosis. Management and visual outcomes: a case series. Int J Retin Vitr 2022;8:1–9.

[15] Cochrane TF, Silvestri G, McDowell C, et al. Acute retinal necrosis in the United Kingdom: Results of a prospective surveillance study. Eye 2012;26:370–8.

[16] Holland GN. Standard diagnostic criteria for the acute retinal necrosis syndrome. Am J Ophthalmol 1994;117:663–6.

[17] Yang P. Atlas of uveitis: diagnosis and treatment. People's Medical Publishing House; 2021; https://doi.org/10.1007/978-981-15-3726-4.

[18] Tripathy K, Sharma YR, Gogia V, et al. Serial ultra wide field imaging for following up acute retinal necrosis cases. Oman J Ophthalmol 2015;8:71–2.

[19] Harper TW, Miller D, Schiffman JC, et al. Polymerase Chain Reaction Analysis of Aqueous and Vitreous Specimens in the Diagnosis of Posterior Segment Infectious Uveitis. Am J Ophthalmol 2009;147:140–7.

[20] Iwahashi-Shima C, Azumi A, Ohguro N, et al. Acute retinal necrosis: Factors associated with anatomic and visual outcomes. Jpn J Ophthalmol 2013;57:98–103.

[21] Meghpara B, Sulkowski G, Kesen MR, et al. Long-term follow-up of acute retinal necrosis. Retina 2010;30:795–800.

[22] Wong RW, Jumper JM, McDonald HR, et al. Emerging concepts in the management of acute retinal necrosis. Br J Ophthalmol 2013;97:545–52.

[23] Taylor SR, Hamilton R, Hooper CY, et al. Valacyclovir in the treatment of acute retinal necrosis. BMC Ophthalmol 2012;12:4.

[24] Emerson GG, Smith JR, Wilson DJ, et al. Primary Treatment of Acute Retinal Necrosis with Oral Antiviral Therapy. Ophthalmology 2006;113:2259–61.

[25] Baltinas J, Lightman S, Tomkins-Netzer O. Comparing Treatment of Acute Retinal Necrosis With Either Oral Valacyclovir or Intravenous Acyclovir. Am J Ophthalmol 2018;188: 173–80.

[26] Tam PMK, Hooper CY, Lightman S. Antiviral selection in the management of acute retinal necrosis. Clin Ophthalmol 2010;4:11–20.

[27] Wong R, Pavesio CE, Laidlaw DAH, et al. Acute Retinal Necrosis. The Effects of Intravitreal Foscarnet and Virus Type on Outcome. Ophthalmology 2010;117:556–60.

[28] Yeh S, Suhler EB, Smith JR, et al. Combination Systemic and Intravitreal Antiviral Therapy in the Management of Acute Retinal Necrosis Syndrome. Ophthalmic Surg Lasers Imaging Retina 2014;45(5):399–407.

[29] Shantha JG, Weissman HM, Debiec MR, et al. Advances in the management of acute retinal necrosis. Int Ophthalmol Clin 2015;55:1–13.

[30] Anthony CL, Bavinger JC, Yeh S. Advances in the Diagnosis and Management of Acute Retinal Necrosis. Ann Eye Sci 2020;1–11; https://doi.org/10.21037/aes-2019-dmu-09.

[31] Choudhury H, Jindal A, Mithal K, et al. Intravitreal triamcinolone acetonide as an adjuvant in the management of acute retinal necrosis. Can J Ophthalmol 2014;49:279–82.

[32] Majumder PD, Biswas J, Ambreen A, et al. Intravitreal dexamethasone implant for the treatment of cystoid macular oedema associated with acute retinal necrosis. J Ophthalmic Inflamm Infect 2016;6:6–9.

[33] Ocieczek P, Barnacle JR, Gumulira J, et al. Cytomegalovirus Retinitis Screening and Treatment in Human Immunodeficiency Virus Patients in Malawi: A Feasibility Study. Open Forum Infect Dis 2019;6:1–7.

[34] Kuo IC, Kempen JH, Dunn JP, et al. Clinical characteristics and outcomes of cytomegalovirus retinitis in persons without human immunodeficiency virus infection. Am J Ophthalmol 2004;138:338–46.

[35] Kempen JH, Min YI, Freeman WR, et al. Risk of Immune Recovery Uveitis in Patients with AIDS and Cytomegalovirus Retinitis. Ophthalmology 2006;113:684–94.

[36] Jabs DA, Van Natta ML, Thorne JE, et al. Course of cytomegalovirus retinitis in the era of highly active antiretroviral therapy: 2. Second eye involvement and retinal detachment. Ophthalmology 2004;111:2232–9.

[37] Wei LL, Park SS, Skiest DJ. Prevalence of visual symptoms among patients with newly diagnosed cytomegalovirus retinitis. Retina 2002;22:278–82.

[38] Colby DJ, Vo DQH, Teoh SC, et al. Prevalence and predictors of cytomegalovirus retinitis in HIV-infected patients with low CD4 lymphocyte counts in Vietnam. Int J STD AIDS 2014;25: 516–22.

[39] Heiden D, Ford N, Wilson D, et al. Cytomegalovirus retinitis: The neglected disease of the AIDS pandemic. PLoS Med 2007;4:1845–51.

[40] Ho M, Invernizzi A, Zagora S, et al. Presenting Features, Treatment and Clinical Outcomes of Cytomegalovirus Retinitis: Non-HIV Patients Vs HIV Patients. Ocul Immunol Inflamm 2020;28:651–8.

[41] Schneider EW, Elner SG, Van Kuijk FJ, et al. Chronic retinal necrosis: Cytomegalovirus necrotizing retinitis associated with panretinal vasculopathy in non-hiv patients. Retina 2013;33:1791–9.

[42] Davis JL, Haft P, Hartley K. Retinal arteriolar occlusions due to cytomegalovirus retinitis in elderly patients without HIV. J Ophthalmic Inflamm Infect 2013;3:1–8.

[43] Kim DY, Jo J, Joe SG, et al. Comparison of visual prognosis and clinical features of cytomegalovirus retinitis in HIV and NON-HIV patients. Retina 2017;37:376–81.

[44] NA; A Controlled Trial of Valganciclovir As Induction Therapy for Cytomegalovirus Retinitis. Infect Dis Clin Pract 2002;11:180–1.

[45] Studies of Ocular Complications of AIDS Research Group. AIDS Clinical Trials Group. Mortality in patients with the acquired immunodeficiency syndrome treated with either foscarnet or ganciclovir for cytomegalovirus retinitis. N Engl J Med 1992;23:213–20.

[46] Wolf DL, Rodríguez CA, Mucci M, et al. Pharmacokinetics and renal effects of cidofovir with a reduced dose of probenecid in HIV-infected patients with cytomegalovirus retinitis. J Clin Pharmacol 2003;43:43–51.

[47] Agarwal A, Kumari N, Trehan A, et al. Outcome of cytomegalovirus retinitis in immunocompromised patients without Human Immunodeficiency Virus treated with intravitreal ganciclovir injection. Graefe's Arch Clin Exp Ophthalmol 2014;252:1393–401.

[48] Jabs DA, Ahuja A, Van Natta ML, et al. Comparison of treatment regimens for cytomegalovirus retinitis in patients with AIDS in the era of highly active antiretroviral therapy. Ophthalmology 2013;120:1262–70.

[49] Santos Bravo M, Plault N, Sánchez-Palomino S, et al. Genotypic and Phenotypic Study of Antiviral Resistance Mutations in Refractory Cytomegalovirus Infection. J Infect Dis 2022;226:1528–36.

[50] Rifkin LM, Minkus CL, Pursell K, et al. Utility of Leflunomide in the Treatment of Drug Resistant Cytomegalovirus Retinitis. Ocul Immunol Inflamm 2017;25:93–6.

[51] Yeo TH, Yeo TK, Wong EP, et al. Immune recovery uveitis in HIV patients with cytomegalovirus retinitis in the era of HAART therapy—a 5-year study from Singapore. J Ophthalmic Inflamm Infect 2016;6; https://doi.org/10.1186/s12348-016-0110-3.

[52] Morrison VL, Kozak I, LaBree LD, et al. Intravitreal Triamcinolone Acetonide for the Treatment of Immune Recovery Uveitis Macular Edema. Ophthalmology 2007;114:334–9.

[53] El-Bradey MH, Cheng L, Song MK, et al. Long-term results of treatment of macular complications in eyes with immune recovery uveitis using a graded treatment approach. Retina 2004;24:376–82.
[54] Fan S, Lin D, Wu R, et al. Efficacy of prophylactic laser retinopexy in acute retinal necrosis: A systematic review and meta-analysis. Int Ophthalmol 2022;42:1651–60.
[55] Ando F, Kato M, Goto S, et al. Platelet function in bilateral acute retinal necrosis. Am J Ophthalmol 1983;96:27–32.

Moving?

Make sure your subscription moves with you!

To notify us of your new address, find your **Clinics Account Number** (located on your mailing label above your name), and contact customer service at:

Email: journalscustomerservice-usa@elsevier.com

800-654-2452 (subscribers in the U.S. & Canada)
314-447-8871 (subscribers outside of the U.S. & Canada)

Fax number: 314-447-8029

**Elsevier Health Sciences Division
Subscription Customer Service
3251 Riverport Lane
Maryland Heights, MO 63043**

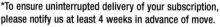